Medical Problems in the Classroom

Medical Problems in the Classroom

The Teacher's Role in Diagnosis and Management

Edited by
Robert H. A. Haslam, M.D.

Professor and Head, Division of Pediatrics,
University of Calgary Medical School, Calgary,
Alberta; formerly Director, The John F. Kennedy
Institute, and Associate Professor of Pediatrics and
Neurology, The Johns Hopkins University School of
Medicine, Baltimore

and
Peter J. Valletutti, Ed.D.

Dean of Extension and Experimental Programs and
Professor of Education, Coppin State College,
Baltimore; Assistant Professor of Special Education
(Pediatrics), The Johns Hopkins University School
of Medicine, Baltimore

Illustrated by
Carolyn V. Jones

University Park Press
Baltimore · London · Tokyo

UNIVERSITY PARK PRESS
International Publishers in Science and Medicine
233 East Redwood Street
Baltimore, Maryland 21202

Typeset by The Composing Room of Michigan, Inc.

Printed in the United States of America by Universal Lithographers, Inc.

Second printing, September 1976

Third printing, January 1978

Library of Congress Cataloging in Publication Data
Main entry under title:

Medical problems in the classroom.

Includes Index.
1. Children—Diseases—Addresses, essays, lectures.
2. School children—Health and hygiene. 3. Excep-
tional children—Education—Addresses, essays, lectures.
I. Haslam, Robert H. A. II. Valletutti, Peter J.
[DNLM: 1. Education, Special. 2. Handicapped.
3. Learning disorders. 4. School health. LC4580
M489]
RJ71. M42   618.9'2'000 24372   75-25776
ISBN 0-8391-0823-0

Contents

Preface

It is hoped that this book will alert readers to the possible existence of various medical problems that may be discovered in the classroom, especially those physical conditions which affect learning and behavior. A teacher who is keenly aware of the importance of medical disorders in the overall development of her students can perform a vital role: that of facilitating delivery of a host of medical and paramedical services to those students who require such specialized attention. Teachers, perhaps second only to parents, come into contact with children and young adults on a sustained basis more often than any other professional group in society. This prolonged contact provides the teacher with an unparalleled opportunity to make a significant contribution to preventive medicine and to assist in obtaining needed medical and other noneducational therapeutic procedures. It is universally recognized that the earlier the identification and diagnosis of a medical condition, the more likely that the disorder may be reversed and/or its effects minimized.

Because of changes in philosophy, educators are placing increasing numbers of special students in the mainstream of education. In addition, judicial decisions and legislative actions are mandating that public education be made available to all children, regardless of the multiplicity or severity of the handicapping condition. As a result of these factors, the teacher will be required to become more sophisticated in the recognition of untoward medical conditions and in providing educational programs designed to meet the special needs of these children. Decisions will have to be made on appropriate curriculum objectives and experiences, on classroom organization and behavioral management, and on methods and materials that will facilitate learning for students with medical problems. The teacher will increasingly be called upon to participate as a member of an interdisciplinary team or network providing total diagnostic and prescriptive services to these students.

This book, then, is intended for all teachers, both in regular and special classes. It is also designed for teacher educators as they provide preservice and inservice education for the novice as well as the experienced teacher. Also, it is for school administrators as they seek to better serve the students in their care. Finally, it is written for the physician and his paramedical colleagues who need to become more familiar with the child and young adult with medical problems as they function within the school setting.

This book does not attempt to outline all diseases and conditions that are peculiar to school age children and youth. It does, however, present the reader with information relevant to those disorders that are more prevalent and those that are more likely to be successfully remediated or reversed. Above all, this work strives to provide a basis for the establishment of meaningful and reciprocal communication between the educator and those responsible for the medical supervision of the student.

List of Contributors

Michael Bender, Ed.D., *Director, Special Education Department, The John F. Kennedy Institute; Instructor in Special Education (Pediatrics), The Johns Hopkins University School of Medicine, Baltimore, Maryland*

Arnold J. Capute, M.D., M.P.H., *Assistant Professor of Pediatrics, The Johns Hopkins University School of Medicine; Deputy Director, The John F. Kennedy Institute, Baltimore, Maryland*

Thomas J. Craig, M.D., *Assistant Professor of Psychiatry, Instructor of Medicine, The Johns Hopkins University School of Medicine, Baltimore, Maryland*

Harold E. Cross, M.D., Ph.D., *Chief, Ophthalmology Division, University of Arizona, Tucson, Arizona*

Gregory C. Fernandopulle, M.D., *Instructor in Child Psychiatry, The Johns Hopkins University School of Medicine, Baltimore, Maryland*

Judith L. Friedman, M.S., *Supervisor of Audiology, The John F. Kennedy Institute, The Johns Hopkins University School of Medicine, Baltimore, Maryland*

Robert H. A. Haslam, M.D., *Professor and Head, Division of Pediatrics, University of Calgary Medical School, Calgary, Alberta, Canada; formerly Director, The John F. Kennedy Institute for Habilitation of the Mentally and Physically Handicapped Child, and Associate Professor of Pediatrics and Neurology, The Johns Hopkins University, Baltimore, Maryland*

Robert B. Johnston, M.D., *Assistant Professor of Pediatrics, The Johns Hopkins University School of Medicine and The John F. Kennedy Institute, Baltimore, Maryland*

Harvey P. Katz, M.D., *Chief of Pediatrics, Columbia Medical Plan and Howard County General Hospital; Associate Professor of Pediatrics, The Johns Hopkins University School of Medicine, Baltimore, Maryland*

Thaddeus E. Kelly, M.D., *Assistant Professor of Pediatrics and Medicine, The John F. Kennedy Institute and The Johns Hopkins University School of Medicine, Baltimore, Maryland*

Beverly A. Myers, M.D., *Assistant Professor of Pediatrics and Psychiatry, The Johns Hopkins University School of Medicine; Director, Division of Pediatric Psychiatry, The John F. Kennedy Institute, Baltimore, Maryland*

David M. Paige, M.D., M.P.H., *Associate Professor of Maternal and Child Health, Assistant Professor of Pediatrics, The Johns Hopkins University School of Medicine and School of Hygiene and Public Health, Baltimore, Maryland*

Alejandro Rodriguez, M.D., *Associate Professor of Pediatrics and Child Psychiatry, The Johns Hopkins University School of Medicine, Baltimore, Maryland*

Charles E. Silberstein, M.D., M.Sc., *Assistant Professor of Orthopaedic Surgery, The Johns Hopkins University School of Medicine, Baltimore, Maryland*

Peter J. Valletutti, Ed.D., *Dean of Extension and Experimental Programs and Professor of Education, Coppin State College, Baltimore, Maryland; Assistant Professor Special Education (Pediatrics), The Johns Hopkins University School of Medicine, Baltimore, Maryland*

Acknowledgments

We are indebted to each of the contributors, who have shared their invaluable experience in the preparation of this book. All of the authors were selected because of their demonstrated interest in nurturing the physical and mental health of children. Their interaction with the educational system in meeting the medical needs of all students has provided an important framework for the presentation of each writer's expertise.

We particularly extend our heartfelt appreciation to Mrs. Lucinda Hoffmaster for manuscript preparation and chapter review.

The Teacher's Role In the Diagnosis and Management Of Students with Medical Problems

Peter J. Valletutti, Ed.D.

Teachers have an unparalleled opportunity to observe the behavior of children on a sustained basis. This prolonged exposure to children provides teachers with the opportunity to identify behaviors which signal possible medical problems in the students they teach. The teacher, in her[1] day-to-day observations and in her more formal evaluations, must be alert to the possibility that deviant classroom performance may be a product of some abnormal physical condition.

Among the physical reasons which might account for student underachievement are impairments in sensory functioning. The teacher is aware that the primary sensory modalities through which learning occurs are those of vision and hearing. It, therefore, logically follows that a student with deficits in visual or auditory acuity might have difficulty in acquiring key academic skills. He might also have difficulty in perceiving the teacher's cues which indicate desired behaviors. The teacher, therefore, must be alert to those behaviors of a student which suggest that a sensory deficit might exist. Such behaviors as failure to respond to oral directions, confusion in execution of oral directions, sound substitutions, omissions, and distortions, faulty voice production, mispronunciations, and the uttering of expletives (Huh? What?) should suggest the possibility of an impairment in auditory acuity (Streng, 1960). If these behaviors occur with a degree of frequency, the teacher should view them as possible reasons for

---

[1] The teacher will be referred to as female because of the larger number of women teaching the elementary grades, while the student will be identified as male because of the larger number of males with learning problems.

further inquiry. It is at this point that the observant teacher performs a significant professional function by referring the student for audiometric and/or otologic examinations.

In the area of vision, such behaviors as abnormal positioning and distance spacing of the student's head and eyes vis-à-vis reading material, squinting, and faulty or peculiar eye movements are some indicators that a visual problem might be present (Lowenfeld, 1971). The student with reddened eyes who squints while tilting his head during reading probably reads that way so that he can see. This constellation of behaviors suggests visual impairment and the teacher must be responsive to its implications. If she is aware of the possibility of visual impairment, she will refer the student for ophthalmologic study. If she is not, she will allow the student to continue without receiving assistance and thus, inadvertently, contribute to his becoming a poor reader.

Since the teacher typically works with students who have only minor medical problems, she is more likely to disregard pathology and seek reasons for academic failure and/or misconduct within the student's intellectual, motivational, and affective systems or within his sociologic history. In part because of her training, which emphasizes the behavioral sciences and minimizes the biologic bases of behavior, and in part because of her experiences with only the normal student, the teacher rarely looks toward the physical domain for an explanation of deviant student performance.

It has become increasingly clear over the past several years that it is essential for the teacher to develop a scientific evaluation strategy if she is to meet the individual needs of students within the traditional group setting of education (Smith, 1969; and McCloskey, 1971). Diagnostic-prescriptive teaching has been identified as a model for the teacher to follow in her efforts to personalize instruction. Teachers have been increasingly called upon to refine their diagnostic skills despite the lack of guidelines. "What is educational diagnosis?" and "How does one diagnose a student?" become significant questions. Little progress has occurred because the individualization of instruction has at its conceptual core the precise and comprehensive appraisal of each student. Because of this failure to precisely and comprehensively diagnose each student, a distinctive program or prescription designed to meet needs or remedy deficiencies cannot be devised. The function of the teacher has taken on new dimensions and she is expected to be an evaluator, a programmer, a classroom organizer, and a manager of behavior for each of the students in her class (Hammill and Bartel, 1971).

The role of programmer, of generating or applying methods and materials, traditionally was assigned the highest priority in the preparation of teachers. The role of evaluator-diagnostician received the least emphasis. The lack of emphasis on the diagnostic function was reinforced by the cookbook approach to instruction, i.e., the use of curriculum guides, prepackaged programs and materials, textbooks and the grade level, age level, intelligence level, and sex preference categorization of materials and subject matter. From this stereotyping orientation, curriculum and methodology have been preordained by group expectations rather than by individual characteristics and performance. The call for individualized instruction has been an intellectual charade.

One way to counteract this is to develop educational programs using a diagnostic paradigm. The diagnostic teaching process may be viewed as having three separate but interdependent aspects: (1) educational evaluation for programming purposes and for developing strategies for classroom organization and behavioral management; (2) a diagnostic awareness of underlying and perhaps reversible medical causes for which treatment may be obtained; and, (3) an appreciation for the special methods of instruction and management needed to meet the educational needs of students with medical conditions.

THE TEACHER AS EVALUATOR-PROGRAMMER

It is not sufficient to identify the objectives of the curriculum without stating these goals in such terms as to allow their achievement to be precisely measured. Out of the need to devise more precise measures for evaluating teaching success and the necessity to provide the teacher with a more explicit focus to her instruction came the practice of stating objectives in behavioral terms (Mager, 1962). The writing of behavioral objectives requires that they be phrased in such a manner so that the behavior's achievement may be clearly demonstrated by the student under previously specified conditions. The recording of behavioral objectives provides the teacher with an evaluative tool after a task is taught. It also supplies the teacher with a list of behaviorally described tasks from which she may evaluate the student before entry into a program and after she has exposed the student to a series of instructional activities. When this approach is pursued, educational evaluation rises above an amorphous, unpredictable, and nonproductive undertaking into the domain of scientific inquiry. The student should be evaluated in relation to the educational task, nothing less and nothing more.

If a student accomplishes an educational task, then he has realized the objective and that is important to know. If a student fails to complete a task, however, that is not enough to know. The teacher must discover what skills or competencies the student possesses which are prerequisite to the achievement of the task. The adept teacher matches with as much precision as possible the student's skills with those skills required to achieve the task successfully. For example, facility in auditory discrimination is a precursor to both speech and reading. If the student is lacking in this faculty, his speech may be characterized by sound substitutions, mispronunciations, and faulty word usage; his reading will be confused and generally poor in quality (Eisenson and Ogilvie, 1971). The teacher should then analyze thoroughly the sequence of events and the prerequisite competencies needed to achieve the desired objective. This cataloguing and charting of an educational task is called a task analysis (Gagne, 1965).

A task analysis is initiated with a statement of a curriculum objective in behavioral terms. This behavioral statement becomes the terminus for the completed task analysis. A desired behavioral objective could be written in the following manner: the student, when shown any phonetic word with the patterns vowel-consonant and consonant-vowel-consonant containing the letter vowel *a* and the consonant letters *b, d , t, g, n,* will word call the words with 95% accuracy.

Once the teacher has identified the desired objective and stated it in explicit behavioral terms, she should then identify the sequence of events and/or prerequisite skills needed to realize the goal. After listing these skills in an ordered arrangement, they should be charted and utilized for evaluation purposes. For the above listed behavioral objective, the task analysis shown in Figure 1 could be considered appropriate.

If student A accomplishes the task successfully as specified in the terminal objective, the teacher records this success (perhaps by checking the terminal objective box in the charted task analysis). If student B, on the other hand, fails to do so, the teacher seeks to find that point on the chart which represents the last area of his success. For instance, if student B were unable to blend sounds but was able to orally sound out a single letter phonogram, the teacher would mark off box 8 on the chart. The teacher would then continue by presenting those activities which would assist student B in progressing from step 8 to step 9. After identifying the highest skill within the student's repertoire of behaviors relevant to a specific educational task, the teacher would then design an educational program or prescription to aid the student in bridging the gap between the achieved and the unachieved.

Before proceeding to this programming, however, the teacher must be cautious. She must be alert to the possibility that an existing physical condition may be interfering with the attainment of the next significant step in the task sequence. She must be sophisticated enough to seek out appropriate medical assistance so that the student's problem may be remedied, if medically possible. The teacher must not merely pinpoint the locus of the behavioral deficit but must question whether there exist any medical reasons which might be etiologically significant. She must pursue this one step further and ask whether there are corrective medical or paramedical procedures which would facilitate learning and improve the general physical and/or psychologic health of the student. It is at this critical evaluation point that the teacher plays a significant role in both the preventive medical process and in assisting the student to obtain various medical services and other noneducational therapeutic procedures.

The teacher must understand that the student's medical status undeniably affects learning. She must recognize that she needs a thorough understanding of normal and deviant development and the effects of physical functioning on the learning process. The early diagnosis of medical problems offers many advantages in that early diagnosis can result in prompt treatment and the increased probability of remediation and/or cure. It also helps to prevent further physical

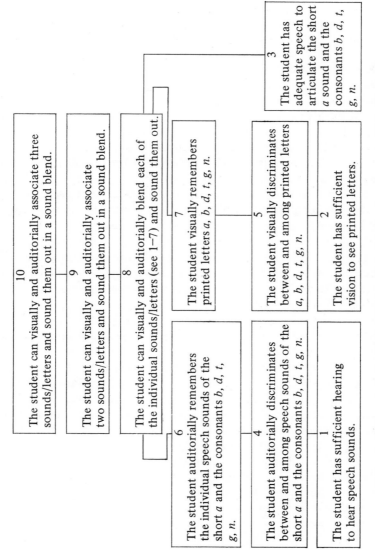
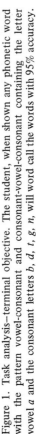

Figure 1. Task analysis—terminal objective. The student, when shown any phonetic word with the pattern vowel-consonant and consonant-vowel-consonant containing the letter vowel *a* and the consonant letters *b, d, t, g, n,* will word call the words with 95% accuracy.

deterioration and permanent damage to the involved organs. Early correction of physical problems will minimize the effects of a pathologic condition on learning. This is especially true when the medical problem affects vision and hearing. The longer the student is sensorially handicapped, the more difficult it will be to remediate learning problems and to facilitate new learning.

As the age of entry into school continues downward, the teacher's role in identifying behaviors which signal medical problems increases in importance and in difficulty. The teacher must be skilled enough to differentiate behaviors which represent normal development and those which are symptomatic of an existing medical problem. As a case in point, the teacher needs to know whether a child's difficulty in fine or gross motor coordination is merely a variation in normal development or whether it indicates some neurologic or orthopedic problem. In order to make this differentiation, she must be skilled not only in observing individual behaviors but also in determining whether there is a pattern to or constellation of these behaviors which, when considered together, suggest a specific physical basis for this pattern of behaviors.

The student who does not appear to listen to daily classroom directions may be bored, may not comprehend, may have a hearing problem, or may have a problem with auditory memory. This conduct, accompanied by other behaviors, such as difficulty in sounding out blends and words with difficult sequences, in remembering details of what he has heard, frequent omissions and transposing of words in short sentences, and the inability to learn words in series including days of the week, months of the year, and counting, more clearly points to a deficit in auditory memory (Farrald and Schamber, 1973).

The teacher's role in diagnosis and management will increase in complexity and in importance as more and more children with severe and profound handicaps are placed in classroom settings. This increase is to be expected as a result of recent legislation and court decisions which mandate free public education for all handicapped children regardless of the degree of handicap (Abeson, 1974; Casey, 1973; and Kuriloff et al., 1974). The diagnosis of a medical problem assumes greater importance with this population not only because of its need for medical and paramedical treatment, but also because the physical condition may have serious implications for educational programming. For example, an educational objective for an individual student might be the elimination of drooling. Before the teacher subjects the student to a rigorous program designed to correct this behavior, she should first find out from the appropriate medical specialist whether the student is physically capable of controlling this drooling.

The effect of medical problems on programming is not limited to the handicapped, but applies equally to the nonhandicapped. Consider the frustration to both student and teacher in attempting to teach a student to articulate the *s, z, sh, ch,* and *j* sounds when he has a significant open bite or missing upper incisors. Besides being frustrating, it would also be a poor use of time because, in most cases, the student will automatically articulate these sounds correctly once his teeth have grown in or have been corrected by orthodontic procedures.

THE TEACHER AS REFERRAL AGENT

The teacher's role in the diagnosis of medical problems should, however, not be limited solely to the identification of behaviors which signal possible pathology. Her role should be expanded to assist in the process of obtaining needed medical and other allied health services, such as occupational, physical, and speech and hearing therapy. Indeed, the teacher often must initiate the referral process because she may be the first adult to observe students over a long period of time. If she fails to detect existing medical problems, they will often go undetected because no one else has this singular opportunity.

In order to carry out the referral process, the teacher needs to be aware of the role of the various professional disciplines in the total treatment-rehabilitation procedure. She must understand the relationship between a specific physical condition and the medical specialty under which that condition's care is subsumed. Knowing the professional scope of such medical specialties as pediatrics, otology, ophthalmology, neurology, orthopedics, endocrinology, and psychiatry will be of incalculable help in determining the direction of the referral process. She must also be familiar with those specific individuals and agencies within her community which provide medical and paramedical assistance. She should be aware of hospital-related programs and those of public and private agencies. Many general hospitals offer a variety of clinics as part of their comprehensive medical services; some also provide itinerant services. State, county, and city departments of health frequently offer clinical diagnostic and treatment services on a regular and often itinerant basis so that all areas of the community, no matter how remote, may receive necessary medical assistance. Private organizations such as the United Cerebral Palsy Association, the Association for Retarded Citizens, the local Speech and Hearing Agency, an agency of the National Society for the Prevention of Blindness, and a center administered by the National Society for Crippled Children and Adults often provide comprehensive diagnostic and treatment programs for individuals with special medical problems. The teacher should know the health services available in her community and should understand the kind of clients they serve, and perhaps, the inclusiveness of their programming, their referral requirements, their fees for service, as well as their usual availability.

To be an effective referral agent, the teacher must become familiar with whatever referral system already exists within her school or school system. Very often, structured referral procedures have not been formulated by either the central office or by the local school administration, and decisions are made on an on-the-spot basis in those instances when the teacher recognizes the need to seek medical or paramedical guidance.

The teacher who is a skilled diagnostician frequently must initiate, on her own, procedures within her school. Before approaching the school principal, she should compile all relevant data which would support the need for referral. Perhaps the best type of supportive data would be anecdotal records which describe in sufficient detail the significant behaviors of the student concerned. These records should be reported in behavioral terms stating the conditions under which they occurred and noting the frequency of occurrence. The teacher should avoid interpreting these behaviors but should suggest that one of the possible explanations for them lies within the medical sphere.

One of the ways in which a referral system can be effective is to have an interdisciplinary team established, consisting of the school principal, referring teacher, school nurse, school psychologist, guidance counselor, school social worker, reading teacher, speech-language therapist, and any other ancillary school personnel. It is recognized that many schools do not have this range of personnel and the referral team would thus be smaller.

After the interdisciplinary group has examined the data supplied by the teacher and other members of the team, a decision as to whether an outside opinion is required is then made. The next step would be to communicate this joint decision to the student's parents, since their cooperation is essential in carrying out the referral plan. It should be noted here that a parent may be reluctant to obtain medical consultation. This reluctance may be due to a variety of reasons: financial considerations, religious beliefs, fear of confirming their own suspicions, and/or a genuine lack of interest. If this resistance occurs, it is urgent that a member of the team be responsible for parental counseling and guidance. In cases in which the problem is financial, this team member must seek out sources of financial assistance.

Whatever referral procedures are followed, the teacher should make sure that they include provisions for having the medical evaluation and recommendations communicated to her as soon as possible. Only in this way will the teacher's subsequent educational programming be consistent with the findings of the physician. The lines of communication must be open between the teacher and the physician. The teacher should be free to report, when necessary, the results in the classroom of the physician's recommendations.

SPECIAL PROGRAMMING AND MANAGEMENT NEEDS OF STUDENTS WITH MEDICAL PROBLEMS

The teacher, in preparing instructional materials, establishing curriculum priorities, choosing methodologic approaches, organizing the classroom's physical arrangement, and managing behavior, must appreciate the special needs of students with medical problems. For example, the student with a moderate to severe hearing loss may require auditory training, speech reading, speech and language development and correction, and special instruction in the use of hearing aids (Keaster, 1967). He may require special seating arrangements and the use of additional visual clues for the management of behavior (O'Neil, 1964). The teacher working with the partially seeing student must be especially concerned with adequacy of classroom illumination, both natural and artificial (Pelone, 1962). She must be aware of the effect that the color of walls and ceilings has on learning among the partially seeing (Kirk, 1972), as well as the need for unique equipment and materials such as special typewriters, pencils and paper, chalkboards, desks, books and other reading materials, and projection and magnifying equipment (Leach, 1971). Because partially seeing students learn a great deal aurally, tape recorders, dictaphones, record players, and talking books are indispensable. The teacher with a blind student in her class must provide him with instruction in the use of the braille system for reading, writing, and arithmetic. Braille writers, braille books, braille slates and styli, specially embossed maps, the abacus, and audio aids are necessary classroom equipment for the blind student (Jones and Collins, 1963). The blind student benefits greatly from instruction in the use of the typewriter as it enables him to communicate through typing with seeing individuals (Scholl, 1967). The blind student requires particular instruction in both physical and social independence. Mobility training and individualized instruction in social competency, including the reduction of mannerisms, are of special importance (Cutsforth, 1951).

The cerebral palsied student frequently requires aids and supports for mobility, in addition to special shoes, braces, walkers, and wheelchairs and specific instruction in their use (Connor, 1967b). He often needs assistance from a host of habilitation specialists including speech, hearing, physical, occupational, vocational, and recreational therapists (Denhoff and Robinault, 1960). He frequently benefits from specially designed and constructed equipment for a wide variety of everyday activities that include eating utensils, writing materials, buses, bathroom equipment, and guard rails along the wall (Blessing, 1968).

The student who suffers from seizures requires that the teacher spend instructional time helping classmates to understand and deal with their own feelings toward their handicapped classmate (Lennox, 1954). The teacher must prepare for the seizure not only in terms of dealing with the student and his classmates during the convulsion but also in terms of procedures to follow after the convulsion has occurred (Connor, 1967a).

In epilepsy, as in other handicapping conditions, it is important to direct the attention of the class to the needs of the handicapped student and to instruct them in the facts of the condition so that the mystery, mythology, and stigma may be reduced (Gulliford, 1971). When a student with a chronic health problem has a terminal illness, the teacher must overcome her own feelings and deal with the student's fears, yet still provide a program that is as normal and pleasurable as possible (Connor, 1964). Most students with chronic health problems require neither a modification in the curriculum nor unusual methods of instruction, but do require special management to take into consideration reduced energy, strength, motivation, and various personality variables. They also require help from the teacher in developing positive self-concepts. Frequent negative reactions to his handicapping condition usually result in lowered self-esteem, fear of school failure, and hostility toward others (Barker et al., 1953).

Whenever a student in her class has a medically related problem, the teacher must determine whether there are any special modifications to be made in the physical environment which would assist the student in obtaining optimum benefits from his school experience. She must examine such things as the relative accessibility of the school to the student. Are there entrance and exit ramps? Are there elevators and walking rails, if needed? She must even check into such items as whether there are special railing bars at urinals and commodes and wide enough doorways for wheelchair-bound students to enter toilet cubicles. Is there a pay phone available at wheelchair level? For the student with seizures and those with unsteady balance, are there cushioned floors and/or padded helmets? Are there standing tables and walkers? Are there soft lead pencils, large print typewriters, and gray-green chalkboards for the partially seeing? Is there a place for a student to rest after he has a seizure? Does the teacher stand so the light illuminates her face and does she speak in such a way that she is an easy subject to speech read?

The teacher must also ask whether a student with a medical problem requires a modification in curriculum and instructional practices. The addition of auditory training and speech reading for the hard-of-hearing is a case in point. The blind benefit from mobility training and social competency training especially to remove mannerisms (Morse, 1965). The retarded often require training in many of the self-care skills, including toilet training, and other social skills generally acquired by most students prior to entry into school programs. Students who are behaviorally disordered require programming concerned with value and attitude development in addition to programs designed to facilitate cognitive development. A great deal of the teacher's time initially may be devoted to preparing the student to be receptive to learning and to function within a group setting. Time must be spent in dealing with the psychologic concomitants of learning problems in that the student's sense of self-worth and/or his anxieties related to the learning task may have to be dealt with before learning will take place. The fact that many behaviorally disordered students strongly resent authority, which they equate with coercion, requires the teacher to devote inordinate time to overcoming this resistance. Because of this, it has been said for this group of students that the teacher is the curriculum (Rabinow, 1964).

EDUCATIONAL IMPLICATIONS OF MEDICAL INTERVENTION STRATEGIES

The teacher needs to become increasingly cognizant of medical intervention strategies so that the effects on learning and behavior may be anticipated. Of special interest to the teacher is the use of drug therapy to control behavior and facilitate learning. Since the physician frequently uses responses to drug therapy as a means of differential diagnosis, the teacher may serve as a vital source of critical feedback to the medical practitioner on the etiology of the condition as well as the efficacy of the medical strategy and/or regimen. On other occasions, students are placed on special diets because of endocrine problems, convulsive disorders, or allergies, and it is essential that the teacher assist the student in meeting the dictates of that diet. In the typical classroom and school this may indeed be a difficult task, since morning milk and cookies and birthday and holiday parties have become routine classroom practices. The addition of soft drink, candy, and cake dispensing machines to school cafeterias makes it difficult for a student to maintain his diet and adds significantly to the teacher's task.

The teacher faces a number of problems when she is expected to aid in the dispensing of medication to her students. There are legal and ethical ramifications and she must thoroughly evaluate them before she agrees to participate in such a program. This is especially true when she is dealing with a student who has been diagnosed as hyperactive and is receiving drugs to control his behavior. Since hyperactivity is a relative and subjective phenomenon, the teacher may find herself in diagnostic disagreement if she views the child's behavior as within normal limits requiring no medication. The use of drugs as a management strategy may be in conflict with the teacher's view of behavior modification. She may feel that the student must develop internal controls rather than having him depend upon external agents such as drugs. If the student is on a drug regimen, does this prevent the teacher from dealing with emotional controls? Does this interference by a medical intervention technique unfairly disrupt the teacher's professional responsibilities? Does the use of medication reduce student activity and, thus, inhibit learning? The answers to these questions are further confounded by the fact that megavitamin therapy has been proposed as an alternative medical treatment procedure (Cott, 1972). The teacher, already confused by the alien jargon of medicine, is further bewildered when physicians and other allied health professionals appear to disagree. Should their students with learning problems learn to crawl all over again? (Delacato, 1966). Should all their students with reading problems receive visual perception training or optometric exercises? (Gearheart, 1973). Should students with nerve deafness obtain acupuncture? (Wensel). Should dyslexic students walk balance beams and wear eye patches? (Goldberg and Schiffman, 1972). Should autistic students be given amphetamines, tranquilizers, and/or megavitamins? (Cott, 1972). A multidisciplinary approach in which all the disciplines communicate and share their expertise can be invaluable in obtaining answers to these perplexing questions (Clements, 1969).

As she interacts with students who are under medical treatment, the teacher must define her role in that process as it affects the students in her classroom and in their life in general. The problem becomes more complex when the student is receiving therapeutic interventions from paramedical specialists. The teacher who for many years has been exhorted to teach the whole child must retain the whole child concept as she shares "parts" of him with others. The speech and hearing therapist is concerned with his oral language and so is the teacher. Oral language is the medium of interchange through which most classroom interaction occurs. Facility in oral communication is the foundation upon which written language, arithmetic, and thought is built (Johnson and

Myklebust, 1967), and the teacher must help to clarify the different roles she and the speech and hearing therapist are to play. The occupational therapist is frequently concerned with the functioning of the upper extremities in activities of daily living (Willard and Spackman, 1971). The teacher cannot ignore educational objectives related to fine motor coordination and to the use of the arms and hands in feeding, dressing, and grooming activities. The occupational therapist is also concerned with the use of arts and crafts as media for the development of arms and hands and for leisure time utilization. The teacher in the twentieth century cannot ignore the importance of leisure time education in a comprehensive educational program. She needs to clarify, with the occupational therapist, the nature and dimensions of interdisciplinary cooperation. The physical therapist is frequently concerned with the mobility training of physically handicapped students, and so is the teacher. She views mobility as not only a physical skill but also a combination of skills involving estimates of space and directionality. The teacher is also viewed by practitioners of each of the above therapies as a carry-over agent. This added responsibility taxes not only her emotional reserves but also depletes the time available to teach those tasks within her own previously established educational priorities.

The teacher must decide what role she is to play in establishing communication guidelines and strategies for effective and efficient interaction with medical and allied health professionals. This must be done so that the student with medical problems may more promptly be discovered and more rapidly and effectively treated.

SUMMARY

The teacher's perspective relevant to the educational implications of medical problems was presented by first clarifying the three separate areas of professional responsibility involved in clinical or diagnostic teaching: educational evaluation for programming purposes and for developing strategies for classroom organization and behavioral management; a diagnostic awareness for referral purposes; and an appreciation for the special methods of instruction and management for students with medical problems.

The role of the teacher as a referral agent and the significance of the referral process in preventive medicine were outlined. The teacher's part in obtaining needed medical and paramedical services was also discussed. Some of the significant behaviors of students which suggest the presence of atypical physical conditions were given and suggestions were offered for establishing viable referral procedures.

Special programming and management needs of students with medical problems were discussed from a teacher's perspective as were the effects of medical and paramedical intervention strategies on learning and behavior. The different roles of noneducational (paramedical) therapists were considered and the need for clarification of these roles, as they overlap the teacher's professional responsibility, was identified.

REFERENCES

Abeson, A. 1974. Movement and momentum: Government and the education of handicapped children. II. Exceptional Child. 41:109–115.

Barker, R. G., B. A. Wright, L. Meyerson, and M. R. Gonick. 1953. Adjustment to Physical Handicap and Illness: A Survey of the Social Psychology of Physique and Disability. Social Science Research Council, New York. 440 p.

Blessing, K. R. 1968. The Role of the Resource Consultant in Special Education. Council for Exceptional Children, Washington, D. C. 127 p.

Casey, P. J. 1973. The supreme court and the suspect class. Exceptional Child. 40:119–125.

Clements, S. D. 1969. A new look at learning disabilities. In L. Tarnopol (ed.), Learning Disabilities: Introduction to Educational and Medical Management, pp. 31–40. Charles C Thomas, Publisher, Springfield, Ill.

Connor, F. P. 1964. Education of Homebound or Hospitalized Children. Teachers College Press, Columbia University, New York. 125 p.

Connor, F. P. 1967a. The education of children with chronic medical problems. In W. M. Cruickshank and G. O. Johnson (eds.), Education of Exceptional Children and Youth. 2nd Ed. pp. 507–566. Prentice-Hall, Inc., Englewood Cliffs, N. J.

Connor, F. P. 1967b. The education of crippled children. In W. M. Cruickshank and G. O. Johnson (eds.), Education of Exceptional Children and Youth. 2nd Ed. pp. 432–506. Prentice-Hall, Inc., Englewood Cliffs, N.J.

Cott, A. 1972. Megavitamins: The orthomolecular approach to behavioral disorders and learning disabilities. Acad. Therap. 7:245–258.

Cutsforth, T. D. 1951. The Blind in School and Society. American Foundation for the Blind, New York. 269 p.

Delacato, C. H. 1966. Neurological Organization and Reading. Charles C Thomas, Publisher, Springfield, Ill. 189 p.

Denhoff, E., and I. P. Robinault. 1960. Cerebral Palsy and Related Disorders. McGraw-Hill Book Company, Inc., New York. 421 p.

Eisenson, J., and M. Ogilvie. 1971. Speech Correction in the Schools. The Macmillan Company, New York. 436 p.

Farrald, R. R., and R. G. Schamber. 1973. A Diagnostic and Prescriptive Technique. Handbook I. Adapt Press, Sioux Falls, S. Dak. 523 p.

Gagne, R. M. 1965. The Conditions of Learning. Holt, Rinehart and Winston, Inc., New York. 308 p.

Gearheart, B. R. 1973. Learning Disabilities: Educational Strategies. C. V. Mosby Company, St. Louis. 233 p.

Goldberg, H. K., and G. B. Schiffman. 1972. Dyslexia Problems of Reading Disabilities. Grune & Stratton, Inc., New York. 194 p.

Gulliford, R. 1971. Special Educational Needs. Routledge & Kegan Paul, Ltd., London. 213 p.

Hammill, D. D., and N. R. Bartel. 1971. Educational Perspectives in Learning Disabilities. John Wiley & Sons, Inc., New York. 420 p.

Johnson, D. J., and H. R. Myklebust. 1967. Learning Disabilities: Educational Principles and Practices. Grune & Stratton, Inc., New York. 328 p.

Jones, J. W., and A. P. Collins. 1963. Educational Programs for Visually Handicapped Children. Government Printing Office, OE-35045, Bulletin No. 39. Washington, D. C. 55 p.

Keaster, J. 1967. Impaired hearing, *In* W. Johnson and D. Moeller (eds.), Speech Handicapped School Children. 3rd Ed. pp. 390–432. Harper & Row, Publishers, New York.

Kirk, S. A. 1972. Educating Exceptional Children. 2nd Ed. Houghton-Mifflin, Boston. 478 p.

Kuriloff, P., R. Truz, D. Kirp, and W. Buss. 1974. Legal reform and educational change: The Pennsylvania case. Exceptional Child. 41:35–42.

Leach, F. 1971. Multiply handicapped visually impaired children: Instructional materials needs. Exceptional Child. 38:153–156.

Lennox, W. G. 1954. The epileptic child. *In* H. Michal-Smith (ed.), Pediatric Problems in Clinical Practice, pp. 245–272. Grune & Stratton, Inc., New York.

Lowenfeld, B. 1971. Psychological problems of children with impaired vision. *In* W. M. Cruickshank (ed.), Psychology of Exceptional Children and Youth. 3rd Ed. pp. 211–307. Prentice-Hall, Inc., Englewood Cliffs, N. J.

Mager, R. F. 1962. Preparing Instructional Objectives. Fearon, Palo Alto, Calif. 60 p.

McCloskey, M. G. 1971. Teaching Strategies and Classroom Realities. Prentice-Hall, Inc., Englewood Cliffs, N. J. 355 p.

Morse, J. L. 1965. Mannerisms, not blindisms: Causation and treatment. Int. J. Educ. Blind 15:12–16.

O'Neil, J. 1964. The Hard of Hearing. Prentice-Hall, Inc., Englewood Cliffs, N. J. 146 p.

Pelone, A. J. 1962. The adjustment of the partially seeing child in the regular classroom. *In* J. F. Magary and J. R. Eichorn (eds.), The Exceptional Child: A Book of Readings, pp. 270–279. Holt, Rinehart and Winston, Inc., New York.

Rabinow, B. 1964. A training program for teachers of the emotionally disturbed and the socially maladjusted. Exceptional Child. 26:287–295.

Scholl, G. T. 1967. The education of children with visual impairments. *In* W. M. Cruickshank and G. O. Johnson (eds.), Education of Exceptional Children and Youth. 2nd Ed. pp. 287–342. Prentice-Hall, Inc., Englewood Cliffs, N. J.

Smith, R. M. 1969. Teacher Diagnosis of Educational Difficulties. Charles E. Merrill, Columbus, Ohio. 226 p.

Streng, A. 1960. Children with Impaired Hearing. Council for Exceptional Children. Washington, D. C. 72 p.

Wensel, L. (Undated.) Introduction to Acupuncture. Washington Acupuncture Center. Washington, D. C. 9 p.

Willard, H. S., and C. S. Spackman (eds.) 1971. Occupational Therapy. 4th Ed. J. B. Lippincott Company, Philadelphia. 551 p.

2

Educational Implications Of Visual Disorders

Harold E. Cross, M.D., Ph.D.

Vision is among the most precious of man's senses. A Gallup poll conducted several years ago found that Americans fear blindness second only to cancer as a threat to good health. Most of us give little thought to the importance of good visual acuity in our daily lives and seldom realize how tedious essential functions such as communication, mobility, education, and even recreation become for those with poor vision.

The real tragedy in the majority of visual handicaps lies in the fact that early diagnosis and treatment often could have prevented permanent damage. This is particularly true of certain childhood ocular problems such as amblyopia, strabismus, and progressive cataracts. It has been estimated that one-fourth of school children have or will develop visual defects. Since teachers and educators have extended contact with children during visual activities, they are in an excellent position to recognize early problems and to ensure that proper medical management is available.

In this chapter, certain common types of visual impairment will be considered with special emphasis on their clinical manifestations and possible influence on the learning process. Aspects of therapy which may involve teacher participation and understanding are stressed in the hope that physician-educator cooperation will lead to improvement in the educational experience of the child with ocular disease.

STRUCTURE AND FUNCTION OF THE VISUAL SYSTEM

The visual system includes the globe (eyeball), the optic nerves and tracts which carry messages to the brain, the occipital lobes of the cerebral hemispheres where the visual messages are projected, and numerous connections throughout the brain where images are interpreted and correlated with other cerebral functions. In addition, numerous accessory structures are present, such as the tear glands, the extraocular muscles which move the eyes, and the eyelids which serve to protect and maintain the peripheral visual apparatus.

The globe itself is remarkably similar to a camera in both function and structure (Figure 1). Incident light rays enter the eye through the pupil and then pass through the lens where they are focused to form a sharp image on the retina. The primary function of the globe is, therefore, a relatively passive one since its major purpose is to receive reflected light from the environment.

The normal eye actively modifies recipient light in several respects, however. Inside the globe are small muscles which change the shape of the lens to maintain the proper focus of images on the retina. Such refractive activity is largely automatic, requiring little conscious effort. With increasing age, there is progressive loss of focusing ability (accommodation) at close distances, resulting in the condition known as presbyopia. Another active function of the globe, as yet poorly understood, is the conversion of light impulses into electrical signals which are transmitted to the brain via the optic nerves. Recent evidence also suggests that some retinal cells actually integrate and interpret certain types of visual data before it is sent to the brain. What role this process plays in visual perception is unclear at this time.

CLUES TO VISUAL IMPAIRMENT

Ideally, visual problems should be diagnosed prior to the development of any functional handicap. Well-designed visual screening programs among preschool children are especially productive since they often detect subclinical defects for which early treatment can lessen the danger of permanent impairment. Most individuals, especially children, who have never experienced normal vision have no reference basis upon which to judge their acuity, and hence, are unlikely to complain spontaneously unless vision is sufficiently limited to impair perfor- mance. In fact, it is not unusual for ophthalmologists to evaluate adult patients who were unaware of subnormal vision until they failed the minimum visual requirements for a driver's license. Thus, it is essential that educators and other adults be aware of the signs and symptoms of ocular disease to prevent develop- mental defects and educational retardation.

Unusual Behavior

Unusual activity patterns in very young children may provide the first clue to a visual handicap. Irritability, inattention, rubbing of the eyes, squinting or closing one eye, and unusual reading positions sometimes suggest an ocular problem. Of course, these signs may also be a product of bad habits or a manifestation of other

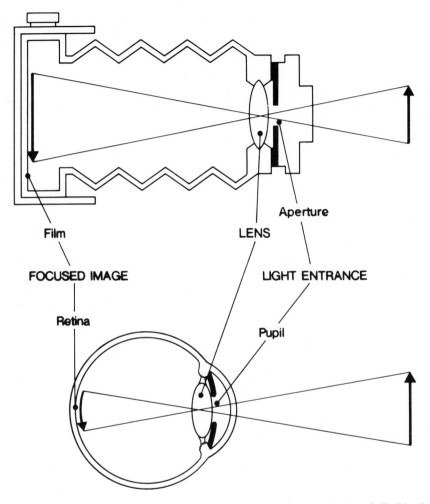

Figure 1. Diagrammatic cross-section of an eyeball and a camera showing similarities in both structure and function.

diseases as well, so professional medical advice is necessary to rule out any physical or emotional problem. Contrary to popular opinion, sitting close to the television set or "burying his nose in a book" does not necessarily imply a significant visual problem in a child. Most children have considerable accommodative (focusing) ability and may prefer to look at near material out of simple habit alone. However, children with a high degree of myopia (near-sightedness) are unable to see distant objects clearly and their preferred proximity to objects is an important clue to a visual handicap. A child who can see letters on the blackboard clearly from the rear of the classroom, even though he tends to hold reading material abnormally close, probably does not have significant myopia. In suspicious or questionable cases, an ophthalmic evaluation should be obtained.

An inadequate school performance may itself result from poor vision, although other etiologies must also be considered. Children possess an amazing ability to adapt to certain visual handicaps. Blurred vision due to simple refractive errors may be partially corrected by adjustment in viewing distance or by squinting, for example. In most cases, however, such compensation is not possible, so that poor learning or failure in school may require an eye examination to rule out ocular problems.

Headaches

Most headaches in children are not caused by ocular problems (see Chapter 4). In fact, blurred vision alone probably does not produce any systemic symptoms. However, one form of refractive error, hyperopia, or far-sightedness, may produce a constellation of symptoms collectively known as eye strain, including the sensation of tired eyes, ocular pain, and even headache. In this condition, the accommodative apparatus must exert unusual effort during close work, causing the muscles controlling accommodation to become overly fatigued. Characteristically, symptoms appear after prolonged close work such as reading, which requires more accommodation. Correction of the refractive error is the only treatment necessary.

Diplopia

Any student with diplopia or double vision should have an ophthalmic evaluation immediately, since this symptom suggests strabismus (squint) of recent onset. If allowed to persist in children, amblyopia (impaired vision) may result, although most children will not spontaneously complain and few admit diplopia even under direct questioning. It should be emphasized that even if crossed eyes are not apparent to the lay observer, diplopia should never be ignored since it is a more discriminating symptom.

Nystagmus and Strabismus

Both nystagmus and strabismus may occur as primary disorders or as a result of poor visual activity. Nystagmus (abnormal, rapid movement of the eyes) is sometimes present as a congenital anomaly and, in such cases, usually causes a permanent reduction in visual acuity. However, in other children, wandering movements result when the eyes are unable to fixate properly due to abnormalities of the retina or optic nerves.

Strabismus, in most patients, is secondary to certain congenital anatomic variations in the eyeball muscles and other orbital structures that are as yet poorly understood. More rarely, strabismus develops as a result of uniocular loss of vision. In children, this type is usually manifested as esotropia (one eye deviating toward the nose). Whatever the etiology, consultation is important to ensure that proper medical and surgical therapy is given.

DETERMINATION OF VISUAL ACUITY

Testing for visual acuity is one of the simplest and most useful determinations of ocular functions. As a screening procedure, it is the single most valuable test for the presence of significant ophthalmic disease. Testing should never be substituted for a diagnostic examination, however, when other evidence of disease is apparent or suspected.

Terminology

The terms used to record and describe the level of visual acuity are often confusing to nonmedical personnel. In this country, vision is usually determined at a distance of 20 ft., using standardized symbols such as those on the Snellen eye chart (Figure 2). These are carefully scaled to subtend uniform visual angles

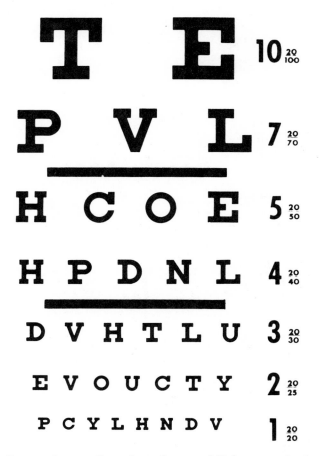

Figure 2. Snellen eye chart usually read at a distance of 20 ft. to test visual acuity. *Right*, the acuity is recorded as the fraction corresponding to the smallest line of letters which the patient is able to read.

corresponding to levels of acuity achieved by "normal eyes." Thus, a person with normal vision should be able to see the series of letters on the 20/20 line at a distance of 20 ft. If he is unable to see any letters smaller than those located on the 20/50 line, it is said that he has 20/50 vision since he is able to see at 20 ft. (the numerator) what a "normal" or average person is able to distinguish at 50 ft. (the denominator). Most states require a minimum vision of 20/40 to qualify for a driver's license, while 20/200 is considered "legal blindness" and entitles the individual to income tax deductions and certain other benefits available to the visually handicapped.

Standardized eye charts for the illiterate are also available (Figure 3). Most youngsters who do not yet know the letters of the alphabet will readily learn the "E game" and indicate their degree of acuity by pointing a finger in the direction that the "E" is oriented. Children as young as 2½ or 3 years of age with normal vision will usually recognize the rough outline of objects depicted on the Allen cards (Figure 4) at a distance of 15 or 20 ft. (Since a normally sighted

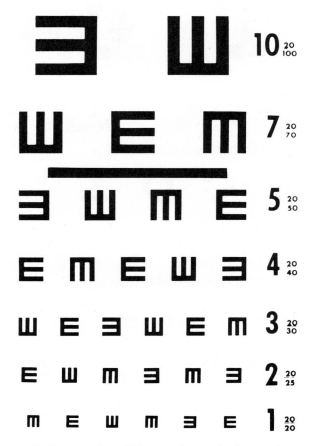

Figure 3. Illiterate Snellen eye chart. This chart is used in the same manner as the one depicted in Figure 2.

adult can distinguish these pictures at 30 ft., the child's vision would be designated as 15/30 or 20/30.)

Methods

Vision testing should always be carried out with each eye separately. Special attention is necessary to ensure that the subject does not look around the occluder covering the eye; children are particularly tempted to peek if vision in the uncovered eye is subnormal. It is also important, whenever possible, to present the entire line of letters rather than only single ones. Amblyopic eyes characteristically are able to distinguish isolated letters more readily than those of identical size present in a linear array.

Effect of Illumination

Too much light, as well as insufficient light, may result in a decrease in visual acuity. This is true not only for people with normal eyes but also for those with certain ocular disorders. For screening examinations, it is possible to use average room illumination. Lighting of the acuity chart (approximately 20 footcandles) is more important than the degree of illumination in the rest of the room, but under no circumstances should the patient area be more brightly lit than the

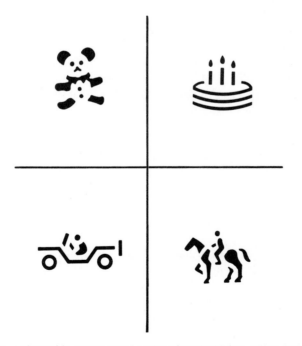

Figure 4. Allen cards used in testing visual acuity of small children. These may be presented at variable distances with appropriate modification of the numerator of the acuity fraction.

chart. Care should be taken to ensure that there is no glare in the patient's line of vision.

Individuals with certain types of early cataracts may be dazzled and complain of ocular discomfort when exposed to bright lights. Persons with exophoria (outward deviation of an eye), especially if they have a large angle, may also complain of photophobia (abnormal intolerance of light) in the presence of intense illumination.

Countless generations of parents have warned their offspring that reading or working in dimly lit surroundings will "hurt your eyes." While this falsehood has probably caused relatively little harm, it is a fact that there is no more danger of damage to the eyes by trying to see in dim illumination than of harming the ears by listening to faint sounds. At the same time, it must be emphasized that reading in poor light can be mentally taxing and, therefore, should be avoided whenever possible in order to achieve and maintain maximum perceptual efficiency.

Certain rare inherited disorders of the retina (e.g., retinitis pigmentosa) cause "night blindness." Individuals with these conditions experience progressive loss of acuity, initially only in dim light, but subsequently under all conditions of illumination. No effective treatment is known, although there is some evidence that too much light increases the rate of deterioration.

Interpretation of Results

Due to the shortened attention span of many children, they often lose interest in the smaller letters on the chart and may not concentrate sufficiently to read the 20/20 or 20/30 lines. Hence, even under ideal testing conditions, one may need to exercise some clinical judgment in the interpretation of the visual acuity of children. Children at 4 years of age should have at least 20/30 vision in each eye, and older students can usually be encouraged to read the 20/20 line. Individuals with an acuity of one or more lines worse should be referred for further evaluation. Likewise, any child with an acuity difference of at least two lines between the two eyes should be examined by an ophthalmologist. Unusual behavior or difficulty during the test should always be noted.

COMMON OCULAR PROBLEMS IN CHILDREN

The diagnosis and therapy of ocular problems should, of course, be directed by a physician and remain under his supervision. Frequently, however, the teacher can provide supportive assistance, particularly in cases requiring short-term intensive therapy. Since psychologic support and adjustment of classroom activities can lessen the emotional trauma in the affected child, it is desirable that teachers have some understanding of the appropriate indications and restrictions of various forms of treatment.

Refractive Errors

Except in rare special instances (e.g., keratoconus) for which contact lenses are necessary, corrective glasses are used to neutralize refractive errors. Today, fortunately, there is little social stigma attached to the wearing of glasses, and many young people actually consider modern styles of glasses to be a cosmetic asset.

Indications for corrective lenses vary. Some patients require them primarily as an aid for distance vision, while others need a correction for near work. Hence, not everyone needs to wear glasses at all times. Flexibility is necessary to avoid the psychologic trauma that may result when a child is harshly forced to wear glasses all the time. It is the physician's duty to set appropriate guidelines which can reasonably be expected to be followed. If no requirements are specified, the patient may be allowed to judge his own need for corrective lenses at specific times.

Visual requirements for various activities will usually determine the appropriate wearing habits. In case there is uncertainty regarding the need for corrective lenses, the prescribing physician should be consulted. With the important exception of patients with hyperopic esotropia, no ocular harm results if glasses are not worn constantly.

Strabismus

Lack of binocular fixation due to abnormal alignment of the two eyes is one of the most frequent and serious of childhood ocular disorders. Between 1 and 2% of children are affected.

Esotropia is the most common type of strabismus in children (Figure 5). Usually it is evident unilaterally, although, rarely, both eyes deviate toward the nose. Some individuals are alternators; i.e., at different times either eye turns in. A minority of strabismic children are exotropes (one eye turns out) or have a large angle exophoria (the eyes are usually straight but one may wander out when fixation is temporarily disrupted, or when the child is tired or daydreaming). Nontraumatic vertical strabismus is rare in children, but any form of misalignment should be referred to the physician for diagnostic evaluation.

A minority of crossed eyes can be straightened with glasses alone, although it is rare even among children that such therapy restores full sensory function (e.g., normal stereopsis). Visual training and eye exercises are seldom either cosmetically or functionally effective. Most children with gross deviations require surgery for permanent correction.

Amblyopia

Perhaps the least understood among all forms of visual handicaps is amblyopia, commonly known as the "lazy eye" condition. This problem is of particular

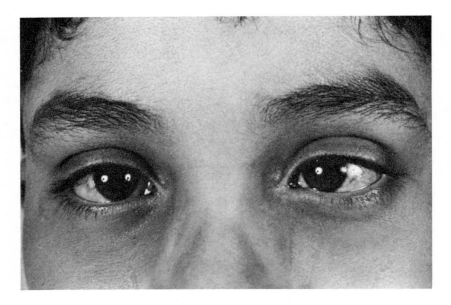

Figure 5. Manifest esotropia in a 12-year-old male. Note the asymmetrical position of the corneal light reflexes, which is often a helpful diagnostic clue to strabismus.

importance among children since its onset occurs sometime during childhood and must be treated before the age of 8 or 9 years. Amblyopia is usually unilateral but, in rare cases, may develop in both eyes. Although a pathophysiologic basis for this disorder is still unknown, ophthalmologists do know something about conditions which may lead to "lazy eye."

Any obstruction to the normal passage of light through the eye will, of course, interfere with the proper display of images on the retina. Light must pass through four ocular components in order to reach the retina (see Figure 1): the cornea (the transparent anterior portion of the eye), the aqueous humor (a clear fluid which fills the anterior chamber between the lens and the cornea), the lens, and the vitreous humor (the gel-like material which normally fills the posterior chamber). These structures may lose their normal transparency as a result of either congenital or acquired diseases, but fortunately opacities of the media (transparent tissues and fluids of the eye) can often be surgically corrected. Interference with the projection of images on the retina, such as opacification of the media or irregular refractive errors, prevents normal maturation of the visual system, and amblyopia may result.

Strabismus may also lead to amblyopia, although a different mechanism seems to be responsible. In this case, the ocular apparatus is usually perfectly capable of focusing images on the retina. However, when the two eyes do not look in the same direction, diplopia and visual confusion result. The brain subconsciously compensates for this by repressing the visual impulses from one eye. If allowed to persist in children, this repression becomes permanent, leading to amblyopia. Not all children with strabismus develop a "lazy eye," but since it can lead to a permanent loss of vision, immediate medical attention is mandatory. Children under 5 years of age with nonalternating esotropia are most likely to develop amblyopia, but it may begin as early as the first 3 months of life or as late as approximately 9 years of age.

The only effective treatment for amblyopia is to stimulate the affected eye with normal visual images. This usually requires occlusion (patching) or blurring (use of various eye drops) of the vision of the good eye in order that the amblyopic (weaker) eye is used. Therapy should begin before 8 years of age in order to effect a significant improvement. Furthermore, results in older children usually are not as favorable as in those in whom treatment was begun at a younger age. In general, the earlier treatment is started, the better the prognosis. All children under treatment for amblyopia must be examined frequently.

Wearing a patch over one eye is a nuisance, and children, like most adults, object to this form of treatment. Fortunately, its use is limited, being utilized primarily in postoperative cases and in the treatment of amblyopia.

Occlusion therapy in the latter case is particularly important in younger children in order to force them to use their "weaker" eye. It is frequently necessary that an opaque patch be worn constantly during waking hours, including school hours. The teacher should, of course, provide psychologic support to such students but should also recognize that since the weaker eye is being used, special educational assistance may be needed. In most cases, full-time occlusion is necessary for brief periods only, and the ophthalmologist can restrict these periods to times when the patient is not in school (Figure 6).

Loss of Stereopsis

Loss of stereopsis is an important form of visual impairment, but its functional significance is often overemphasized. Stereo vision is, of course, necessary in order to perceive the environment in three dimensions. But loss of stereopsis should not be equated with poor visual acuity since each eye may see objects clearly. However, since both eyes must simultaneously perceive the same object in order to achieve proper spatial perception and distance judgment, it is apparent that loss of one eye, significant unilateral loss of vision, or misalignment of the optical axes (e.g., strabismus or crossed eyes) can all lead to a defect in stereopsis.

Any abnormality that interferes with normal binocular fixation will reduce depth perception. While it is technically true that one of the parameters of ocular health is normal stereopsis, loss of stereo vision is not a serious handicap. Even people who suffer total loss of vision in one eye learn to utilize other visual clues that enable them to function normally. Absence of stereopsis does make certain tasks such as catching a ball or reaching for objects more difficult since

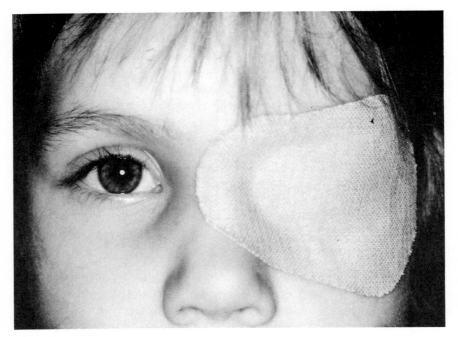

Figure 6*A*. Patching for treatment of amblyopia. In order to be effective, the occlusion must be total by using an adhesive bandage.

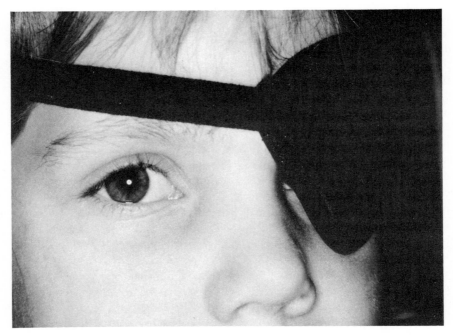

Figure 6*B*. Other techniques such as the "pirate's patch" allows the child to "cheat" by looking around the occluder.

judgment of distance is impaired, but individuals with natural athletic ability may even play professional sports in spite of such a handicap. Loss of normal depth perception alone should never be blamed for lack of physical coordination, although, obviously, poor vision in both eyes can lead to problems in mobility.

Trauma

Ocular trauma occurs all too frequently in children. Careless use of sharp pointed instruments, splashing of chemicals or poisonous substances into the eye, and blunt trauma can cause serious damage. Proper safety precautions should be constantly stressed in the classroom, but the presence of safety-conscious adult models is probably more beneficial in the long run than an organized safety program.

It must be emphasized that any apparent or suspected trauma to the eye should receive immediate ophthalmologic attention. In many cases, prompt attention and treatment significantly reduce the risk of complications.

Visual Field Loss

Only a very small portion of the human retina is actually utilized for most visual tasks. The macular area located in the posterior portion of the eye contains the fovea which is the visually sensitive region of the retina used for fine point discrimination tasks such as reading. The remainder of the retina, often called the peripheral retina, nevertheless, serves a useful function as it broadens one's field of vision.

Diseases of the macula usually cause reduced central vision which, unfortunately, decreases the ability to perform most near tasks. Affected individuals frequently complain of a black or dark spot in the center of their vision and are unable to see any but the very largest letters and objects. Locomotion may be unimpaired, however, since peripheral vision is intact. Other diseases selectively destroy the peripheral retina with preservation of central vision. Loss of peripheral vision usually produces few complaints since it progresses so slowly that patients may be unaware of their constricted side vision. In extreme cases, however, patients may compare their field of vision to the effect produced by looking through a tunnel or a gun barrel.

It is important to distinguish between these two types of visual field loss since the degree and type of educational handicap differ greatly. Children with *abnormal central vision* often require special large print books or even instruction in braille, depending on the degree of loss. However, those with good central vision but *peripheral field loss* are usually able to compete with their peers in educational activities, although they may be handicapped to some extent in athletic and other physical functions.

Dyslexia

Processing of visual symbols and coordination with other functions of the brain take place in the central nervous system. Defects in image recognition and inability to read with understanding are, therefore, not due to a problem in the eye itself but are usually secondary to some anomaly of the more central connections in the brain. Ignorance of this fact has, unfortunately, led to occasional exploitation by otherwise well-intentioned therapists.

Today, fortunately, most educators realize that children with reading problems or learning disabilities due to a defect in the processing of visual symbols do not have a primary visual problem. Several studies (Goldberg, 1959; and Goldberg and Drash, 1968) have failed to find any responsible ocular defect. However, since the slow learner or poor reader may also have associated ocular disease, it is important that such a child's evaluation include a thorough diagnostic examination.

The magnitude and significance of reading and learning problems have recently led the American Academy of Pediatrics, the American Academy of Ophthalmology and Otolaryngology, and the American Association of Ophthalmology to review the scientific evidence supporting the various modes of therapy. Their joint statement (American Academy of Pediatrics, 1972) on the function of the eye and the role of visual training in the treatment of dyslexia and associated learning disabilities may be summarized as follows.

1. The several forms of academic underachievement, including dyslexia and reading disabilities, are complex problems requiring therapeutic input from a variety of disciplines, such as medicine, education, and psychology.

2. There is no known peripheral eye defect which causes reversals of symbols such as letters and numbers, nor is there any evidence that such abnormalities produce any other signs of dyslexia and associated learning disabilities. Existing ocular abnormalities such as refractive errors or strabismus should, of course, be corrected but this should be done only if medically indicated and not as the primary or sole treatment of the dyslexic child.

3. There is no scientific evidence that visual training (e.g., muscle exercises, ocular pursuit, or special glasses) or neurologic organizational training (e.g., laterality training, balance board, or perceptual stimulation) by themselves improve the academic abilities of dyslexic children.

4. Since the treatment of dyslexic and learning-disabled children is a problem of educational science requiring multiple approaches, application of a single mode of therapy such as special glasses or vision training may create a false sense of security and delay more effective treatment.

Ophthalmologists, as well as other physicians such as neurologists, psychiatrists, and endocrinologists, should assist in the evaluation of the poor achiever and institute appropriate therapy for specific problems. The educator must realize, however, that remedial procedures for learning disabilities remain the ultimate responsibility of the entire education team.

SURGICAL AND MEDICAL MANAGEMENT

Surgery

Surgery to correct strabismus is the most frequent type of operative procedure performed upon eyes of children and young adults. Since the operation is performed on muscles located on the outside of the globe, the visual apparatus itself is not disturbed and should remain functionally normal. There may be some mild postoperative discomfort and irritation, particularly from bright lights, but this rarely persists for more than 48 hrs. although the eye may appear red and inflamed for several weeks. As long as the patient feels comfortable and is anxious to return to school, there is no reason why he should not be allowed to resume normal activities with 24–48 hrs. following a strabismus operation.

Other types of ocular surgery, such as removal of cataracts, repair of retinal detachments, or transplantation of the cornea, are considerably more rare in the pediatric age group. Postoperative management is highly individualized and the surgeon's advice should be followed carefully.

Medications

The vast majority of ocular medications are topically applied and prescribed for short periods only. These are dispensed in the form of ointments or drops. They may be used for diagnostic purposes to induce cycloplegia (paralysis of accommodation) prior to refraction, for the therapy of acute illnesses such as infections, or to reduce postoperative inflammatory reactions. Application schedules usually are sufficiently flexible that medications need not be given during school hours. Rarely, however, more intensive utilization is necessary and the teacher may have to assist in the application of such medications.

Most adults are familiar with the technique of applying topical mediations to the eye. Perhaps the simplest method is to have the child sit with his head extended back and look up as far as possible. Then, by simply pulling down the lower lid, a drop or small amount of ointment is instilled on the inside of the lid. This is much easier and less irritating to the patient than the technique of applying medication directly on the eye itself. It has the further advantage of avoiding the blink reflex that sometimes interferes with the instillation of medications.

Most topical medications do not seriously interfere with ocular function. Consequently, the advisability of continued school attendance during treatment depends primarily on the nature of the underlying eye disease. Cycloplegic drugs, such as atropine, homatropine, or scopolamine, are important exceptions to this generalization since they cause blurred near vision by inhibiting the accommodative mechanism. These medications also dilate the pupils, providing a useful clue to their utilization in patients who complain of sudden onset of blurred near vision. Fortunately, they are usually applied for only the short period of time needed to determine refractive errors. The cycloplegic effect of these drugs generally wears off within about 24 hrs., with the exception of atropine in which the effect may last a week or two.

REFERRAL OF CHILDREN WITH VISUAL DISORDERS

Because the educator occupies such a central and influential position during the formative years of childhood, he or she can evaluate visual handicaps earlier and often more objectively than immediate members of the family. Thus, the teacher plays a vital role in the referral of ocular problems, and, by working closely with the physician, may provide valuable assistance in the evaluation of the degree of functional handicap.

The first step in a suspected visual problem should always be a complete diagnostic evaluation, followed, of course, by appropriate medical and surgical therapy. The teacher can and should suggest such a course to the parents if the child is not already under treatment.

In cases where poor vision is uncorrectable, special training and equipment may be needed. Most states have excellent programs for the blind and visually handicapped, including facilities for the counseling of families beginning soon after the affected child is born. Where such contacts have not been established, the teacher should suggest to the physician or parents the advisability of doing so. Close liaison between educational institutions and agencies for the visually handicapped should be established whenever possible.

No arbitrary level of acuity automatically precludes a child's attendance in regular classes. Individual levels of motivation and aptitude vary, and, therefore, the ability to perform in the face of handicaps cannot be arbitrarily determined. For this reason, an ophthalmologist cannot always advise the teacher regarding a specific student's need for special educational facilities. The educator should learn to judge the degree to which a visual handicap interferes with scholastic achievement and to draw upon available resources when necessary.

Many communities and states have active organizations dedicated to the problems of the visually impaired. Educators should be familiar with referral procedures of state educational institutions for the blind and visually handicapped. Much valuable and informative material is available in numerous publications distributed by the National Society for the Prevention of Blindness, 16 East 40th Street, New York, New York 10016.

SUMMARY

Visual handicaps can lead to serious difficulties in educational achievement and can best be avoided by early detection and treatment. The prolonged and pivotal role of educators during childhood and adolescent development thereby places on this segment of the professional community a vital responsibility in eye care.

The teacher should have an understanding—both scientifically and emotionally—of certain basic aspects of ocular dysfunction and the manner in which they may be expressed. By recognition of the signs and symptoms of ocular disease, as well as continued observation for evidence of disability or improvement, the teacher can make important contributions to the management of visual handicaps. The teacher should be able to determine the degree of scholastic impairment caused by the visual handicap and, if necessary, work closely with the parents, child, and physician to ensure that all available resources are utilized. Through such cooperation, the visually handicapped can mature academically to become well-adjusted and productive members of society.

REFERENCES

American Academy of Pediatrics. 1972. The Eye and Learning Disabilities. Joint Organizational Statement. Prepared by an ad hoc committee of the American Academy of Pediatrics, The American Academy of Ophthalmology and Otolaryngology, and The American Association of Ophthalmology, and approved by the executive committees and councils of these organizations. J. School Health 42:218.

Goldberg, H. K. 1959. The ophthalmologist looks at the reading problem. Am. J. Ophth. 47:67—74.

Goldberg, H. K., and P. W. Drash. 1968. The disabled reader. J. Pediat. Ophth. 5:11—24.

SUGGESTED READING

Patz, A., and R. E. Hoover, 1969. Protection of Vision in Children. Charles C Thomas, Publisher, Springfield, Ill. 172 p.

Scholz, R. O. 1960. Sight—A Handbook for Laymen. Doubleday & Company, Inc., Garden City, N. Y. 166 p.

Vision Screening in School. Publication No. P-257, National Society for the Prevention of Blindness, Inc., 16 East 40th Street, New York, N.Y.

3

Teacher Awareness Of Hearing Disorders

Judith L. Friedman, M.S.

Few would disagree that the most vital aspect of the teacher-pupil relationship is communication. Since the processes of speaking and hearing are the primary vehicles by which teachers and students impart information and exchange ideas, a clear explanation of the various disorders of hearing is an essential part of any concerted effort to alert educators to medical problems that may have significant effects on the ongoing education of hearing-impaired children. This chapter will define essential terminology, give pertinent details of the anatomy and physiology of the ear, and discuss some etiologies of hearing loss. In addition, descriptive elements of behavior common to children with hearing deficits, suggestions for meaningful teacher referral and classroom management of these children, and procedures for coordination of follow-up services will be discussed.

While the educator is not expected to perform as an audiologist or a physician, the efficacy of his or her role in detection of hearing loss, in making proper referrals, and the ability to conduct appropriate and creative classroom activities to teach the impaired child will hopefully be enhanced by the information presented here. It is the function of the audiologist to diagnose the type, degree, and probable anatomic site of the lesion giving rise to the hearing loss and to initiate and follow up on management, while the physician, with the information provided by the audiologist, may intervene medically. Yet these professionals are only two members of the team that deal with the hearing-impaired youngster. The educator who is in contact with the child for a good

This paper was supported in part through Project 917, Maternal and Child Health Services, United States Department of Health, Education, and Welfare.

The writer wishes to express appreciation for the suggestions and editing assistance given by Malcolm Preston, Ph.D., former Director, and Stephen Shevitz, M. A., Assistant Director of the Hearing and Speech Division, The John F. Kennedy Institute.

portion of his waking day also bears considerable responsibility, and only the informed cooperation of all concerned can assure that this special child is provided for in the most effective manner.

BASIC ANATOMY OF THE EAR

To further the reader's understanding of the discussion of hearing loss, a summary of the anatomic structures of the ear is presented below.

Outer Ear

The *pinna* or *auricle* is readily visible. It serves a vestigial function of sound gathering, although the capacity for directional aiming is no longer present as it is in dogs and horses. The pinna increases one's sensitivity to sound slightly by funneling the incoming sound waves into the *external ear canal,* which is a short tunnel between the exterior and the *eardrum* or *tympanic membrane.* The sound waves strike the eardrum and make it vibrate. These structures are shown in Figure 1.

Middle Ear

The *middle ear* is an air-filled space in the skull which lies beyond the eardrum and contains three tiny articulated bones: the *malleus* (hammer), *incus* (anvil), and *stapes* (stirrup), which act as a lever system to conduct the movement of sound waves from the eardrum to the inner ear. Collectively, these bones are referred to as the *ossicles.* The middle ear also has a ventilation duct, the *Eustachian tube,* which permits passage of air into the cavity each time it is inflated by swallowing or yawning. It should be noted that equal air pressure on either side of the eardrum is necessary for optimal function of the middle ear structures, and, when this pressure is disturbed, as is the case with ear infection, temporary hearing loss results. Also, if the ossicles are malformed or attached to each other incorrectly, abnormal patterns of hearing will result. Figure 2 shows the structures of the middle ear.

Inner Ear

Medial to the middle ear and separated from it by a bony wall with two membranous windows (the *oval* window and the *round* window) is the *inner ear,* which is a fluid-filled cavity containing the end organs of equilibrium (*vestibular* portion) and of hearing (*cochlear* portion). We shall be concerned only with the cochlear portion. The *foot plate* of the stapes is seated on the membrane of the *oval window.* The stapes vibrates when sound strikes the eardrum since it is linked to the other ossicles. The vibrations of the foot plate against the oval window in turn produce vibrations in the fluid contained in the cochlea. The

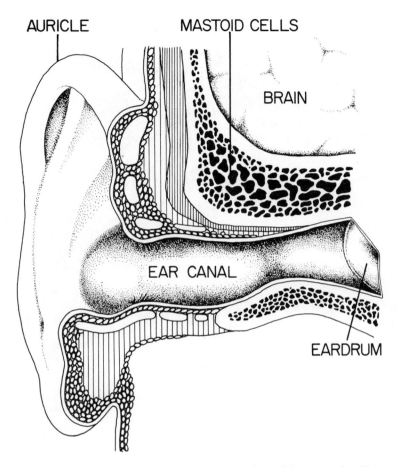

Figure 1. Cut-away view of the external ear showing the auricle, external auditory canal, and tympanic membrane (eardrum).

cochlea closely resembles a snail shell, hence its name. It may also be described as a "winding staircase" structure that contains microscopic sensory cells which line up along the spiral. When the sensory cells are stimulated by movement of the fluid that surrounds them, they transmit a chemical electric impulse to the higher cortical centers via the auditory nerve and the other nerve fibers connecting the auditory nerve to the brain. The impulse is then interpreted in the auditory cortex. Figure 3 shows the structures of the inner ear.

PHYSIOLOGY OF THE EAR

When all the structures described are operating normally, one may summarize the overall function of the ear briefly as follows. When airborne sound waves reach the outer ear, they are ushered to the eardrum where they are changed

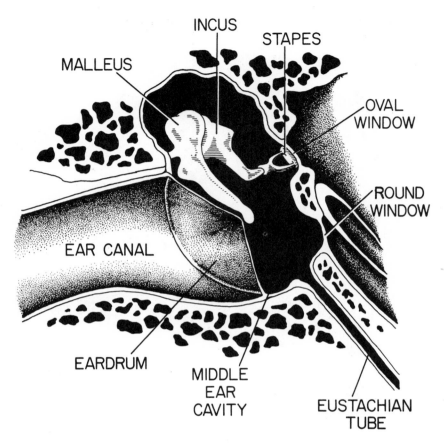

Figure 2. The middle ear structures.

into mechanical energy resulting in movement of the ossicles of the middle ear. The ossicles conduct the energy, in a chain reaction fashion, to the fluid of the inner ear through the movement of the stapes against the oval window. When changes occur in the sensory cells of the cochlea because of the motion of the inner ear fluid, chemical electric energy is produced and transmitted via the auditory nerve to the brain. If we accept that the brain can accurately interpret the various impulses it receives, we can see that the function of the outer, middle, and inner ear structures is to translate an environmental event (sound) into a form that is meaningful to the brain. A cutaway view of the entire ear is shown in Figure 4. A breakdown in the system, be it in the outer, middle, or inner ear, results in a reduction in the amount of information that reaches the brain; or if the brain does not perceive and interpret incoming information correctly, perhaps due to a central nervous system anomaly, the function of the ear itself if not affected but the end result is that the child's communication system is still not adequate.

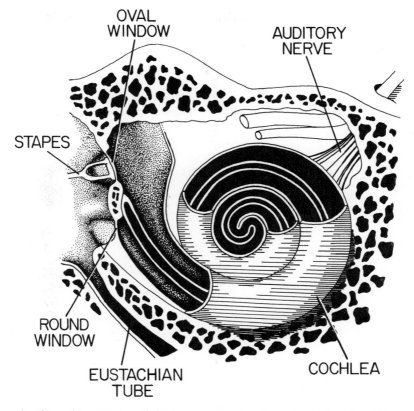

Figure 3. The cochlear portion of the inner ear showing the multichambered cochlea, oval and round windows, and auditory nerve.

CLASSIFICATION OF HEARING LOSS

Loss of hearing is not synonymous with deafness. Actually, sometimes the presence of hearing loss is not empirically obvious. Of the estimated 5–10% of the school age population who demonstrate significant hearing impairment, few are in fact deaf (Newby, 1971). The term "deaf" is generally restricted to those individuals who have insufficient residual hearing to learn language from the speech of others and who cannot learn to speak or understand the spoken word, even with the use of hearing aids. Silverman (1971a) estimates this population to number approximately 39,000 among the school age children in this country.

Terms such as "hearing impaired" or "hard-of-hearing" describe those whose loss of auditory acuity is mild enough to permit them to acquire at least some language and speech, sometimes requiring the aid of amplification. According to the United States Health Interview Survey of 1962–1963 (Human Communication and Its Disorders, 1970) approximately 360,000 individuals under the age of 17 have hearing losses "less severe than deafness but which impair communi-

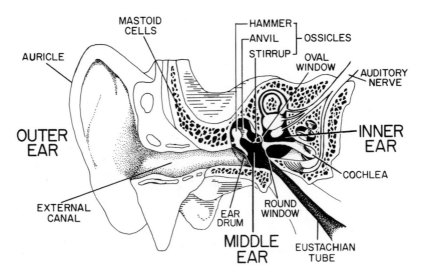

Figure 4. The external, middle, and inner ear structures. Note the pathway of sound inward from the environment.

cation and hence social efficiency." As one might guess, there is no absolute cutoff in terms of degree of loss to distinguish these two groups, although the following generalizations may be offered.

Functional descriptions of degrees of hearing loss may be more useful to the educator than mere grouping into classifications such as "deaf" or "hard of hearing." First, the normal hearing population has, as its best sensitivity (threshold), an intensity range of 0–20 decibels (dB) for pure tones and speech, according to established standards. The decibel is a relative measure of intensity of sound and not an expression of percentage of hearing loss. The audiogram, which is a graph on which hearing thresholds are recorded, shows the minimal intensity level in decibels necessary to elicit a response to a tone of specified frequency. The normal human ear can detect sounds ranging in frequency from 20–20,000 cycles/sec (or Hertz, Hz). Audiometric testing, however, concentrates only on several frequencies which span the range of those found in human speech. These include 125, 250, 500, 1,000, 2,000, 4,000, and 8,000 Hz presented as pure tones. The audiogram will show how intense (dB measure) each test tone (frequency) must be for the ear to just barely hear it. The dB level at which detection of a given tone takes place is called the threshold for that frequency.

An example of an audiogram indicating thresholds falling within the normal range of hearing is shown in Figure 5. For each test frequency, an intensity level of 0 dB is the faintest sound that most persons with no auditory deficit can hear and respond to under standard test conditions which require a special sound insulated chamber of the kind found in a hearing and speech center. Please note that Figure 5 shows a pattern within the normal range of hearing for both ears, although for the left ear the intensity of the test tone must be set at 20 dB to

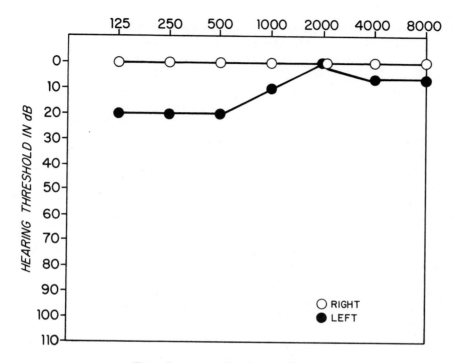

Figure 5. An example of normal hearing.

produce a response at certain frequencies. While one may speak of a 20-dB loss at those frequencies, thresholds up to 20 dB are considered normal and would not significantly affect the communication processes under most circumstances.

A mild (Class 1) hearing loss refers to a loss ranging between 21 dB and 40 dB (Silverman, 1971b). With best hearing in this range, a child will experience difficulty hearing faint or distant speech. His own speech patterns may be unremarkable or reflect only minor distortions and omissions.

A moderate (Class 2) hearing loss falls in the range between 41 dB and 55 dB, and when it is bilateral it significantly impairs the child's ability to follow conversation of normal intensity levels at a distance of more than 3–6 ft. from the speaker. This child's speech usually has noticeable articulation errors, particularly in consonant sounds such as sue, shoe, and chew.

A moderately severe (Class 3) loss means the loss is in the range of 56 dB to 70 dB. A child who hears only this well cannot follow conversation unless it is loud and very close. He will not function in group work and will probably have limited vocabulary and language skills. His speech patterns will be poor with many articulation errors and he may have a swallowed or hollow vocal quality. He generally wears a hearing aid with successful results.

A severe (Class 4) hearing loss lies between 71 dB and 90 dB. With bilateral impairment of this type, the child cannot follow conversation, although he may hear single words at a distance of about 1 ft. and he may hear some loud environmental noises. Even with hearing aids, this youngster will not hear speech clearly and usually has difficulty following even simple spoken sentences. His own speech production is often unintelligible with an abnormal voice quality and he will require specialized help to produce recognizable speech.

A profound (Class 5) hearing loss exists when thresholds lie above 90 dB. A child with this degree of bilateral loss may react on occasion to very intense sound. He cannot rely on hearing for communication even with hearing aids and is usually trained by specialists in deaf education, often employing manual (sign language) or total communication (sign language while talking) techniques. His speech, if he has any, is unintelligible although he may produce some recognizable words with training.

Figure 6 presents examples of audiograms for each of these five classes of hearing loss. In actual practice, a child may exhibit a distorting loss in which hearing is relatively good for some frequencies and may be poor for other frequencies. One example of this is also illustrated in Figure 7. In this case, classification of hearing loss is difficult. The most commonly used classification method involves calculating the average threshold for the frequencies 500, 1,000, and 2,000 Hz. For the case presented in Figure 7, this three frequency pure tone average (PTA) would be 50 dB for both ears, thus putting the child into Class 2. However, this child may have greater difficulty than other Class 2 children in understanding words with phonemes (sound units), such as "s," "sh," "ch," that have high frequency components because his loss at frequencies above 1,000 Hz is severe. His speech may also show abnormalities in the production of these sounds. Thus, in preparing educational programs for the hearing impaired child, the educator should be familiar not only with the classification of hearing loss but also with the general slope or configuration of thresholds presented in the child's audiogram.

TYPES AND ETIOLOGIES OF HEARING LOSS

Conductive Hearing Loss

In a given sample of a school population, the most common causative factor in hearing loss is an upper respiratory infection (URI) and related ear pathologies. The resultant loss is called a conductive hearing loss because there is interference with the mechanisms of the outer or middle ear that serve to conduct the sound inward toward the brain. When secondary to URI, this type of impairment may be associated with ear infections, but it may also occur with excessive ear wax (cerumen), foreign objects in the auditory canal, or structural abnormalities. Depending on the medically diagnosed etiology, conductive losses are generally temporary and require medical treatment. Regardless of etiology, conductive losses do not exceed 60 dB and generally only rarely require the use of hearing aids.

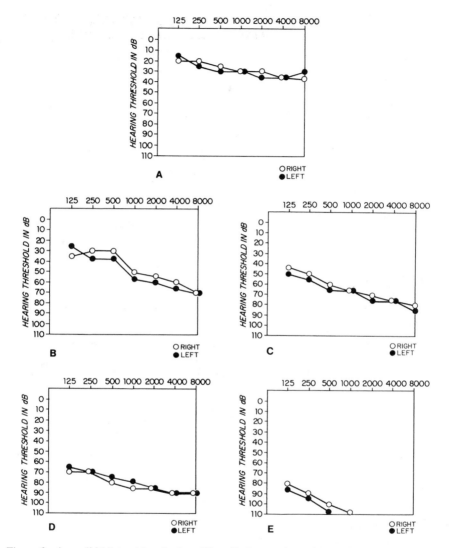

Figure 6. *A*, a mild bilateral hearing loss (Class 1); *B*, a moderate bilateral hearing loss (Class 2); *C*, a moderately severe bilateral hearing loss (Class 3); *D*, a severe bilateral hearing loss (Class 4); and *E*, a profound bilateral hearing loss (Class 5).

Sensorineural Hearing Loss

Hearing losses of this type are caused by damage to the sensory cells in the cochlea or the neural pathway between the cochlea and the brainstem (Goodhill and Guggenheim, 1971). Sensorineural losses are secondary to factors such as maternal rubella which can damage the fetus if contracted during the first trimester of pregnancy, severe illness and high fever in a child, ototoxic drugs

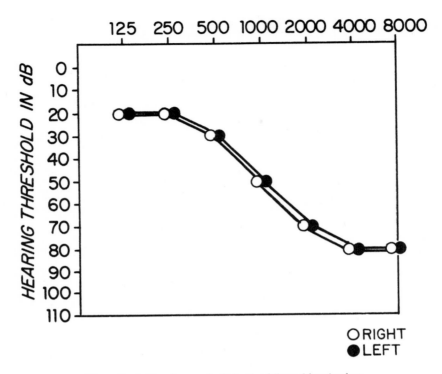

Figure 7. A Class 2 severely distorting bilateral hearing loss.

such as kanamycin (an antibiotic), traumatic injury, a tumor of the middle or inner ear, congenital or inherited abnormalities, oxygen deprivation at birth or thereafter (anoxia), or Rh blood group incompatibility between the mother and the fetus. These hearing losses are permanent and may be progressive. Depending upon the degree of the loss and the signal distortion it causes, use of hearing aids may be required.

Mixed Hearing Loss

Occasionally a child demonstrates a two-in-one hearing impairment, that is, a sensorineural impairment is present with a conductive overlay. This is a mixed hearing loss. Before the sensorineural loss is dealt with, the conductive component should be treated by a physician.

Central Auditory Problems

Central hearing losses are rather rare and present a complex of diagnostic and remediation problems. To oversimplify for the purpose of illustration, the central or perceptive loss may be thought of as one in which the incoming signal is not properly sorted and associated, or possibly, as Myklebust (1954) states, the disorder is one of "symbolic functioning" in which the child hears the signal but attaches no meaning to it. The point of breakdown can be anywhere in the brain and it is often impossible to determine just where it is. Conditions which affect brain function, such as anoxia or trauma, are probably the easiest to connect with central auditory problems.

TEACHER DETECTION OF HEARING LOSS

Often, hearing impairment is detected before a child enters school, but, unfortunately, this is not always the case. Sometimes, too, a child of school age may acquire a hearing loss adventitiously. Once the undiagnosed child is in the classroom situation, it often falls to the teacher to detect and deal with the problems that may have their origin in a hearing deficit. Although hearing-impaired children behave in a variety of fashions, depending on many factors such as degree and duration of loss, etiology, intelligence, socialization, etc., common patterns may be seen by the informed observer. The following descriptions of behavioral patterns are necessarily general, but are nevertheless applicable to many children who have hearing impairment.

Children with Conductive Hearing Loss

Most conductive hearing losses are of a severity no worse than Classes 1 or 2. Since many conductive hearing losses are secondary to upper respiratory infections, the child's behavioral responses to sound may change for the worse when he is congested or has a cold. Improvement is often noted as the infection clears. The child with such a loss will hear the teacher adequately when he is standing or sitting within a few feet or 1 or 2 yds. However, as the teacher moves away or turns his back, the child will be less likely to hear his voice. Spoken to from across the room, the child may look up belatedly with "Huh?" or often answer with "I don't know." When beyond the range that permits him to hear and follow conversation, the child may daydream or appear to be inattentive, or he may sit straining unusually hard to watch the face of the speaker. Sometimes, especially if the loss has been present for a prolonged period, the child's voice will be very soft, overly nasal or denasal, high pitched, and monotonous. Obvious clues to ear pathology are behaviors such as rubbing or pulling at the ears or complaints of pain, particularly in the presence of the other symptoms just mentioned.

Children with Sensorineural Hearing Loss

There is no rule of thumb to describe the usual severity of a sensorineural loss. These losses range from Class 1 through Class 5. The severe and profound losses (Classes 4 and 5) are usually obvious at an early age in that the child does not respond to most sounds and has not acquired speech. Such children often require extensive specialized training within the public school system or placement in a special school for the hearing impaired or deaf. The following discussion will concentrate on Classes 1 through 3.

One characteristic rather common to sensorineural losses as opposed to conductive losses is that the incoming signal is not only reduced in intensity but is also distorted in various ways so that sound may seem both softer and muffled or tinny to the listener. As with the conductive hearing loss, the child who has a sensorineural loss responds less well when he is farther from the sound source. His ability to understand what is said to him may be dramatically reduced with only a slight increase in his distance from the speaker. In some cases where the hearing loss severely distorts the incoming signal, the child may consistently respond by looking up or around when addressed but be unable to discriminate the words well enough to follow even simple commands without some gestural or visual cue given by the speaker. These children often present behavior problems and may be very difficult to handle unless one is aware of the possibility that a signal-distorting hearing impairment lies beneath the exasperating behavior. They are often described as stubborn, inattentive, and incorrigible—which, indeed, they may become if frustrated by the inability to comprehend auditory signals and the behavior of others.

In many instances, significant sensorineural hearing losses are accompanied by distortion or omission of certain sounds in the child's speech, particularly sibilants (e.g., "s" and "sh") and fricatives (e.g., "f"). The youngster is, in effect, speaking as he hears. Usually the more severe hearing losses are associated with poorer speech; severe and profound losses are reflected in hollow sounding voices with very imprecise articulation and poor control of pitch. In some cases, where the child's articulation is not greatly impaired and his hearing loss is mild and only slightly distorting, the teacher may be unaware of its existence except that the child may confuse similar sounding words or consistently miss the endings of words and plurals. The errors increase as the child moves away from the speaker.

Many children with significant hearing impairment demonstrate unusual sensitivity to visual and vibratory stimuli. They learn at an early age to scan the environment for additional clues to what is happening around them, and they often watch the facial expressions and gestures of others very closely for their communicative content. However, in spite of a child's attempts to absorb information, he may lag in language and speech development. This is even more probable if his hearing loss is nearer the severe to profound categories and if the loss were present from birth or early childhood before he learned much of the language around him.

Children with Central Auditory Problems

Of all the types of hearing loss, perhaps the most difficult to detect and manage involves the receptive or associative portions of the auditory cortex and/or lower brain structures. Generally, the audiologist or physician cannot determine the nature of a central auditory problem without exhaustive testing and observation. The educator can help in this process by being aware of some key behaviors that may be related to central auditory dysfunction. For example, the child's reactions to repeated presentations of the same sound are often highly irregular and unpredictable. He may respond to a novel sound but often only once. That is, his ability to listen in a sustained fashion is disturbed. The child may demonstrate poor ability to attend to important foreground sound in the presence of distracting background noise. Surprisingly, he often ignores loud sounds but will react quickly to very soft sounds. Also, the child may seem to have no recognition that a particular sound and event go together. And finally, his language function is usually severely disturbed. He might be able to parrot words, sometimes sentences, but may have limited capacity to utilize spoken language communicatively. Children with such disorders are found in a multitude of diagnostic categories ranging from autistic to severely retarded, and more often than not demonstrate a multiplex of problems besides the central auditory dysfunction. Such a child will rarely reach the public school undetected except under extraordinary circumstances.

TEACHER REFERRAL OF A CHILD SUSPECTED OF HAVING A HEARING LOSS

Once the educator has reason to believe that a child in the classroom may have a hearing loss, a number of options are available for initial referral. Depending upon the school's procedure for referral of children for evaluation, the teacher may request that the school nurse or physician screen the child's hearing with a portable audiometer. Sometimes the principal, the speech therapist, or pupil personnel service worker may perform the screening. If the screening test indicates a loss or is inconclusive, the child's parents should be contacted as soon as possible by the proper authority and a full explanation given for the suspicion of hearing loss, including a description of his classroom behavior. In many school systems, the parents may be advised to take their child to their physician for examination. Realizing that many physicians do not have the necessary equipment for further hearing testing, the school spokesman should also inform the parents that audiologic services may be required following physical examination. Hopefully, the internal referral and evaluation procedures of most schools are designed to deal quickly and efficiently with teacher-initiated referrals.

TEACHER FOLLOW-UP

After initial referral of a child with possible hearing impairment, the teacher should be informed of the results of the evaluation and what methods have been utilized in the observation and questioning of the child. The teacher's effectiveness in coping with hearing-impaired children will be enhanced only when he is fully aware of what is happening. Ideally, the final diagnosis of the nature and degree of hearing loss, proposed intervention procedures, and recommendations for educational placement should reach the referring teacher as soon as possible, thus insuring that the teacher's follow-up will be coordinated with that of the audiologist and/or physician. Furthermore, the daily contact of the teacher with the child can provide an invaluable link between the child, his parents, and the other professionals involved because the teacher has a unique opportunity to carry out specific recommendations in a long-term structured situation and is easily accessible for feedback to others.

Enabling the teacher to receive diagnostic and management information about a child will necessitate the use of specific procedures of referral by the school. A special form which states the problem as viewed by school personnel and requests a return form from the other professionals who evaluate the child is useful. The return portion of such a referral form should include a space for a brief description of the deficit, functional effect, plan of action, and immediate and long-range recommendations for management in the individual classroom. If reports are to be returned to the principal or personnel other than the teacher, they should be routed to the teacher for his or her consideration. Most importantly, the teacher should have access to the individual who evaluated the child and wrote the report. No matter how efficient a referral system may be, if the persons critically involved with the hearing-impaired child are not in communication, the effectiveness of management of the child may be seriously hampered.

TEACHER MANAGEMENT OF THE HEARING-IMPAIRED CHILD

It has already been noted that children whose hearing losses fall in Classes 4 or 5 are not usually found in the public school system. Occasionally, a child with a Class 3 loss attends public school, but generally requires the additional specialized services of a speech, language, or hearing therapist who works closely with the classroom teacher.

For those hearing-impaired youngsters who do attend public schools and whose needs require special considerations, some very practical changes in the classroom procedure can make the teaching and learning processes much more satisfactory. Essentially, the teacher has to be concerned that the hearing-impaired student is hearing, seeing, and understanding what is being said. Simply alerting him in an inconspicuous manner that something *is* being said is a start. Preferential seating closest to the teaching situation is an ideal way to manage this task. Suppose that Johnny is hearing impaired, that he is seated next to the teacher, and that someone in the rear of the classroom wants to speak. The teacher can alert Johnny of the fact by calling on and pointing to that child. Then she can paraphrase or repeat back to the whole class the statement or question being asked, thus allowing Johnny to use her as a signal to listen and a source of information in case he missed what was said.

Preferential seating helps to minimize the strain of listening while maximizing the opportunity to fill in with visual cues. It is very important that the hearing-impaired child be seated close to the teacher, but, at the same time, as far away from noise sources as possible because ambient noise often interferes with listening even if the child can see the speaker clearly. If the teacher teaches from her desk but the desk is next to the open door or heating register, the noise may make listening very difficult for the student. Furthermore, if the child has a better ear, it should be toward the teaching situation and away from noise. Usually the audiologist's report will state which is the better ear to assist the teacher in proper seating. If no such statement is made, the teacher may assume that the ears are equally impaired and attempt central preferential seating, possibly directly in front of her desk rather than on one side.

Another important aspect of preferential seating is visibility. The hearing-impaired child will rely heavily on visual cues, speechreading, and facial expressions to assist him in comprehension. He cannot utilize these skills well if he is forced by seating to look directly into a light source such as a window or door. Even when he is seated directly opposite the teacher's desk, if the desk has its back to the window, the child will not be able to see her face clearly without excessive strain because of glare. Light that shines from behind the student and illuminates the teacher's face is preferred unless interfering shadows are cast.

Full-face speechreading is much easier than reading from a turned face or the back of someone's head! The teacher should avoid turning away from the hearing-impaired child as much as possible while talking. Supplementary gestures and vivid facial expressions are also helpful. If at all possible, the teacher should emphasize the mouth area—brighter lipstick for women and shaved faces or smaller moustaches for men. Other visual cues that can be helpful are sequential pictorial explanations and illustrations, especially when presenting new material or when making assignments. Creation of cartoon characters which pantomime assignments on a bulletin board can make understanding required homework less traumatic for any child, but especially the hearing-impaired youngster.

If the structure of the class is such that the hearing-impaired child can move around to hear better when others are reciting, this freedom will be very helpful to him. This may have to be handled very diplomatically or the entire class may want to share this activity. Perhaps moving would be allowed only during certain kinds of activities in which the speaker changes frequently and teacher paraphrasing would be difficult. Johnny may need several seats reserved for him in the classroom with one as his home base. The teacher can help minimize the need to move the child by being as stationary as possible. While it is difficult and rather boring to teach in one place, the teacher can avoid excessive pacing, particularly when giving new material, assignments, or oral work.

Once the teacher has taken as many wise precautions as he or she can so that the hearing-impaired child can hear and see maximally, he should check frequently to make sure the child has understood. A teacher may ask Johnny inconspicuously to repeat the assignment that has just been made, or put him in charge of the assignment bulletin board. The teacher should be ready to reword statements if simple repetition of what was said does not improve understanding. The rest of the class can be taught to do the same. "Mary, can you say that in a different way?" may be a subtle way of helping Johnny to understand.

A considerable degree of the hearing-impaired child's success may depend on the teacher's skill in directing the attention of the rest of his class to the needs of that child. Class discussion centered on the functions of the ear, on sound, and listening may be a good way to illustrate to the class what it is like to have a hearing loss. Simply announcing that Johnny is somehow different is certainly not the best way to elicit help from the rest of the class or to make him feel comfortable, but frank and sensitive discussion can.

One very important aspect of being hearing impaired in a regular classroom is the strain imposed on the student in keeping alert during verbal communication. The child may have to remain constantly vigilant for long periods and he will be literally exhausted by the effort. Shorten lesson periods if possible, or intersperse oral and written work with frequent rest periods. Send Johnny on errands routinely; he might be asked to go to the lunchroom a few minutes early to reserve tables for the class, to take the teacher's daily report to the principal, or to feed the fish in the afternoon. The nature of the task is not so important as the relief from strain. Johnny may even need a short nap during rest period.

It is often the case that the hearing-impaired youngster does not participate in many class activities like music or dancing because it is assumed he cannot. At first he may be unable to, but the child should be encouraged to continue because such activities help improve his sense of rhythm and discrimination. Likewise, he is often excluded from social activities and functions. Again, he should be encouraged to participate. If he and others can accept the simple concessions that will have to be made to get him involved in clubwork or games, the child will benefit considerably.

One extremely important question that arises many times is the management of a child's hearing aid. The youngster may be unable to handle even the simple act of taking the aid off correctly without the teacher's help. Since different hearing aids operate in various ways, the teacher must ask the audiologist or the parent how to use a particular aid. The teacher should make sure she knows how to load and unload the batteries, turn the aid on and off, check for proper functioning, and insert earmolds. Although the hearing aid, earmolds, wires, and receivers may seem excessively complex, they are simple parts of an amplifying system (see Figure 8). Certain common sense precautions must be taken to ensure their proper function, but they are not the fearful machines for which they are often taken. One basic step any teacher of young children can take is to make an attractive and soft-lined storage box for each child's hearing aid (or glasses). It should be kept in a locked place known to the child. The rule should be that whenever the hearing aid is taken off, it is placed in its box with the battery removed and the drawer or cabinet locked. If a schedule for wearing the aid is given by the audiologist, the teacher alone can make it work in the classroom. He or she should be in contact with the audiologist to make sure the

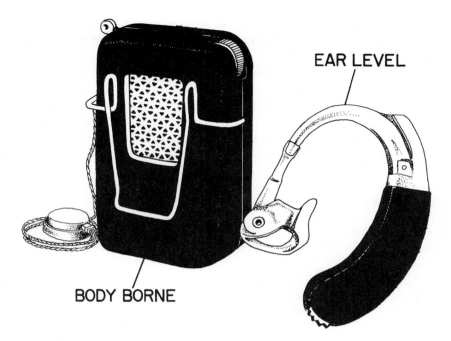

Figure 8. Two of the most commonly used types of hearing aids are the body-borne aid and the earlevel aid. The component parts of both are essentially the same, although the body-borne models are generally more powerful.

schedule is correctly understood and to give progress reports. This is especially important if the child is a new wearer.

Another important individual in the hearing-impaired child's life may be the special therapist who works with him in a resource capacity. Regardless of whether the specialist is a speech, language, hearing, or reading therapist, the teacher should work closely with him to coordinate classroom activities and material content. The professionals working with a hearing-impaired youngster perform best when they cooperate as a team to make sure that their individual efforts are relevant to the child's total educational and social function.

CONCLUSION

The child with a hearing loss is often misunderstood and managed badly as a result. Probably the most important factors in his mismanagement are lack of knowledge about hearing impairment on the part of the persons who are involved in his treatment and education, or their failure to understand each other when they exchange information. The educator is a member of a professional team who has a unique opportunity to influence the child over a long period of time. Thus, if he is informed about types and degrees of hearing loss, associated functional effects, etiology, and prognosis, he can contribute immeasurably to the total education and adjustment of the hearing impaired. Furthermore, the educator can contribute to the professional effectiveness of audiologists and physicians by making them aware of what goes on in the classrooms and schools where their patients are placed, and how their intervention and recommendations may or may not be producing desired results. Exchange of technical information is necessary and must be understood across professions. Hopefully, the end result will be better, more effective service to the hearing-impaired child and his family.

REFERENCES

Goodhill, V., and P. Guggenheim. 1971. Pathology, diagnosis, and therapy of deafness. In L. E. Travis (ed.), Handbook of Speech Pathology and Audiology, pp. 279–346. Appleton-Century-Crofts, Inc., New York.

Human Communication and Its Disorders: An Overview. 1970. United States Department of Health, Education, and Welfare, Bethesda, Maryland.

Myklebust, H. R. 1954. Auditory Disorders in Children: A Manual for Differential Diagnosis. Grune & Stratton, Inc., New York. 367 p.

Newby, H. A. 1971. Clinical audiology. In L. E. Travis (ed.), Handbook of Speech Pathology and Audiology, pp. 347–373. Appleton-Century-Crofts, Inc., New York.

Silverman, S. R. 1971a. The education of deaf children. In L. E. Travis (ed.), Handbook of Speech Pathology and Audiology, pp. 399–430. Appleton-Century-Crofts, Inc., New York.

Silverman, S. R. 1971b. Hard-of-hearing children. In L. E. Travis (ed.), Handbook of Speech Pathology and Audiology, pp. 431–438. Appleton-Century-Crofts, Inc., New York.

SUGGESTED READING

Carrow, M. A. 1968. The development of auditory comprehension of language structure in children. J. Speech & Hearing Disorders 33:99–111.

Education of the Deaf: The Challenge and the Change. 1967. United States Department of Health, Education, and Welfare, Washington, D. C.

Hardy, W. G. 1952. Children with Impaired Hearing. Children's Bureau Publication #326. Superintendent of Documents, United States Government Printing Office, Washington, D. C.

Learning to Talk: Speech, Hearing, and Language Problems in the Pre-School Child. 1969. United States Department of Health, Education, and Welfare, Washington, D. C.

Myklebust, H. R. 1964. The Psychology of Deafness. 2nd Ed. Grune & Stratton, Inc., New York. 423 p.

Palmer, C. E. 1961. Speech and Hearing Problems: A Guide for Teachers and Parents. Charles C Thomas, Publisher, Springfield, Ill. 137 p.

Teacher Awareness Of Some Common Pediatric Neurologic Disorders

Robert H. A. Haslam, M.D.

The intent of this chapter is to outline three rather prevalent neurologic disorders in children which may be encountered by the teacher: headaches, seizures, and head injuries. The presenting symptoms are stressed in order to familiarize the educator with the clinical composition of these common conditions. In particular, certain neurologic features are emphasized to illustrate the interaction of the child, school, and learning process. Unfortunately, because of a lack of understanding and information on the part of some educators, children with these disorders may be hampered to a degree in attaining realistic educational goals.

This brief account of common neurologic conditions in children does not propose to create medical diagnosticians or therapists among educators, but hopefully will alert the teacher to the inherent complexities associated with disorders of the child's central nervous system. Cooperation on the part of the educator and physician in sharing knowledge and concerns about these sorts of problems will accomplish a mutual understanding for the ultimate benefit of the child.

HEADACHES IN CHILDREN

Headache is a common condition in children and young adults. One study suggested that 48% of children had headache, albeit infrequently (Bille, 1962).

This paper was supported in part through Project 917, Maternal and Child Health Service, United States Department of Health, Education, and Welfare.

Another found an incidence of approximately 15% in young adolescents (Hughes and Cooper, 1956). And finally, Øster (1972) suggested a prevalence of 20% in children of school age. The effect that headaches have on a child's academic performance, personality, memory, and interpersonal relationships, as well as school attendance, depends upon their etiology. Thus, if headaches are more than a casual encounter, it is probable they may interfere with intellectual fulfillment and occasionally pose as a life-threatening symptom, and for that reason, deserve careful medical scrutiny.

There are a host of reasons for headache in the school-aged child, but oftentimes their delineation is difficult. Refractive errors of vision, sinusitis, and malocclusion of the teeth, contrary to popular belief, are not common causes. Any child who develops a high fever, for whatever cause, or who has a systemic illness (e.g., pneumonia) may develop a headache which tends to parallel the severity of the illness. The headache, however, in the latter situation, always disappears with recovery from the primary sickness.

For the purpose of this discussion, three major types of headache will be outlined: migraine, tension (or muscle contraction headache), and headaches due to increased intracranial pressure. The interested reader may refer to a text for a comprehensive discussion of other possible sources of headache in children (Friedman and Harms, 1967).

MIGRAINE (SICK HEADACHES)

Incidence

Migraine headaches are relatively common in children. Fortunately, they are usually not severe so that medical advice is not always sought. The youngest child known to develop migraine was approximately 1 year of age (Vahlquist, 1955). Migraine accounts for about 25% of all cases of headache in children. In an extensive well-organized study in Uppsala, Sweden, Bille (1962) noted a 4% incidence of migraine in school children between the ages of 7 and 15. Prior to adolescence, the sex distribution is equivalent; however, later in life, girls are more frequently affected by migraine headache.

Definition

Migraine is difficult to define. It certainly has many variable presentations, and the accompanying symptoms and severity of its manifestations make diagnosis arduous. No two children have common symptoms or complaints referable to their headache. The headaches of migraine tend to be recurrent with intervals free of symptoms. Migraine may be associated with warning signs (or aura), the headache is most often one-sided (or hemicranial), nausea and vomiting are prominent features, and there is usually a family history of migraine.

Precipitating Factors

Migraine headaches tend to have many characteristics in children that set them apart from adults. Migraine attacks are precipitated by a multitude of factors: tension, bright flashing lights such as a movie or a television screen, physical exertion, excessive noise, hunger, and excitement have all been incriminated. One interesting observation is the finding that many children develop their migraine headaches following a stressful event such as an examination, presenting a speech, participating in an athletic activity, or performing in a school play. In contrast to tension headaches, migraine in children frequently occurs on weekend days. Migraine develops in children from all social strata and appears to be more common in compulsive, highly competitive children. Contrary to many reports, migraine attacks the normal or handicapped child, as well as the very bright and intelligent student.

Prodrome (Aura)

One possible reason for the difficulty in diagnosis of migraine in children is the fact that they would not appear to have warning signs (prodrome) as frequently as do adults. An alternative explanation may be that the child misinterprets these symptoms or gives little significance to them. The prodromal symptoms, when they occur, are brief and most commonly visual, such as bright, flashing, often colored lights in the form of stars, zigzag lines, or circles. Various crude visual shapes and distortion of body images may be perceived as well. A graphic description of visual misinterpretation was depicted by Lewis Carroll, a migraine sufferer, in his *Alice's Adventures in Wonderland* (Carroll, 1960). As Alice is explaining to Caterpillar, "'I'm afraid I am, Sir,' said Alice. 'I can't remember things as I used—and I don't keep the same size for ten minutes together!'" Other precursory symptoms may include numbness and tingling sensations in the extremities, dizziness, and aphasia.

Symptoms

The prodromal symptoms are soon followed by the onset of the headache. It may begin in the posterior region of the skull, but the headache almost immediately tends to radiate to the forehead, often over an eye or the temple. It is described as pounding, pulse-like, or throbbing. The headache is frequently not as severe in children as in adults and is usually of shorter duration. During this stage of the migraine attack, the child may be extremely confused and belligerent. The child prefers to lie in a quiet, darkened room. Characteristic features of childhood migraine are the rather severe nausea and vomiting that accompany the headache (i.e., sick headaches). The gastrointestinal symptoms are usually more intense in children. Oral medication to alleviate the headache is, therefore, of little benefit to many children with migraine. The vomiting may be associated with abdominal pain and fever so that other conditions such as appendicitis and infection may be incorrectly entertained.

The entire migraine attack is usually less than 6 hrs. in duration and is almost always much shorter than what is commonly found in older patients. The child often awakens from a rather deep sleep quite alert, asking to be fed and ready to resume normal activities as if nothing had transpired.

If migraine attacks are frequent, significant absenteeism from school may result. This of course can produce anxiety for the child, particularly if the school performance diminishes.

Treatment

Treatment of migraine in children can be a challenge to the pediatrician. Prior to prescribing medication, he must rule out other significant causes of headache. Because some of the symptoms of migraine are similar to epilepsy, he may wish to perform an electroencephalogram (EEG). The occasional patient may require more specialized studies to rule out abnormalities of blood vessels (arteriovenous malformation). A very thorough history and physical examination are mandatory. Unfortunately, there is no laboratory aid that ensures the diagnosis of migraine. Radiographs of the skull (x-ray), the EEG, and blood tests are normal. Although a thorough psychologic examination may demonstrate a compulsive, deliberate, and perhaps insecure student, these findings are obviously not diagnostic of migraine as they are found in many headache-free children.

The initial step in a treatment regimen should be an attempt to alter or diminish any significant positive causative events. If television or movies clearly enhance or provoke migraine, other pleasurable activities should be substituted for them. Sometimes prolonged parental counseling is necessary in order to relieve pressures at home or ensure that their expectations for the child are realistic. Occasionally, children with migraine are placed in too highly competitive classrooms so that reassessment of school placement must be considered. Ideally, a conference between physician, teacher, and parents would ensure a satisfactory arrangement in most cases. Obviously, the physician and teacher must be cognizant of the occasional pupil who utilizes his headaches as an excuse for not partaking in physical education or other activities that are disliked by the student.

Many headaches of migrainous origin in children may be simply treated by the judicious use of salicylates (aspirin), particularly if the headaches are relatively mild, infrequent, and of short duration. The child with more severe, disabling headaches poses a therapeutic challenge. The ergot preparations, which include Cafergot, must be considered for these children. They are most efficacious during the early stages of the migraine attack, and for that reason are less beneficial in children than in adults, as children are often unaware of the earlier discussed preliminary symptoms or fail to communicate them to their parents.

In addition, the severe nausea and vomiting so often observed in children preclude the use of orally administered medication.

There are additional drugs which may be used to abort the frequent, severe, or cluster attacks that occasionally occur in children unresponsive to other forms of medication, but this is done under close supervision by a physician anticipating possible side effects. Finally, some children with incapacitating migraine episodes respond favorably to the prolonged use of drugs such as phenobarbital or diphenylhydantoin (Dilantin). Needless to say, any child on medication should be frequently reevaluated by the physician, searching for possible harmful drug reactions, but just as importantly reassessing the possibility of discontinuing the drug. Communication with school personnel may be helpful in this decision.

The teacher may assist the pupil during an acute migrainous attack by providing a secluded area in which to rest. In addition, reappraisal of the child's curriculum may demonstrate that undue pressures are being placed. Frequent absenteeism is uncommon in childhood migraine, and if present, steps should be initiated for medical reevaluation of the student.

TENSION, FUNCTIONAL, OR PSYCHOGENIC HEADACHES

Tension headaches are the most common type of head pain in children as they are in adults. For most children, this headache is a rare occurrence and so clearly related to a stressful situation of short duration that treatment is not necessary. Others are not so fortunate.

Symptoms

Psychogenic or tension headaches infrequently appear in the morning, but more commonly are bothersome during school hours, particularly during a test or other similar anxiety-provoking circumstances. They rarely occur on weekends and usually have abated by the evening. Some children with tension headaches are found to have parents whose expectations are far too high, whether for academic or athletic achievement. The most common cause of tension headaches would appear to be unrealistic scholastic goals for the child developed by the parents, teacher, or the child himself. If a child complains of headaches characteristic of the tension type more commonly during a vacation period when he is in greater contact with his parents, parental marital discord or related phenomena are often found as a cause for the child's anxiety. The student with severe psychogenic headaches frequently has a parent with very similar headaches.

Tension or psychogenic headaches are poorly described by children. They are usually located in the temples, over the forehead, or even in the base of the skull and neck muscles. The headache is usually a steady, dull, aching pain and is sometimes described as a pressure band constricting the skull. The student may complain of scalp tenderness, particularly prominent during hair combing. These headaches are likely the result of prolonged, unconscious contraction of the muscles of the neck or temples which so often accompanies states of anxiety or tension. Unlike migraine, tension headaches are not associated with nausea or vomiting.

Diagnosis

The diagnosis of tension headache is only made after exclusion of other possible causes of head pain following a very careful history, physical, and neurologic examination. Once again, the physician may require a skull x-ray, EEG, and perhaps a brain scan to aid him in reaching a diagnosis. The physician must then search for possible stressful situations. The teacher may be of great assistance during this phase of the evaluation. Most children have considerable insight as to the origin of their emotional derangement and, if given the opportunity in confidence with a teacher or pediatrician, will often share their concerns. Poor self-image, fear of school failure, and lack of confidence are often repeated apprehensions. Occasionally, a child who is very depressed will only complain of headache (Ling, Oftedal, and Weinberg, 1970). Further questioning may suggest mood change, lack of energy or excessive fatigue, poor appetite and weight loss, crying spells, and withdrawal from social activities. These children are in need of psychiatric care.

Treatment

The physician's and educator's major responsibility in treatment is to explain to the child how stressful events may culminate in a headache. Efforts should be taken to alter obvious anxiety-provoking situations. The teacher should be very much aware of her role in this regard. By careful interaction with the child, certain stressful situations can be circumvented in order that tension-provoking episodes are minimized. Finally, the child and his family must be reassured that the tension headaches are not serious and that a healthy, normal life is to be expected.

HEADACHES DUE TO INCREASED INTRACRANIAL PRESSURE

Headache may be the earliest symptom of increased pressure within the skull. The causes of increased intracranial pressure in children are many, including brain tumor, chronic lead poisoning, brain abscess, or an abnormal collection of blood clots over the surface of the cortex. In addition, elevation of intracranial pressure may result from hydrocephalus, infection of the central nervous system (meningitis), vitamin A poisoning, water intoxication, or, rarely, as a complication of drug therapy, particularly tetracycline (an antibiotic) in young children, and occasionally oral contraceptive agents in adolescent females. The characteristics of the "pressure" headache vary somewhat, dependent upon the age of the child and the underlying pathologic condition. Sooner or later, other symptoms or neurologic signs appear, implying a progressive, destructive process.

The headache of increased pressure is probably the result of abnormal tension or stretching of the cerebral blood vessels and dura, the thick membranous covering of the brain. The headache tends to occur in the early morning hours or shortly after arising. It is poorly localized by most children, but tends to be a diffuse, generalized, often throbbing pain which may be more prominent over the forehead or the occipital region of the skull. Its onset is usually insidious, and, in the beginning of the disease process, there may be days or even weeks when the child is pain-free. The headache is often made worse by activity which normally raises the intracranial pressure such as coughing, sneezing, exercise, or straining during a bowel movement. Certain positions tend to influence the headache of increased intracranial pressure; lying down may enhance the pain and sitting up or standing may relieve it. Later, the headache becomes more frequent and intense. With increasing intracranial pressure, the child becomes lethargic, uncooperative, and finally comatose.

The headache may be associated with vomiting. Thus, the child may awaken with a headache and vomit shortly thereafter. The child usually does not complain of nausea and may very well eat a normal breakfast immediately following the episode of vomiting and remain symptom-free for the duration of the day. Unfortunately, some children who complain of morning vomiting and who appear normal in every other respect are accused of malingering or are thought to display a school phobia. These children more appropriately require careful medical attention.

Diagnosis and Treatment

The treatment of "pressure" headaches, of course, depends upon the cause. Every child suspected of increased intracranial pressure must have a thorough examination including a history, blood pressure determination, and neurologic evaluation, including inspection of the eyegrounds. In addition, certain tests are mandatory. A skull x-ray may show an abnormality suggestive of elevated intracranial pressure (Figure 1). The EEG may demonstrate a focal disturbance which demands further study. And a brain scan in certain conditions will outline a specific lesion (Figure 2). The decision as to whether to proceed with further investigation, such as special dye tests or air studies, is dependent upon the outcome of these routine tests in conjunction with the patient's clinical findings. If an organic disease process is found, the appropriate medical or surgical therapeutic techniques can be utilized.

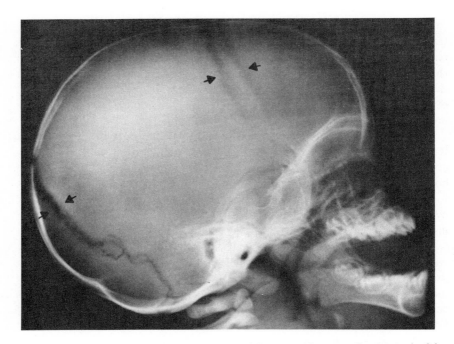

Figure 1. Skull radiograph of an 8-month-old child demonstrating separation (*arrows*) of the sutures (the line of junction of adjacent cranial bones), a reliable sign of increased intracranial pressure.

HEADACHES: EPILOGUE

The investigation and management of headaches in children can be a taxing experience for the physician. A thorough understanding of the child is a must, particularly if migraine or tension headaches are to be treated successfully. Information brought forth by school officials concerning change in personality, decline in school performance, or the observation of unusual behavior can be crucial in assisting the physician. The teacher can often initiate a referral to the pediatrician in cooperation with the parents, if worrisome symptoms are noted.

Generally speaking, recurrent episodes of headache over a *prolonged* period suggest a benign process, such as migraine or tension headaches. The characteristics of the headache, including the inciting factors, location, duration, and associated symptomatology, usually differentiate the two. Many pupils in this category do not require medical attention because of the sporadic nature and insignificant consequences of their headaches. The educator must be aware of provoking events in the child with more troublesome headaches. Improvement can be expected if the appropriate causative factors can be established and reconciled. Simple maneuvers, such as excusing a migrainous pupil from observing a movie or from participating in functions productive of loud noises (for example, excusing a member of the school band), may serve to abort many headaches. Migraine headaches tend to be less severe in adolescence if their onset

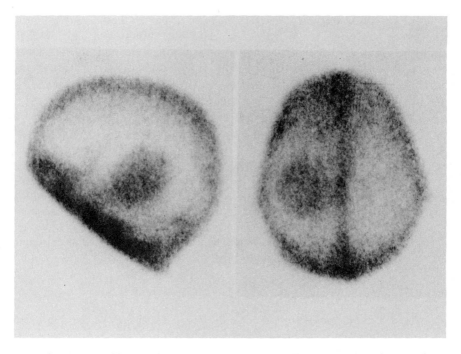

Figure 2. The area of increased density in the brain scan outlines a tumor in a 12-year-old boy (lateral and vertex views).

is prior to 10 years of age. Tension or psychogenic headaches respond favorably to the relief of anxiety-provoking situations and the factors that promote them. Some patients must be taught how to live with their headaches.

There are some headaches that are worrisome and require prompt medical attention. A sudden excruciating onset of head pain suggests an underlying organic disorder, particularly if there is no past history of headache. Any headache that occurs in association with or shortly after head trauma may be extremely serious (see Head Injuries in Children), no matter how trivial the injury may appear. All headaches suggestive of increased intracranial pressure justify immediate evaluation. They tend to become more frequent and intense, often associated with other neurologic symptoms in a relatively *brief period.* The prognosis of headaches due to increased intracranial pressure depends upon the underlying abnormality. *Early diagnosis and treatment are extremely important as many of these conditions are life-threatening illnesses.*

CHILDHOOD EPILEPSY

Convulsions or epilepsy is a common disorder of school-aged children. Most teachers have been confronted by a student with epilepsy; many are fearful of the condition and develop a negative relationship with the child, while still others become overprotective and solicitous. Even in these modern times, epilepsy is considered by many well-educated but misinformed individuals to represent a host of incredible conditions and aberrations including mental illness, mental retardation, evil spirits, and perverted thoughts. Unfortunately, therefore, the patient with epilepsy is oftentimes thwarted, shamed, and abused by friends, fellow students, teachers, and even parents.

The term epilepsy (or convulsion, seizure, or fit) is utilized to describe a wide variety of disorders due to many different causes. The clinical picture of epilepsy is partially dependent upon the age of the child, the etiology of the convulsion, and the area within the brain that is malfunctioning.

Epilepsy occurs in approximately 0.5% of the population, thus affecting about one million Americans. The initial presentation commonly occurs during the latter half of the first decade, or at the time of adolescence. The causes of convulsions are numerous, and include genetic factors, high fever, head injury, infections of the central nervous system, metabolic diseases, as well as poisoning by exogenous substances (Livingston, 1963).

Classification of Epilepsy

Grand Mal (Major Motor)   Major motor convulsions are the most common and, to the uninitiated, the most frightening form of epilepsy. On occasion, the patient can anticipate a seizure minutes or hours prior to its occurrence. A severe headache, tired feeling, or clouding of the sensorium may be premonitory symptoms.

The convulsion is usually initiated by a sudden loss of consciousness. The child may fall, the eyes roll upward, respirations momentarily cease, and the face becomes slightly dusky. At this point, rhythmic synchronous movements of the extremities and face develop, which usually persist a few minutes but, in the rare situation, may continue for hours. During this phase of the convulsion, the patient's arms and legs are rigid. Within minutes, the child usually becomes relaxed, moans, and may begin to move spontaneously. In most instances, the patient is drowsy following a convulsion and prefers to sleep, although he can readily be aroused.

If a patient has repetitive seizures without regaining consciousness in the interval, a medical emergency exists. The child must be immediately transported to a hospital for treatment of this rare complication of epilepsy coined *status epilepticus.*

Petit Mal (Absence Attacks)   The investigation of children with petit mal epilepsy is often initiated by the teacher. The onset of this type of convulsion commonly occurs between the ages of 5 and 10. The seizure is manifested by brief episodes of staring. The child momentarily appears to be disinterested and out of contact with reality. There may be lapses of speech and fluttering of the eyelids, but the child does not fall. Petit mal seizures may occur so frequently that they interfere with a child's concentration, and, thus, school performance may decline (Freemon, Douglas, and Penry, 1973). Frequent seizures undoubtedly interfere with memory. The physician may enhance or demonstrate these seizures by asking the child to take deep breaths (hyperventilate) for diagnostic purposes (Figure 3). Unfortunately, many children with this type of epilepsy are not recognized but rather are castigated for their general lack of academic interest and enthusiasm. The condition must be differentiated from daydreaming which is more frequently the result of a boring classroom environment, a tired student, or, more appropriately, a longing anticipation for the events of the coming weekend.

Psychomotor (Temporal Lobe) Psychomotor seizures may be extremely difficult to identify because of their bizarre nature and variable modes of presentation. They rarely begin before 2 years of age, but more commonly become evident during the elementary school years. The seizure may begin with vague hallucinations, either visual, auditory, or gustatory. These sensations can be very frightening and, because they are difficult to interpret, the child rarely relates these experiences. Some children complain of abdominal discomfort or headache during the onset of their seizure. Shortly thereafter unusual movements of the tongue, smacking of the lips, or repetitive motor movements, such as buttoning and unbuttoning a sweater, may be observed. Some children appear frightened and are noted to run after and clutch a parent or friend. Most children demonstrate signs such as perspiration, salivation, rapid pulse, pallor of the face, or marked blushing during a psychomotor seizure. For the most part, its duration is a matter of a few minutes, but on occasion a psychomotor seizure may progress to a major motor convulsion (Figure 4).

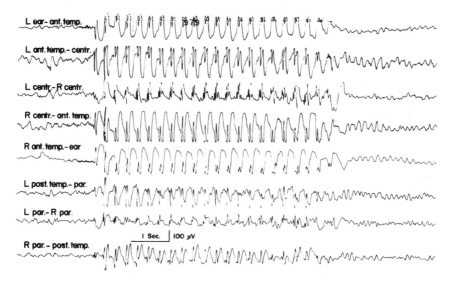

Figure 3. An electroencephalogram showing the typical three per second discharges of petit mal epilepsy. Note the sudden return to normalcy at the termination of the recording.

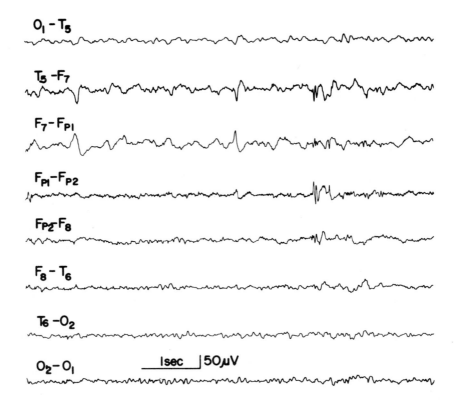

Figure 4. An abnormal electroencephalogram supporting the clinical diagnosis of psychomotor epilepsy in a 10-year-old boy. Note the spikes in T_5-F_7 and F_7-Fp_1.

Some students with this type of epilepsy are at high risk for learning disorders. They may display a shortened attention span or the inability to concentrate. A few children tend to demonstrate temper tantrums or acting-out behavior, requiring psychiatric consultation. Fortunately, with appropriate medication and counseling, the behavior outbursts can usually be controlled.

Minor Motor (Akinetic Seizures)   Minor motor seizures are perhaps the most severe form of epilepsy and, accordingly, are associated with a guarded prognosis. As a rule these seizures are evident during infancy. They are characterized by brief lapses of consciousness and loss of body tone so that the infant or child falls (Figure 5). These seizures may occur as frequently as several hundred times daily. Usually the child has no preliminary warning of an impending convulsion, and cut lips or bruised foreheads are often the result. Minor motor seizures have many causes. The treatment and prognosis of this type of epilepsy depend, to a great extent, upon the underlying disorder. A thorough medical investigation is mandatory in order to intelligently treat these children.

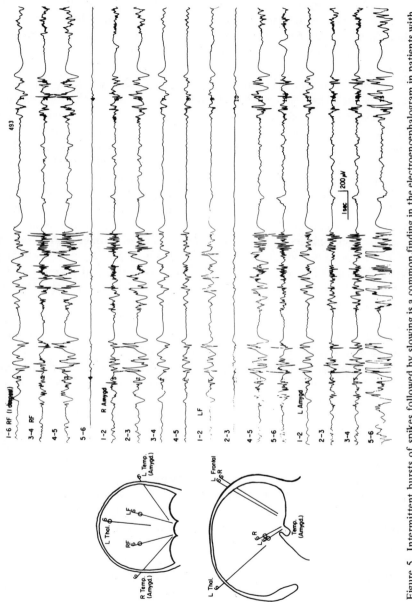

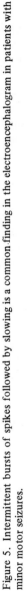

Figure 5. Intermittent bursts of spikes followed by slowing is a common finding in the electroencephalogram in patients with minor motor seizures.

Management

The successful management of a child with epilepsy is dependent upon many factors. The patient who has a clear understanding of his disorder is in a better position to cope with frustrations as they occur. The child, physician, parent, and educator must appreciate the many facets of epilepsy in order to ensure a normal, happy existence.

Emergency First Aid The only type of epilepsy that warrants emergency assistance is the grand mal variety. The others are often unrecognized and are rarely associated with complications. If a patient is actively convulsing, he should be moved from potentially dangerous areas, such as the Bunsen burner in the chemistry lab or the kitchen stove in the home economics department. The child should be placed in a horizontal position, preferably lying on his side, and tight, confining garments should be loosened. The patient *must have a free airway*, so the mouth and nose should be uncovered and any objects in the oral cavity removed (including candy, chewing gum, or food). If the convulsive movements are vigorous, the patient can be gently restrained. Some children tend to bite their tongues during a major motor convulsion, and a padded object (handkerchief wrapped around a stick or spoon) gently inserted between the teeth may obviate this injury. The majority of major motor convulsions may be managed in this fashion and complete recovery is anticipated. If the seizure is prolonged, the child must receive further care.

Medical Investigation The physician initiates a course of management by taking a careful history and performing a physical examination, seeking a cause for the seizure. A complete description of the convulsion by a parent or teacher is an essential component of the investigation, as the seizure activity has ceased, in most instances, by the time the child reaches the hospital or doctor's office.

Following the completion of the examination, the pediatrician may perform a variety of blood tests, including a serum glucose, calcium, and, perhaps, lead determination. In addition, he may obtain a skull x-ray. These tests are carried out to seek a specific cause for the seizure, enabling a direct approach to its treatment.

The interpretation and value of a brain wave test (EEG) are greatly misunderstood by most individuals. The physician orders this examination only to confirm his clinical impression. The EEG, however, can be quite useful as a diagnostic tool when utilized in the proper context (Figure 6).

During the past three decades, significant advances have been made for the treatment of epilepsy with the discovery of effective anticonvulsant drugs. The majority of children with grand mal, petit mal, and psychomotor epilepsy can be expected to become seizure-free by the employment of specific anticonvulsant drugs.

Failure to direct therapy to the "whole child" eventually results in lack of cooperation, erratic intake of medication, and gradual recrudescence of seizures.

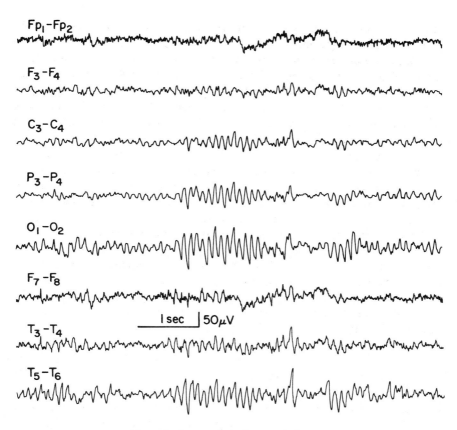

Figure 6. A normal electroencephalogram.

The physician must be in contact with the patient at regular intervals to readjust the anticonvulsant medication, attempt to answer questions, and alleviate fears and assume responsibility for discontinuing the drug when medically feasible.

Long-Term Care It is well recognized that certain events tend to precipitate or enhance seizures. The child with seizures who is under undue emotional stress or who is ill and not sleeping well is at a greater risk for worsening of the convulsive disorder. Some physicians feel that puberty is a particularly vulnerable period in an epileptic child's life.

A concerted effort must be made to allow the child with epilepsy to lead as normal a life as possible. Both parents and patient must understand the essence of epilepsy. The reasons for long-term anticonvulsant medication should be stressed. It must be explained that anticonvulsants are not addictive or "dope." Many children may be reassured that they will eventually outgrow their epilepsy and lead perfectly normal lives. Children who have seizures that are well controlled should be allowed to engage in activities of all types, with the exception of swimming unattended.

The Educator's Role Many parents do not inform school officials of their child's seizure disorder because of the concern that the child may be ostracized and treated as less than normal. Some schools resist the responsibility of dispensing the child's midday anticonvulsant medication. Thus, the pupil with epilepsy often faces the embarrassment of his mother personally delivering his noontime medication.

The school and educators must take a more positive attitude. Teachers must be aware of the fundamental principles of epilepsy and its management. Furthermore, *the educator is in a unique position to normalize the life of an epileptic child.* The astute educator may utilize this opportunity to teach the facts of epilepsy to the entire class so that the social stigma of seizures will be lessened and epileptic children will be allowed to truly function as normal individuals.

Finally, the educator may play an active role in the management of a child with convulsions. It is difficult for the physician to accurately prescribe the proper quantity of an anticonvulsant drug for a given child. Severe seizures may be adequately controlled in the hospital, but with a change in activity at home or at school, the seizures may reappear. An educator's observations could be of considerable assistance. Is the child excessively drowsy, suggesting too much medication? Has the pupil become hyperactive, combative, or recalcitrant, perhaps indicating an adverse reaction to the drug? Or is the child alert, cooperative, and apparently seizure-free?

Most children with epilepsy are well controlled on medication, have normal intelligence, and can be expected to lead normal lives. Cooperation between patient, parent, physician, and educator provides a ready avenue for this goal.

HEAD INJURIES IN CHILDREN

Head injury is an inordinately common phenomenon in infants and children. It is the rare child who reaches adolescence without experiencing a blow to the head which produces a momentary loss of consciousness, a brief period of dazedness, or, in some cases, more significant trauma requiring hospitalization. It is not the purport of this chapter to discuss the physiology, pathology, or acute management of cerebral injury in children, but rather to classify the various types of head trauma and highlight possible complications which may potentially interfere with satisfactory achievement at home and at school.

Accidents, including ingestion of poisons and acute trauma, are the leading cause of death in infants and children (Vital Statistics Report, 1973). It has been estimated that approximately 200,000 children are hospitalized annually in the United States because of head injury, and 5–10% have long-standing mental or physical impairment as a result (Mealey, 1968).

Children are particularly disposed to head injury because of their various activities, many of which take place in the school yard. Blows to the head from a ball or baseball bat, falls from a swing, bicycle, or tree are all frequent accidents. Children tend to be injured as pedestrians more commonly than do adults. Male children experience head injury at least twice as commonly as girls, perhaps resulting from their innate desire to climb and jump from dangerous heights, or from lack of fear and concern for the consequences of their actions. The child with the latter behavior may in fact be accident prone and, thus, be subjected to recurring injury. Often, these children participate in dangerous activities to counteract their serious subconscious fears; others are found to be substantially depressed and in need of medical care. Most accident-prone children are nervous, temperamental individuals who for some unknown reason are committed to intense activity. Frequent accidents in children may superficially be reported as numerous falls or clumsiness on the part of the child, when, in fact, they are due to abuse on the part of the parent or guardian.

The mechanism of head injury and the resultant damage to the brain are only partially understood, and it is clear that much is yet to be learned. Various studies have demonstrated that it requires much more force to produce unconsciousness when the head is held in a fixed position than when the skull is freely moving at impact (Denny-Brown and Russell, 1941). The degree of brain trauma is extremely variable and is dependent upon the age of the individual, the velocity of the fall or blow, the presence or lack of protective head gear, and whether the injury was a closed or opened skull wound.

Classification of Head Injury

Concussion   Concussion is the most frequent closed head injury in children. This syndrome is characterized by a brief, but variable and reversible, alteration in the level of consciousness, transient paralysis of reflexes, and amnesia for the surrounding events of the injury. There are no permanent neurologic sequelae.

The duration of abnormal behavior associated with a concussion may be as brief as a few minutes, but frequently persists for several hours. The child is apt to be lethargic, irritable, and pale. The patient may be confused and disoriented. Vomiting is one of the most common symptoms accompanying a concussion in children, and at times may be severe and out of proportion to the apparent mild head trauma. The child may also complain of transient dizziness and headache. The patient prefers to sleep, and when he awakens a few hours later usually appears and feels perfectly normal. *If a child loses consciousness as a result of a head injury, he should probably be admitted to a hospital for careful observation.* A worsening of the level of consciousness or the evolvement of focal neurologic signs (e.g., one-sided weakness) suggest the possibility of a complication, and warrant further investigation and possible surgical intervention.

The rapid, complete recovery from concussion suggests an evanescent injury to the brain. Bleeding or significant injury to the central nervous system has not been observed as a result of a concussion. It is probable that the symptoms of a mild, closed head injury are the result of stretching of fibers within the brain stem or perhaps the momentary interruption of transmission of chemical substances through the reticular activating system so vital for the normal, alert, awakened state.

It is imperative that the child and parents be reassured that the concussion will not produce intellectual deficiency or a physical handicap. The child should be encouraged to return to school and engage in normal activity within a few days.

Contusion   Contusion is a term utilized to describe an injured brain when rather extensive damage has occurred, including bleeding, bruising, or laceration of the brain. The lesion may be very circumscribed, but, more commonly, is widespread. Contusion, therefore, is a more serious injury than concussion.

The clinical findings are dependent on the location or extent of injury, but deep stupor or coma is common. In addition, abnormalities of the pupils, weakness, disturbances of sensation, abnormal body posture, and seizures are frequently encountered signs of brain injury. Needless to say, these children are hospitalized immediately for emergency medical and surgical management.

Skull Fractures   The presence of a skull fracture following head trauma does not necessarily imply injury to the underlying brain. A child may die following a serious brain injury, although the skull may be completely intact.

The most usual skull fracture is linear (Figure 7). It does not, as a rule, interfere with the integrity and function of the brain, and, thus, the outcome is excellent. If, however, the fracture traverses underlying blood vessels or other important structures, serious complications may result requiring immediate medical care. Only an experienced physician, following examination of the child and study of the x-ray, can predict the consequences of a linear skull fracture.

Fractures of the skull may be depressed so that bony fragments may be incarcerated within the substance of the brain. Immediate surgical exploration is necessary in an attempt to elevate the fracture and minimize localized damage to the cerebral cortex.

Finally, the base of the skull may be fractured, often the result of a severe injury. Unfortunately, these breaks are difficult to demonstrate radiographically. The physician is concerned about the possibility of a basilar skull fracture when cerebrospinal fluid is noted to be dripping from the nostril or blood is observed behind the ear drum, or when a bruise develops over the mastoid region of the child who has recently had a head injury. The major concern from a fracture of the base of the skull is the potential for an infection of the central nervous system because of the open entry provided by the break.

Epidural and Subdural Hemorrhage   Bleeding into the spaces that cover the brain may be potentially fatal, so early recognition and therapy are extremely important.

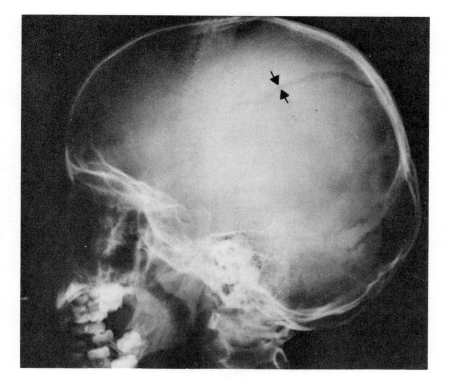

Figure 7. Skull radiograph. *Arrows* point to a linear skull fracture.

Epidural hematoma is the result of disruption of an artery that traverses a potential space (Figure 8), usually due to a fracture of the overlying bone. The child may very suddenly develop focal neurologic signs, with rapidly progressive dulling of the sensorium. The outcome is very favorable if the correct diagnosis and surgical therapy are carried out immediately; if treatment is significantly delayed, the child may die.

Subdural hematoma is the consequence of the rupture of bridging cortical veins that drain the cerebral cortex (Figure 9). Large collections of blood interfere with normal cerebral function, may cause herniation (squeezing) of the brain, and can result in death. Although any form of head trauma may produce subdural hematoma, the physically abused child is particularly susceptible to this type of head injury.

Complications of Head Injury

The nature and severity of complications are dependent upon the degree and location of the injured portions of the brain. Brief periods of blindness have been observed in children following head trauma, often manifested by rest-

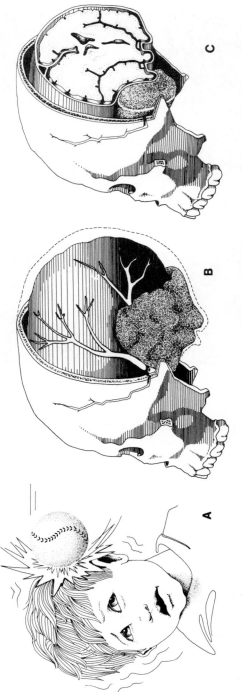

Figure 8. Epidural hematoma. *A*, a forceful injury in the region of the temple is the most common cause. *B*, the trauma may result in a fractured skull causing disruption of the middle meningeal artery. Blood collects in the area between the skull and the dura, a tough membrane covering the brain (epidural space). *C*, the collection of blood acts as a mass, producing pressure upon vital structures within the brain.

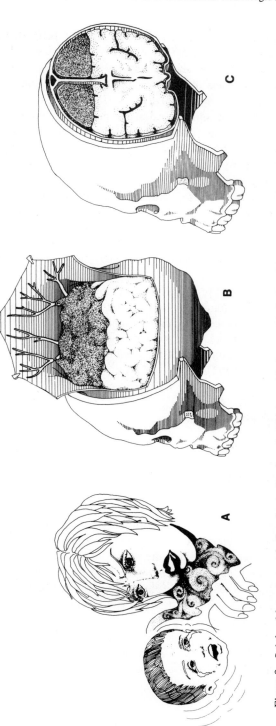

Figure 9. Subdural hematoma. *A*, the physically abused child is at risk for a subdural hematoma. *B*, the trauma results in rupture of bridging cortical veins. *C*, venous blood aggregates in a space between the dura and brain (subdural space), often bilaterally. A marked increase in intracranial pressure may result.

lessness and irritability (Griffith and Dodge, 1968). Fortunately, this phenomenon is reversible. Convulsions are common at the time of the accident,
but their presence does not signify long-lasting epilepsy. For the majority
of children, the convulsions disappear a day or two after the accident, never
to return.

With more severe head injury, a variety of persistent neurologic deficits may
result, including hemiparesis (one-sided weakness), disturbances in speech (including aphasia), intellectual deterioration, or behavioral disturbances. As noted,
in rare instances, epilepsy may result, but its control is usually very satisfactory
by the use of appropriate anticonvulsant drugs.

Many observers have noted that children with personality disorders following
serious head injury in fact had unusual behavioral traits prior to their injury that
seemed to be enhanced by the accident. Mealey (1968) noted that culturally and
environmentally deprived or emotionally disturbed children tend to have more
significant posttraumatic personality disturbances than do well-adjusted normal
children.

Following periods of prolonged coma, the student may display modest
changes in intellectual function. A few children may be left significantly retarded, however. The greatest disability on formal intelligence tests appears to be
aberration of rote memory. The pupil may also show variable scatter on the
subtests of formal intelligence testing, which was not present prior to the
accident (Richardson, 1963).

Prognosis of Childhood Head Injury

The most reliable clinical index for assessing the degree of underlying brain
damage in retrospect is termed *"posttraumatic amnesia."* The period of memory
loss prior to the accident is referred to as retrograde amnesia, and the stage
following the injury is referred to as anterograde amnesia. The sum of retrograde
and anterograde amnesia corresponds to the entire time span of posttraumatic
amnesia. The longer this period is, the more severe the initial injury.

Children have an amazing capacity to recover even from very serious head
injuries. The explanation for this potential is not completely understood, but
children, unlike adults, appear to have unutilized areas within the cerebral cortex
(brain reserve) that can readily and functionally replace damaged portions of the
brain. By the end of 1 year, most neurologic return of function has occurred.
However, on occasion, gradual improvement has been noted for as long as 3 years
following the accident.

Some pupils who experience a grave head injury may require special education facilities. These children may display impulsive behavior, a shortened
attention span, and deficits in memory and cognitive abilities (Hjern and Nylander, 1962).

Conclusions

Most head injuries of childhood are inconsequential. Complete recovery is to be expected. A child's premorbid personality often predicts his behavior following the accident. During the time of the accident, expert medical judgment is necessary to assess the child and to provide medical or surgical care if complications arise (DeVivo and Dodge, 1971; and Jennett, 1972).

It is conceivable that various drugs may be employed in children following a serious head injury. Anticonvulsants may be utilized for prolonged periods for the prevention and/or treatment of seizures or amphetamines for the management of severe hyperactivity or incapacitating inattentiveness. The educator may impart to the parent or physician the apparent benefits or possible detrimental side effects of these drugs following close observation in the classroom setting. Furthermore, specific rearrangements may be necessary within the class to accommodate the pupil, particularly if a persistent deficit is encountered, such as diminished visual acuity, disturbances of posture, or aberrant speech.

It is extremely important that a child return to school as soon as medically feasible. *The stimulation of the educational experience and the companionship of colleagues and peers are the most important prescriptions for full recovery.*

REFERENCES

Bille, B. 1962. Migraine in school children. Acta Paediat. Scand. 136 (Suppl.): 13–145.

Carroll, L. 1960. Alice's Adventures in Wonderland and Through the Looking-Glass. The New American Library, Inc., New York, p. 48.

Denny-Brown, D., and Russell, W. R. 1941. Experimental cerebral concussion. Brain 64:93–164.

DeVivo, D. C., and Dodge, P. R. 1971. The critically ill child: Diagnosis and management of head injury. Pediatrics 48:129–138.

Freemon, F. R., Douglas, E. F. O., and Penry, J. K. 1973. Environmental interaction and memory during petit mal (absence) seizures. Pediatrics 51: 911–918.

Friedman, A. P., and Harms, E. 1967. Headaches in Children. Charles C Thomas, Publisher, Springfield, Ill. 151 p.

Griffith, J. F., and Dodge, P. R. 1968. Transient blindness following head injury in children. N. England J. Med. 278:648–651.

Hjern, B., and Nylander, I. 1962. Late prognosis of severe head injuries in childhood. Arch. Dis. Childhood 37:113–116.

Hughes, E. L., and Cooper, C. E. 1956. Some observations on headache and eye pain in a group of school children. Brit. M. J. 1:1138–1141.

Jennett, B. 1972. Head injuries in children. Develop. M. Child Neurol. 14: 137–147.

Ling, W., Oftedal, G., and Weinberg, W. 1970. Depressive illness in childhood presenting as severe headache. Am. J. Dis. Childhood 120:122–124.

Livingston, S. 1963. Living with Epileptic Seizures. Charles C Thomas, Publisher, Springfield, Ill. 348 p.

Mealey, J., Jr. 1968. Pediatric Head Injuries. Charles C Thomas, Publisher, Springfield, Ill. 243 p.

Øster, J. 1972. Recurrent abdominal pain, headache and limb pains in children and adolescents. Pediatrics 50:429—436.

Richardson, F. 1963. Some effects of severe head injury. A follow-up study of children and adolescents after protracted coma. Develop. M. Child Neurol. 5:471—482.

Vahlquist, B. 1955. Migraine in children. Internat. Arch. Allergy 7:348—355.

Vital Statistics Report, Annual Summary for the United States, 1972. (HSM) 73-1121. 21:No. 13, June 27, 1973.

5

Important Endocrine Disorders Of Childhood

Harvey P. Katz, M.D.

Endocrinology is a complex medical science which refers to that diverse assortment of highly specialized glands which are bound together by the unique ability to manufacture and secrete hormones, the chemical substances which are capable of acting upon and influencing the function of other tissues and organs. Some examples of these endocrine glands and their hormonal products are the *pituitary* (secreting at least 10 hormones) which is under the controlling influence of *releasing factors,* made in the *hypothalamus; thyroid* (secreting thyroxine); *pancreas* (secreting insulin); *adrenal* (secreting adrenalin and cortisol); and the *sex gonads* (secreting estrogen and testosterone). Their anatomic locations are depicted in Figure 1.

Why include endocrinology in a discussion of school health? There are basically two reasons. First, these glands and their hormones may exert a profound influence over the learning process, such as the brain's dependence upon thyroid hormone for normal development during infancy. Second, when these glands malfunction, the result may produce an individual who is in some way different from other children, as with children who manifest the severe growth retardation associated with pituitary growth hormone deficiency. A sound understanding of the basis for this difference may assist the educator in helping the child and family achieve the healthy emotional adjustment so essential for success and joy in learning.

Several specific endocrine disorders and the associated problems which may be encountered in the classroom have been selected for discussion. Wherever applicable, each endocrine subject will include a definition of terms, the basic physiology of the involved gland, the major symptoms associated with the disorder, selective aspects of evaluation and treatment, and the relevance of the problem to the classroom.

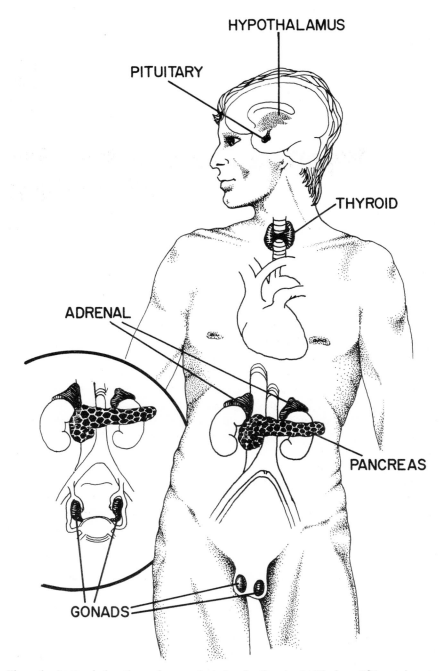

Figure 1. Anatomic locations of some selected endocrine glands. The hypothalamus is not a gland, but rather an area in the brain which exerts a profound influence upon the pituitary gland by means of releasing factors for specific pituitary hormones.

DISORDERS OF CARBOHYDRATE METABOLISM

Diabetes Mellitus (Hyperglycemia)

Juvenile diabetes mellitus is a genetically determined metabolic disorder in which hyperglycemia, or a high level of blood glucose, results from either an absolute or relative deficiency of insulin, the internal secretion of the pancreas. The pancreas is a small organ located adjacent to the stomach (Figure 1), and, although approximately 90% of pancreatic activity is for the production of digestive juices, the pancreas also contains the beta cells of the islets of Langerhans, where insulin is manufactured. Diabetes is a term derived from the Greek word meaning siphon, appropriately descriptive in that "fluid does not remain in the body, but uses the man's body as a ladder whereby to leave it" (Veith, 1971). Although the disorder is 4,000 years old, its exact cause remains obscure. The modern history of diabetes began in the seventeenth century when Thomas Willis described the honey taste of urine and used this taste as the first diagnostic laboratory test. It was not until 1921 that insulin was discovered by Frederick Banting and his medical student, Charles Best, who, on January 11, 1922, first attempted insulin therapy in a 14-year-old boy at the Toronto General Hospital.

Juvenile diabetes represents the most common endocrinologic abnormality of childhood, affecting approximately 1 out of every 1,000 school age children, and accounting for 5% of all cases of diabetes in the United States. A characteristic of juvenile diabetes, in contrast to adult or late onset diabetes, is the total lack of insulin. For this reason, juvenile diabetes must be treated with insulin, rather than using oral medication or diet alone. There are two exceptions to this for which no treatment is indicated because these forms of diabetes are initially asymptomatic. They are stress diabetes, in which sugar appears in the urine only at times of stress, such as with infections, and chemical diabetes, in which only abnormal laboratory determinations indicate the presence of some carbohydrate intolerance. Often, these forms of diabetes are the earliest sign that insulin-requiring diabetes may develop at some future time.

When diabetes does develop, the consequences of insulin lack produce the classic symptoms associated with this disorder: (1) polyuria (excessive urination); (2) polydipsia (excessive thirst); (3) polyphagia (excessive hunger and appetite); and (4) weight loss.

Since insulin is necessary for cells to convert carbohydrate (sugar and starches) into energy, its lack causes the blood sugar to rise. If no insulin is provided, a condition similar to starvation develops, and the body turns to other energy-producing fuels, fats and protein. These fuels are far less efficient energy sources and, as fats are burned in large quantities, acetone or ketone bodies, which are an end product of fat metabolism, appear in the urine along with large amounts of sugar. The sugar, as it passes through the kidney, also takes with it large quantities of water and salts, turning the body chemistry acid. This condition is known as diabetic ketoacidosis. If this process continues unabated, dehydration, shock, and coma will ensue. The administration of insulin and salts in carefully calculated amounts quickly reverses the state of ketoacidosis.

As the emergency situation subsides, attention must turn to the more difficult long-term matter of the impact of this chronic disease on the child, parents, siblings, relatives, community, and school. Education of the child and family about this disorder and its management is of critical importance, and is usually conducted by the team of a physician and nurse (Diabetes Mellitus, 1973). The objectives of good management are the following: (1) normal growth and development; (2) a mature sense of independence and acceptance; (3) no restrictions to normal activity; (4) no or minimal low blood sugar reactions; (5) no or minimal hospitalization; and (6) acceptable small amounts of sugar in the urine, monitored by urine testing at home.

The components of management are: *insulin,* usually as one injection in the morning, self-administered by the child; a balanced nutritious *diet* using the exchange system; and the adjustment of these according to exercise (which lowers the need for insulin) and to the presence of an illness (which increases the need for insulin). Regular progress evaluations provide the physician with the forum for continuing health education. This is aided by larger group discussions with interested families and children, by summer camps for juvenile diabetics, and by supplying families with educational literature (Travis, 1973). All children are instructed to wear an identifying bracelet or necklace, in the event emergencies develop away from home.

In school, teachers may play a vital role by treating the student with diabetes as any other child, recognizing that certain aspects of the child's day may require special attention. Symptoms of both low and high blood sugar should be understood by all teachers (Table 1). There have been several instances where an alert teacher, observing a child's excessive thirst and frequency of trips to the bathroom, has been the first to suspect the diagnosis. In a known juvenile diabetic, delays in mealtime may have to be supplemented by snacks, and a quick energy source such as a candy bar or fruit juice should always be available, if needed, particularly on excursions. These should be used whenever the possibility of a low blood sugar reaction is considered. *If there is doubt, the situation should always be managed as a low sugar insulin reaction*, since the administration of sugar will cause no harm, while withholding sugar could have serious consequences. The overall goal should be for the teacher to work closely with the family to make the child's life as normal and active as any other child's, since there is no activity in which a child with diabetes should not be able to participate. It is this close working relationship between the family, educator, school nurse, and physician which most effectively helps achieve a healthy emotional balance. The school nurse should be encouraged to consult as frequently as is needed with the family's physician, and keep the physician informed of pertinent developments at school. Prolonged absenteeism and tardiness associated with juvenile diabetes have been well documented (Laron, 1970). When this occurs, school work at home is essential as with any chronic disorder.

Table 1. Symptoms of High and Low Blood Sugar

High blood sugar
  Usually develops slowly
  Dry skin
  Sweet or fruity odor to the breath
  Thirst and polyuria
  Deep breathing
  Coma

Low blood sugar
  Usually develops suddenly
  Restlessness
  Sudden change in behavior
  Sweating
  Pallor
  Tired and weak feeling
  Headache
  Extreme hunger
  Convulsions
  Coma

Much research in diabetes is currently taking place, and the possibility of a breakthrough in treatment is anticipated during the next decade. Work in the fields of transistorized insulin-releasing devices and pancreatic transplantation are in their earliest stages, and it is premature at this time to predict their success, but the degree of hope and promise is high.

Hypoglycemia

Hypoglycemia is a term which means an abnormally low level of sugar in the blood, and is, therefore, only a laboratory finding, not a clinical diagnosis. The clinical diagnosis of hypoglycemia depends on the association of specific symptoms with the low blood sugar level. Furthermore, these symptoms should disappear when the level of sugar returns to normal, either spontaneously or after glucose administration, in order to confirm the diagnosis. Hypoglycemia has multiple causes and, as seen in Table 1, may produce a wide variety of symptoms, including irritability, sweating, throbbing headache, twitching of the arms and legs, convulsions, and coma.

Because hypoglycemic symptoms may at times be subtle, the diagnosis of hypoglycemia has been imprecisely extended to maladies of all types. In reality, true hypoglycemia is very rare. Of particular importance to educators, *there is absolutely no evidence that low blood sugar causes either developmental hyperactivity, dyslexia, or other specific learning disabilities.* The overdiagnosis of hypoglycemia and its attendant unnecessary treatment must be viewed critically (Levine, 1974; and Yager and Young, 1974). Since true hypoglycemia is a serious disorder, it is important to establish a firm diagnosis. Whenever vague symptoms are suspected of being caused by hypoglycemia, the matter should be discussed with a competent physician and endocrinologist. The diagnosis of hypoglycemia can only be confirmed by exacting hormonal assays and other specialized testing, and the term should not be used loosely.

DISORDERS OF GROWTH

Short Stature

Growth disturbances constitute the most common referral to the pediatric endocrinologist. Unfortunately, our society has placed a high premium on height, and created problems for those who, in the eyes of others, "don't measure up." What is short stature? The definition applies to an individual who differs from the average or mean height by greater than two standard deviations, a statistical term which separates 97% of the population from the remaining 3%. Therefore, any child who falls below the third percentile for height compared to others of the same age and sex, should be considered significantly short and requires an evaluation to determine if there is a treatable cause.

Another parameter which is important in evaluating growth patterns is the growth velocity, or rate of growth per year. A 7-year-old boy who is of average height, but is growing at a rate of less than 2 in./year, also requires an evaluation. Parents can assess growth velocity by observed changes in shoe and clothing sizes, but previous measurements of height are essential. For this reason, it is important for periodic heights and weights to be recorded and plotted longitudinally on a growth graph, either by the physician or school nurse, as a continuing health screening test.

Growth is a dynamic process which begins at the time of conception, and is the product of complex genetic, nutritional, hormonal, and psychologic factors. The evaluation of children who present with growth problems begins with a detailed history of the family. Although there are certainly exceptions, small parents as a rule beget small children. A review of all previous height measurements by plotting heights on a longitudinal growth curve may reveal specific diagnostic patterns (Figures 2 and 3). A meticulous physical examination may then detect a clue to the cause of the short stature.

Selective laboratory determinations, such as thyroid or pituitary function tests, frequently are necessary to establish a diagnosis. The skeletal or bone age (Figure 4) is an x-ray assessment of developmental age by means of the radiologic study of the growing centers of the bones, comparing the bones of a child to normal standards. This extremely helpful diagnostic tool can detect a delay in bone age which is characteristic of thyroid and pituitary growth failure, among others. A careful consideration of emotional adjustment to the short stature by the child and family is also an integral part of the evaluation.

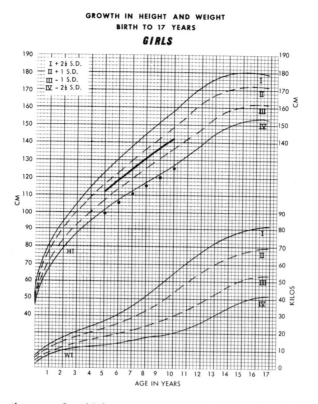

GROWTH IN HEIGHT AND WEIGHT
BIRTH TO 17 YEARS
GIRLS

Figure 2. Growth curve of a girl from age 5 to 10. The *dots* represent a height slightly below the third percentile (greater than two standard deviations), and illustrate a slow but constant rate of growth of about 2 in./year, a pattern consistent with genetic shortness. The *solid line* depicts the mean height for girls of a similar age.

If the examination excludes major systemic abnormalities, there are several remaining diagnostic categories (Gardner, 1969; and Wilkins, Blizzard, and Migeon, 1965) which constitute the vast majority of etiologies for growth retardation (Figure 5). The most common type is *genetic short stature,* the form that runs in families. In this instance, one or more relatives are less than 5 ft. 2 in. tall, the growth rate is slow but constant, and the bone age is normal. *Constitutionally delayed growth* is the pattern where pubertal development and growth lag behind, but eventually catch up. In this type, it is common for 13-year-olds to have the growth, development, and bone age of a 10-year-old. Frequently there is the history of delayed menarche in the mother, who, for example, may not have menstruated until she was 15 years old. Psychologic problems are not uncommon in this group. Another very important cause of short stature is *iatrogenic,* in which medication, such as cortisone, may stunt growth as an adverse side effect of prescribed treatment (Figure 3).

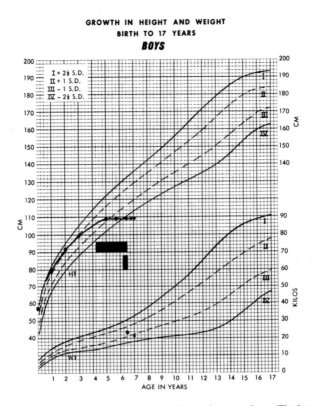

Figure 3. Growth curve of a boy who ceased growing at 5 years of age. The larger dark block under the curve represents a time when he was receiving cortisone injections for an allergy. This is an example of an unrecognized iatrogenic problem. Growth returned to normal when the medication was discontinued.

Two principal hormones which are essential for normal growth are thyroid hormone and growth hormone. *Thyroid deficiency,* which will be discussed separately, may result in markedly delayed growth, as will *pituitary growth hormone deficiency.* The pituitary or master gland is a tiny, pea-sized gland located at the base of the brain. It accounts for at least 10 different hormones, including growth hormone. The pituitary gland is under the control of specific releasing factors, chemical substances located within a higher center of the brain, the hypothalamus (Figure 1). As recently as 1958, scientists isolated and purified human growth hormone, making it available for the treatment of hypopituitary patients. Growth hormone is extremely scarce, since it can only be obtained from pituitary glands which are donated from autopsies. Between 50 and 200 pituitary glands are needed to treat a single child for a period of 1 year. Since the pituitary also contains hormones which control the thyroid, adrenal, and sex glands, some patients may require the replacement of several hormones in addition to growth hormone for normal function. In many children, the severely retarded growth and bone age can be vastly improved in

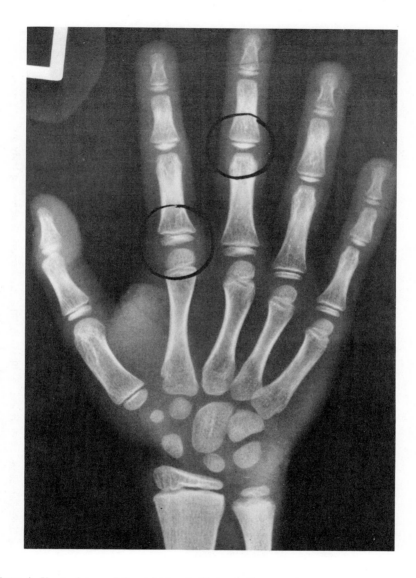

Figure 4. X-ray picture of the right hand. *Circles* outline growth centers (epiphyses) which are studied to determine bone age, here measured to be 7 in a boy who was 11 years of age.

response to growth hormone therapy, which is administered by the parent by means of three intramuscular injections weekly. Other patients may be resistant to therapy. It should be noted that most short children are not deficient in growth hormone.

Psychosocial deprivation is a disorder in which reversible growth hormone deficiency may occur secondary to emotional deprivation. This syndrome's three main features are: (1) a severely disturbed parent-child relationship and a strong

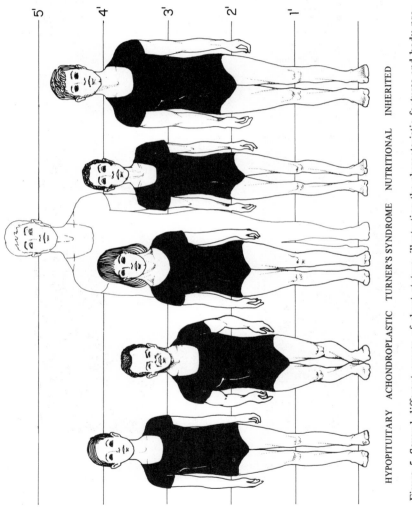

HYPOPITUITARY   ACHONDROPLASTIC   TURNER'S SYNDROME   NUTRITIONAL   INHERITED

Figure 5. Several different causes of short stature, illustrating the characteristic features and body proportions associated with each. All children are the same chronologic age.

history of marital strife; (2) bizarre eating habits such as gorging, eating from garbage cans, and drinking from toilets; and (3) developmental retardation. These unfortunate children must be removed from the home. When the environment is improved, growth increases dramatically, as much as 6 in. in the first year, and intellectual development may improve significantly. Psychosocial deprivation is sometimes combined with malnutrition, another cause of growth disturbance, in which short stature may result from inadequate caloric intake.

Other causes of short stature are: *Turner's syndrome,* the result of absent ovaries in the female, and, in most cases, a missing X chromosome (Figure 6), discussed in Chapter 10; bone disorders such as *achondroplasia* in which the arms and legs are short compared to the trunk; and *intrauterine growth retardation,* where stunted growth develops before birth, secondary to disturbances in the placenta. In this instance, babies are born small and may never attain a normal size. Growth may also be seriously retarded in children with *chronic infections, severe kidney disease, gastrointestinal disturbances, cystic fibrosis,* and in some children with *congenital heart disease.*

Regardless of the cause, the child who is abnormally short is often singled out by others. Children may be cruelly taunted at school by other children and called "pee wee," "shrimp," and "midget." There may also be practical prob-

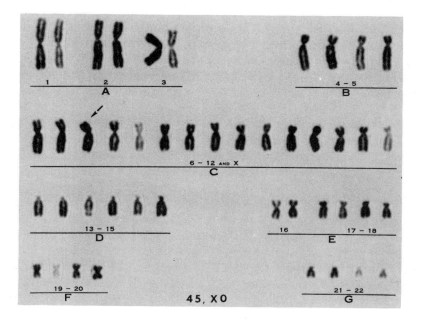

Figure 6. Chromosome analysis showing only one X chromosome in Group C (*arrow*) for a total number of 45. This girl with Turner's syndrome had marked short stature, a webbed neck, a congenital heart defect, and learning disabilities which are common in this disorder.

lems (Figure 7). The short child may have difficulty getting doors open or reaching the water fountain like his peers. In school, fighting the crowds in the cafeteria, or being asked to line up according to size, may produce emotional symptoms, such as withdrawal, aggressiveness, or depression. The child's strongest support should be in the form of parental guidance and acceptance, with the realization that size is really a false standard by which to be measured. Encouragement to participate in sports such as tennis, swimming, and soccer (rather than football and basketball) may be helpful. Here, too, the teacher may be vitally important, recognizing the need to treat children according to their mental and chronologic age, not size. In addition, teachers should anticipate the need for special education in disorders such as Turner's syndrome, where these girls may have serious perceptual problems and learning disabilities, and in some cases of hypothyroidism where treatment began late. Positive reinforcement at all levels assists the child in developing confidence and a healthy body image. Joining groups such as the Human Growth Foundation may be very supportive to many families. If a child feels truly accepted and receives the support of his family and teacher, few serious problems will arise.

Tall Stature

During the past 50 years, approximately 3 in. has been added to the average adult height in the United States. Tall stature is rarely a problem in boys, but the tall adolescent female may well have difficulty adjusting to height in relation to her peers, selecting clothes, and, in later adolescence, dating. Although no uniform definition exists for tall stature, a girl with a predicted adult height in excess of 71 in., or one whose height is above the ninety-seventh percentile, may need evaluation and, in selected instances, treatment because of associated psychologic difficulties.

There are several causes of excessive growth, but the vast majority fit into the category of constitutional or familial tall stature. Conditions such as pituitary gigantism, resulting from excessive pituitary secretion of growth hormone, must be ruled out along with other disorders, but this usually can be done rapidly by a meticulous medical history and physical examination. After the diagnosis is established, the ultimate adult height may be predicted according to the bone age and the child's current height, using special (Bayley-Pinneau) tables. This predicted height must then be discussed at great length with the girl and her parents. After careful consideration of all pertinent emotional factors, as well as the advantages and disadvantages of treatment, a decision is then made by the child and family regarding hormonal therapy. Because of possible adverse side effects, hormonal therapy is discouraged unless a serious emotional disturbance is present, or might be anticipated because of an excessive predicted adult height. Treatment with large doses of female sex hormone (estrogen) may effectively reduce the ultimate adult height by rapidly advancing puberty until the growth centers of the long bones fuse and growth ceases prematurely.

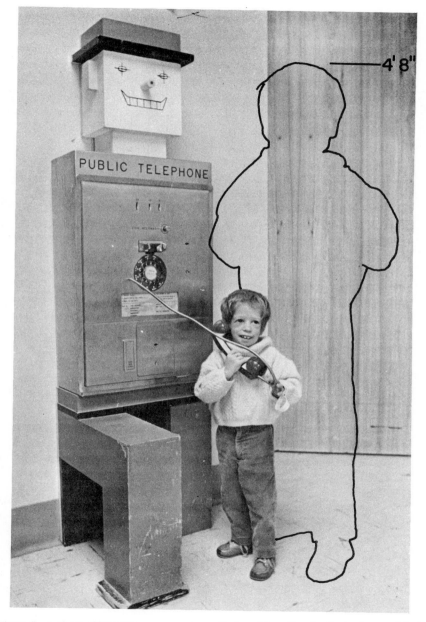

Figure 7. A short child with a very real practical problem. Boy in the background is the same age, 11 years, but of normal stature.

Regular periodic assessments, with continued psychologic support, are important facets of total management.

DISORDERS OF THE THYROID GLAND

Hypothyroidism

The term hypothyroidism means an underactive thyroid gland. Symptoms are caused by a deficiency of thyroxine, or thyroid hormone, and are dependent upon two major factors: (1) the age at which the thyroid deficiency first develops, and (2) the severity of the deficiency, namely, whether it is partial or complete (Gardner, 1969; and Wilkins, Blizzard, and Migeon, 1965). There are multiple causes of hypothyroidism. The most severe form is cretinism, a term which designates those infants who are born with a congenital absence of thyroid hormone. The cretin's face is puffy, round, and the facial features are dull and coarse. The lips are thick and a large tongue may protrude. The skin is cool and dry, frequently mottled because of poor circulation. An umbilical hernia is often present upon a protuberant abdomen. The cretin's cry is hoarse and weak, and there is little activity. Mothers often report that their baby is exceptionally good because there is "hardly ever a cry."

If cretinism progresses and remains untreated, hopeless mental deficiency, along with severe dwarfism, will develop. The early diagnosis of cretinism is urgent and must be established as soon as possible by measuring the level of thyroid hormone in the blood. If treatment is instituted within the first 2 months of life, the prognosis is considerably improved and mental development may be normal (Raiti and Newns, 1971). The developing brain's need for thyroid hormone during the first 18 months of life is great. In fact, if thyroid deficiency develops after this time, there is no adverse effect at all on mental development, although symptoms may develop, facial characteristics may change dramatically (Figure 8), and growth will be retarded (Figure 9). The symptoms and signs of thyroid deficiency are: stunted growth and delayed bone age; sluggish activity; cold intolerance; delayed dentition; slow pulse and low blood pressure; hair loss and dry, scaly skin; delayed tendon reflexes; puffy face and coarse facial features; constipation; mild obesity; menstrual irregularities; muscular hypertrophy (uncommon); and precocious puberty (uncommon).

As mentioned, there are causes of hypothyroidism other than cretinism. An inherited form of the disorder may exist in which one of several enzymes needed to make thyroxine is absent. One of these inherited forms is also associated with nerve deafness and is termed Pendred's syndrome. The gland may sometimes be abnormally small and located in an ectopic position, such as the base of the tongue, as a result of a defect in embryologic development. Additionally, inflammation may occur within the gland, a condition known as thyroiditis, the most common cause of hypothyroidism and goiter in older children. Certain

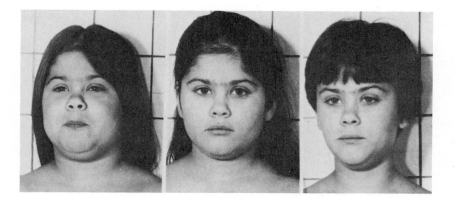

Figure 8. Facial appearance of a child with untreated hypothyroidism (*left*), after 6 months of treatment (*middle*), and 1 year later (*right*).

drugs, as well as iodine deficiency, may interfere with the thyroid gland's ability to perform its role—the manufacture of thyroxine. Whenever this occurs, regardless of cause, a goiter, or enlargement of the gland may develop. The etiology of goiter formation is best understood on the basis of thyroid physiology.

The thyroid gland represents one of the endocrine system's best examples of a feedback mechanism by which the body maintains a particular hormone in balance with its need. The thyroid gland skillfully converts ingested iodine (as in iodized salt) into a protein-iodine molecule by means of a series of enzymatic steps. The final product, thyroxine, is liberated into the blood stream and carried to the cells where it assists in the regulation of metabolism. If more thyroxine is required, a message goes to the pituitary gland which responds by secreting thyroid stimulating hormone (TSH). TSH then acts upon the thyroid gland to produce more hormone. When the amount needed has been reached, TSH is, in a sense, turned off and a new balance achieved. If, for any reason, the thyroid gland cannot manufacture sufficient thyroxine, it continues to be stimulated by TSH and may enlarge and give rise to the appearance of a goiter. When such a patient is treated with thyroxine, TSH is suppressed and the goiter will recede. Goiters may be small or very large, particularly those occurring in areas of the world where iodine deficiency is common and medical care scarce.

Regardless of the cause of hypothyroidism, treatment consists of thyroid replacement. Special education can be of vital help to the child who has either mental retardation or specific learning disabilities, both of which are common when untreated hypothyroidism occurs in early infancy. Placement in an early childhood education program with well-trained teachers is also important, and makes it possible for families to feel that they are doing all they can to help their child as early as possible. Psychometric evaluation prior to entering school is also recommended to assist in correct placement and individualization of the educational program. Some children with treated cretinism are also hyperkinetic and

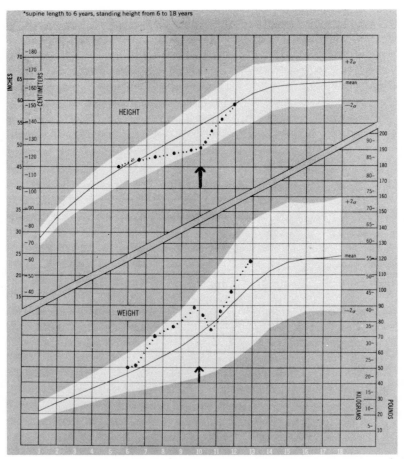

Figure 9. Typical growth curve of a patient with hypothyroidism (patient shown in Fig. 8). The onset of hormone deficiency corresponds with a decline in linear growth and an increase in weight. Catch-up growth occurs in response to treatment. The *arrow* indicates the initiation of replacement therapy with thyroxine.

may require treatment with psychoactive drugs in conjunction with psychiatric counseling for the family. With strong educational support, many retarded hypothyroid children have been shown to improve considerably (Cameron and O'Connor, 1964).

Hyperthyroidism

Hyperthyroidism or Grave's disease, an overactive thyroid gland, results from the excessive production of thyroid hormone (Gardner, 1969; and Wilkins, Blizzard, and Migeon, 1965). Its precise cause is unclear, but the hallmark of this disorder is an autonomously functioning, enlarged thyroid gland often associated with protruding eyes. The increased amounts of thyroxine may cause a wide array of symptoms and signs, such as nervousness, irritability, insomnia, sweating, weakness, palpitations, heart failure, diarrhea, menstrual irregularities, and weight loss in the face of increased hunger, since the basal metabolic rate is increased. But the primary reason why educators should be aware of this disorder is that frequently the major symptom in hyperthyroid children is emotional lability and deterioration of school performance. Often these children are thought to have a primary psychiatric disorder, and, because some of the other symptoms may be overshadowed by the behavior disturbance, the diagnosis of hyperthyroidism frequently is considerably delayed. Once the diagnosis has been established by appropriate tests, treatment is accomplished by the administration of drugs that block the gland's formation of thyroid hormone. Occasionally, surgical removal of the gland is required if drug therapy is unsuccessful.

CHILDREN WHO TAKE CORTISONE MEDICATION

Children, on occasion, have disorders for which large doses of cortisone medication, a product of the adrenal glands, may be prescribed. The adrenal glands are triangular shaped organs that sit on the upper portion of each kidney and produce many essential hormones; however, the major product is cortisol, a hormone similar to cortisone. Although there are many known disorders of the adrenal, only the effect of taking cortisone medication upon the adrenal gland will be discussed. The adrenal, like the thyroid described previously, is also under a feedback control mechanism from the pituitary gland. In this instance, the pituitary hormonal messenger is adrenocorticotrophin (ACTH). The adrenal cortex, or outer layer of the adrenal gland, manufactures cortisol, and, if the body needs additional hormone, pituitary ACTH stimulates it to do so. However, if an individual is taking cortisone medication for the treatment of disorders such as allergy, nephrosis, regional enteritis, cancer, or adrenal insufficiency, the body loses its internal control through ACTH, and the increased need for cortisol which results from accidents or infection must be anticipated by increasing the dose during the period of stress. This is always discussed carefully with families, who readily learn how to regulate the dose. Any serious illness must be reported immediately to the physician. Vomiting is particularly dangerous, since oral medication may not be retained and intramuscular medicine must be substituted. If cortisone medication is not supplied in the necessary amounts, shock may develop. This is one reason why cortisone should never be prescribed indiscriminately and without very strict indications in each individual case (see Chapter 6).

PRECOCIOUS AND DELAYED PUBERTY

Both the normal physiology and the disorders of puberty have long fascinated endocrinologists and biochemists (Wilkins, Blizzard, and Migeon, 1965). The female and male sex gonads manufacture and secrete their sex hormones, estrogen and testosterone respectively, from the time of early infancy. Within the pituitary gland and its controlling hypothalamic releasing factors, there is a "gonadastat" which shifts to a different threshold at a critical developmental age, and, for reasons still unclear, puberty is initiated. The average female in the United States begins breast development as the earliest sign of puberty at an average age of 10 years, with menstruation occurring between 12 and 12½ years. The male begins his pubertal development about 2 years later than the female. Interestingly, the age of menarche is moving backward at the rate of approximately 2–3 months every decade. Adult height 50–100 years ago was reached at 25 years of age; now boys attain adult stature at age 18 to 19, and girls at age 16 to 17. Since variation rather than standardization of these events is more the rule, the ages stated above are the average. Development 2–3 years before, or delay greater than 2 years after the average, may be considered an indication for evaluation by an endocrinologist. For example, a boy with no signs of sexual development at the age of 15, or a girl with breast development at age 7 would be considered delayed or precocious respectively, and require an evaluation. Similarly, a girl who has not begun to develop by age 12 or 13 should be examined. It is beyond the scope of this discussion to deal with all of the disorders of puberty, but sexual precocity in the female and delayed adolescence may be of special interest.

Precocious sexual development with ensuing menses may be seen as early as within the first 6 months of life. There are multiple causes of precocious puberty, ranging from tumors of the ovary to specific brain disturbances, but 90% of all cases of sexual precocity in the female are constitutional, with no specific physical cause demonstrable. A number of specialized hormonal tests may be needed to establish a diagnosis, but once serious organic reasons have been ruled out, management over a long period of follow-up becomes important. If the girl is menstruating, this can be terminated by monthly hormone injections, and breast size can be reduced. These young girls experience a growth spurt which is normally seen in the early teens, and are, therefore, quite tall as children and almost always short as adults, since bone growth ceases prematurely. Intellectual precocity is also an accompanying finding, and frequently because of this and their increased statural development, school acceleration should be seriously considered (Money and Neill, 1967). A close working relationship between the physician, family, and school should lead to an excellent adjustment and good outcome for the future.

In cases of delayed adolescent development, hormonal treatment may also be indicated because of serious psychologic difficulties, such as depression and refusal to participate in any activity where undressing is required. This problem occurs far more frequently in boys. Following a thorough evaluation by an endocrinologist to rule out organic disease, delayed puberty with or without short stature may respond favorably to monthly injections of testosterone for 6 months. Since there are potential adverse effects, the decision to initiate puberty artificially should be weighed carefully.

OBESITY

Obesity is a term that is derived from the Latin "obedere," "obesus"—"to devour." It is a serious nutritional, behavioral, and metabolic disorder which affects between 15 and 25% of American children. It is also one of the most frustrating medical problems, since our current approaches to the management of obesity have been almost completely unsuccessful, and the cause of the disorder remains obscure.

The precise diagnosis of obesity in children lacks standardized criteria, but can best be accomplished by using growth curves to detect a weight greater than two standard deviations from the mean, also taking height into consideration, and by the use of skinfold caliper measurements of subcutaneous fat around the triceps muscle (see Chapter 13). Once obesity has developed, and particularly when it is of long-standing duration, the prognosis for successful weight control is poor. The reason for this may be that excessive weight gain in children under 2 years of age may largely be due to an increase in the total number of fat cells, possibly secondary to overfeeding in infancy. Once the number of cells increase, weight reduction can occur only by a decrease in cell size rather than number, a situation which makes long-term weight reduction difficult. Approximately 90% of obese 6-year-old children in a recently reported series had highly significant increases in fat cell number, indicating that the optimal time for treatment might already be too late.

One high risk factor which might select out children for closer observation and early treatment is the familial nature of the disease. If neither parent is obese, there is a 7% probability of a child developing obesity, 40% if one parent is obese, and an 80% chance if both parents are obese. The natural history of obesity in childhood is such that the majority of children do not outgrow their obesity, but remain overweight as adults. It is these individuals who have the severest form of the disease and the least favorable prognosis.

Some investigators propose the theory that childhood obesity is a disorder of the number of fat cells within the body, while adult onset obesity is a disturbance characterized by increased fat cell size. Other scientists believe that obesity is not a disorder of metabolism but rather a result of human behavior. Both lean body mass as well as adipose tissue mass are increased, possibly due to the effect of increased insulin production and the early initiation of the obesity cycle. Children with obesity of long duration have been shown to have a metabolic pattern characterized by increased insulin levels and low growth hormone production. It should be stressed that the cause of obesity is unknown and that there are many complex genetic, endocrine, and metabolic factors involved.

The dilemma of the management of obesity may explain why Consumers Union (Reducing Drugs and Devices, 1971) has critically reviewed fad diets, "instant skinny" products, before meal candies, appetite depressant drugs, bulk producing products, and slenderizing machines. Hormone treatment with human chorionic gonadotrophin (HCG) injections or thyroid medication is similarly ineffective and also potentially dangerous. There are reviews which attempt to place both the etiology and treatment of obesity into a reasonable perspective (Mayer, 1966; and Winick, 1974).

Since weight gain occurs when the number of calories ingested exceeds the number of calories expended, the most rational approach to therapy involves both diet control and increased exercise, with special consideration of factors which can improve compliance with dietary intervention. This may mean group sessions for adolescents, regular visits at frequent intervals to the family physician, or belonging to weight reduction clubs. There is no place for drug therapy in the management of obesity in any age group. Since there are a number of analogies between obesity and arteriosclerosis (hardening of the arteries), the realistic fear of long-term complications may effectively serve to increase compliance with diet therapy.

Whatever the cause may be, children who are obese frequently develop psychologic problems and deviant behavior because of ridicule by their peers. Educators may play an important role by working closely with the child, family, and physician in developing health education programs directed at early detection and prevention. Instruction in nutrition and the need for exercise should begin in preschool programs, and help for obese young children in nursery and elementary school should be advised at the earliest possible age. If obesity is at least recognized as a true health hazard, much can be done to mobilize the necessary support to carry on the attack against the most prevalent nutritional disease in the United States today. At the present time, the essential ingredients for any therapeutic program are summarized in a recent conference on the topic of obesity: motivation, realistic goals, nutritional education, and the provision of psychologic support (Obesity in Pediatric Practice, 1970).

SUMMARY

Endocrine abnormalities are not uncommon in children of school age. Unless they are detected promptly and treated adequately, enduring effects upon a student's learning process may result because of alterations in physical features, hormonal activity, and emotional stability of the child.

The purpose of this chapter is to familiarize the educator with the symptoms, signs, investigational techniques, and management regimens of the various endocrinologic conditions, including disorders of carbohydrate metabolism, thyroid function, adrenal insufficiency, and deviations in growth. In addition, the features of precocious and delayed puberty are discussed. Finally, the pathophysiology and treatment modalities of obesity are presented, as obesity represents the most common and potentially most severe nutritional and endocrinologic problem among today's school aged children.

The educator is in an unequaled position to suspect and detect certain pediatric diseases, including endocrine disturbances. A firm understanding of normal growth parameters and their accepted variation is important if abnormal conditions are to be uncovered. Following the onset of treatment, the teacher more than anyone can provide the emotional support and guidance which are prerequisites for total recovery.

REFERENCES

Cameron, M., and M. O'Connor. 1964. Brain-Thyroid Relationships. Ciba Foundation Study Group No. 18. Little, Brown & Company, Boston.

Diabetes Mellitus. 1973. Eli Lilly Company, Indianapolis. 201 p.

Gardner, L. I. 1969. Endocrine and Genetic Disease of Childhood. W. B. Saunders Company, Philadelphia. 1072 p.

Laron, Z. 1970. Habilitation and Rehabilitation of Juvenile Diabetes. The Williams & Wilkins Company, Baltimore. 202 p.

Levine, R. 1974. Hypoglycemia. J. A. M. A. 230:462—463.

Mayer, J. 1966. Some aspects of the problem of regulation of food intake and obesity. New England J. Med. 274:610—616; 662—673; 722—731.

Money, J., and J. Neill. 1967. Precocious puberty, I. Q., and school acceleration. Clin. Pediat. 6:277—280.

Obesity in Pediatric Practice. 1970. Ross Roundtable on Critical Approaches to Common Pediatric Problems, Chicago. 48 p.

Raiti, S., and G. H. Newns. 1971. Cretinism: Early diagnosis and its relation to mental prognosis. Arch. Dis. Childhood 46:692—694.

Reducing drugs and devices. 1971. In The Medicine Show, pp. 103—116. Consumers Union, Mt. Vernon, New York.

Travis, L. B. 1973. An Instructional Aid on Juvenile Diabetes Mellitus. University of Texas Medical Branch, Galveston, Tex. 124 p.

Veith, I. 1971. Four thousand years of diabetes. Mod. Med. November 1, p. 118—125.

Wilkins, L., R. M. Blizzard, and C. J. Migeon. 1965. The Diagnosis and Treatment of Endocrine Disorders in Childhood and Adolescence. 3rd Ed. Charles C Thomas, Publisher, Springfield, Ill. 619 p.

Winick, M. 1974. Childhood obesity. Nutrition Today, May-June, p. 6—12.

Yager, J., and R. Young. 1974. Non-hypoglycemia is an epidemic condition. New England J. Med. 291:907—908.

6

The Child with a Chronic Illness

Beverly A. Myers, M.D.

In the past 40–50 years, the scope of health problems in children has changed remarkably. Whereas acute infectious illnesses such as diarrhea, pneumonia, poliomyelitis, diphtheria, and meningitis once posed grave threats to a child's life, modern medicine has dramatically improved the outlook for these diseases. Improved public health measures and refrigeration have decreased the danger of food and water-borne illnesses, such as typhoid fever. Immunization has led to the prevention of poliomyelitis, diphtheria, whooping cough, tetanus, measles, and German measles. The development of many antibiotics, particularly penicillin, has significantly decreased the mortality of such dreaded diseases as meningitis and pneumonia. Thus, the pediatrician's attention has increasingly focused upon chronic illnesses.

A chronic illness or handicap may be defined as a condition that affects one or more organ systems of the body and persists for many months or perhaps for a lifetime. Many such conditions in children are secondary to an inherited disorder or are the result of harmful events that occurred during pregnancy, leading to birth defects. On the other hand, a chronic disorder may be acquired at birth or may be the residue of an acute illness or injury (e.g., head trauma) later in childhood.

It has been estimated that 20% of children in the United States have some form of chronic illness or handicap (Green and Haggerty, 1968) (Table 1). Fortunately, there are fewer children now with chronic disorders that are so seriously incapacitating (such as those with heart disease or residual polio) as to require long-term hospitalization or maintenance at a separate school facility. The majority of children with chronic illness or handicaps can function in a normal school settting and can be expected to lead fruitful lives as adults. While

This paper was supported in part through Project 917, Maternal and Child Health Service, United States Department of Health, Education, and Welfare.

Table 1. United States Children's Bureau (1964) Estimates of Children with Handicapping Conditions

Condition	Year	
	1960	1970
Eye conditions needing specialist care including refractive errors (5–17 yr)	10,200,000	12,500,000
Emotionally disturbed (5–17 yr)	4,000,000	5,400,000
Speech (5–20 yr)	2,580,000	3,270,000
Mentally retarded (under 21 yr)	2,180,000	2,720,000
Orthopedic (under 21 yr)	1,925,000	2,425,000
Rheumatic fever	891,000	1,063,000
Hearing loss (under 21 yr)	360,000–725,000	450,000–900,000
Cerebral palsy (under 21 yr)	370,000	465,000
Epilepsy (under 21 yr)	360,000	450,000
Cleft palate, cleft lip	95,000	120,000
Congenital heart disease	About 25,000 born each year, of whom 7,000 die in the first year	

it was once thought that children with chronic disorders required separate settings, it would appear now that the optimal development of such a child is best fostered by normal school settings, wherever possible. Separate classrooms or schools are indicated for those with more severe handicaps or those whose problems significantly interfere with a teacher's responsibility to his or her other pupils. Thus, teachers must expect to have children or adolescents with chronic illnesses or handicaps in their classrooms.

The ultimate goal for parents, physicians, and educators should be to work in unison toward the optimal physical, intellectual, psychologic, and social maturation of each child. Since the probability of emotional or social maladjustment appears to increase in association with chronic illnesses or handicaps, the total development of such children must be considered and fostered in their daily existence. Such an ideal objective requires not only the skillful use of factual knowledge but, in addition, a keen awareness of and sensitivity to the attitudes and feelings of parents and children. To this end, it may prove instructive to explore those factors which are common to the child with either a life-threatening illness or a less severe, but nevertheless chronic, condition.

LIFE-THREATENING AND FATAL ILLNESSES

Until the past 50 years, fatal illnesses in children were common events. The mortality rate for children aged 1–4 has dropped from 5 per 1,000 in 1935, to 1 per 1,000 in 1960, and for children aged 5 to 14, the mortality rate has dropped from 1.5 per 1,000 to 0.5 per 1,000 population (Cooke, 1968; and

Green and Haggerty, 1968) (Figure 1). However, modern medicine has not established a cause or specific therapeutic regime for many chronic diseases, so that disorders such as cystic fibrosis, leukemia, and muscular dystrophy are relatively common and ultimately lead to a fatal outcome over an extended period of years. Thus, it is a distinct possibility that a teacher may be confronted with such a child at some point.

It is obvious that being the parent of a dying child can be one of the most excruciating experiences a person can endure. The parent requires every available resource to cope with the situation, including the extended family, if available, as well as the community, if aware. Some parents find support in meeting with other parents with the same experience; others find their religion and church a source of strength. A continuing and supportive relationship with a physician enables a parent to continue to provide the needed medical care to sustain a child's life and to provide for the child's physical and emotional needs.

Humans possess several adaptive mechanisms that enable them to cope with extreme stress so that they can continue to function in a relatively normal fashion. Such mental defense mechanisms as denial can serve to protect parents from overwhelming pain and extreme disorganization, so that they can continue to provide the daily care the child requires. Many parents seek to master their anxiety by gaining as much knowledge of the disease as possible. These defense mechanisms of denial and intellectualization (and others) are usually adaptive and should not be discouraged, except when parental denial leads to the refusal to admit that a problem exists, and interferes with adequate medical and emotional care for the child. Other adaptive behaviors commonly observed in these parents are activities seeking to reduce the threat of their child's disorder. Over the years, various parent groups have been the most productive, and often most successful, in changing legislation or seeking funds on behalf of their affected children (e.g., parents of retarded children).

Yet, despite all these efforts to deal with a painful situation, most parents experience periods of anxiety, depression, grief, anger, and guilt. Some may have mental breakdowns; even stable marriages are severely threatened. Some are driven to fruitless searches for faith healers or magic cures. Those professionals who are involved with caring for families who have children with a fatal illness must try to encourage parents to continue to function without constant incapacitating distress and to participate effectively in the medical and psychologic care of their child.

A child with a fatal illness may have varying perceptions of what is happening to him, depending on his age, his familiarity with the disorder (a sibling may have died from the same illness), his personality resources, and his parents' attitudes. Very little is known about a dying child's concept of death. From observations of normal children, it would appear that children under 4 years of age conceive death as a separation from parents, while those under the age of 9 do not comprehend the irreversibility of death. Yet some young children who are dying appear to have some awareness of their impending demise.

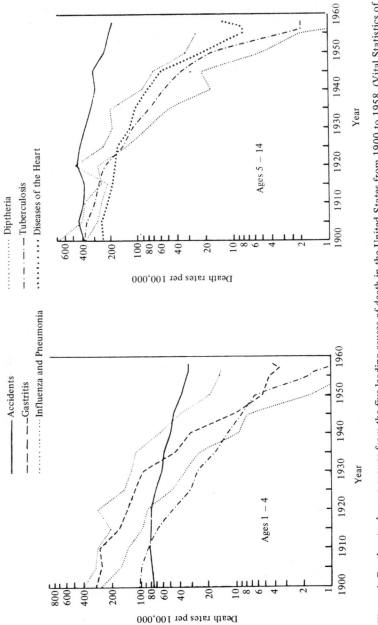

Figure 1. Death rates by age groups from the five leading causes of death in the United States from 1900 to 1958. (Vital Statistics of the United States as shown in American Public Health Association, Accident Prevention, McGraw-Hill Book Company, New York, 1961).

While there has been a major change in the willingness of many medical personnel to explore the phenomenon of dying with their adult patients, as discussed by Kubler-Ross (1969), attitudes and approaches toward children are somewhat different. Most physicians do not discuss dying with children who have a fatal illness, even though they may feel it is important to be as honest as possible in explaining to a child, in a supportive manner, what is happening to him. Nevertheless, many children eventually become aware of their illness by overhearing parents and medical personnel or by observing television programs or commercials. They will give clues to those around them of this awareness but they may or may not be heard. It is indeed difficult for adults to talk with children about dying, and those who have interactions with such children must seek to listen and to be supportive without being overly optimistic.

A child's reactions to a fatal illness are similar to those of his parents, and perhaps more intensified. Anxiety may lead to regression, increased dependency, loss of appetite, apathy, restlessness, and uncooperative behavior. The child may experience guilt, depression, and anger. Preoccupation with death may be seen in drawings and essays (Figure 2). Among adolescents, denial of the existence of the illness may lead to lack of cooperation in treatment.

The goal for all concerned with a fatally ill child is to enable him to enjoy his life as long as possible. In conditions such as muscular dystrophy and leukemia, this period may persist for several years, so that expectations should be as close to normal as possible. Such children require support but not indulgence. Someone listening with an interested ear, but without excessive cheerfulness, can do much to make each day worthwhile.

It is indeed disturbing for a teacher to be confronted in the class by a child with a fatal illness. The wish to flee or to avoid the child is an understandable reaction. For some, it is difficult to avoid overidentifying with the student and becoming paralyzed with despair. Yet the teacher can do much to make the pupil's attendance at school a pleasurable and beneficial experience. In this atmosphere, while associating with normal healthy children, the fears and concerns of pain, death, or hospitalization may be temporarily forgotten. But at the same time, drawings, stories, and essays may provide a means of expression of these fears. A child with a fatal illness demands hope, even if this simply results in his knowing that those around him—his parents and his teachers—will not abandon him.

CHRONIC ILLNESS OR HANDICAP

A society's attitudes toward its members who are deviant produce powerful influences upon their behavior and their role within that community. Those with chronic disabilities usually develop attitudes about themselves through their interactions with those with whom they are in closest contact. Continuous negative reactions from society can influence an individual's sense of self-esteem. Thus, a child's adjustment to his handicap will be heavily influenced by his

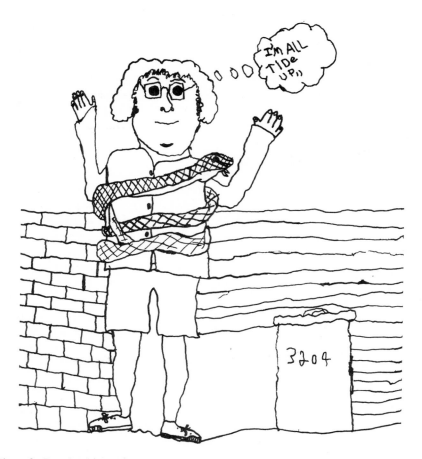

Figure 2. Drawing by a teenager with hemophilia. The encircling snake and the positioned arms depict the adolescent's emotional makeup.

family's and his school's attitudes toward him. For example, expectations that are excessively above or below a child's actual capabilities may lead to significant difficulties. A closer examination of the child's relationship with his parents and teachers may clarify some influences on a handicapped child's development.

The Parents

The discovery of an illness or handicap is bound to have a significant impact on the parents' relationship with their child. Acute illnesses are stressful and frightening at the time but, with recovery, they tend to recede in one's memory. A chronic illness cannot readily be forgotten, however. Initially, parents usually experience the shock and numbness of discovering that their child is abnormal. Through a gradual process of adaptation, this initial feeling develops into mourning or grieving for the loss of their formerly normal child. This is particularly acute in parents of mentally retarded children where their expectations for the child's future must be significantly altered. It is likely that most parents experience a deep sense of mourning or grief. Other feelings are aroused by such a handicap. Many parents feel anger—anger at the physicians for not curing their child, annoyance at the child for inconveniencing them, rage directed toward their spouses for not providing emotional support, and indignation at teachers and other professionals for not comprehending. Many parents suffer overwhelming guilt that their actions, thoughts, or bodies may have been responsible for the child's disability. The feelings most predominant in any one parent will depend on his personality, values, or relationship with the particular child. Some emotional response is inevitable but may change with the years, depending upon the parent's ability to find some acceptable mastery of, and thus acceptance of, an unwelcome event.

Such feelings may significantly interfere with child-rearing practices, leading parents to become overprotective and indulgent, thus fostering excessive dependency. To discipline a sick and helpless child is unacceptable to them, and thus some handicapped children are not exposed to the standards of behavior expected from their peer group. Such overprotection may also lead to unnecessary restrictions upon the child's activities and experiences. Some parents establish rigid expectations and excessive demands to demonstrate that the handicap "doesn't make any difference," even when it does. Children of such parents may become anxious or depressed as they fail to meet their parents' objectives. Frequently parents' expectations are inconsistent; they may feel discouraged, confused, inadequate, or ambivalent and are uncertain as to how they are to handle the child.

Professionals dealing with families in which there is a child with a handicap should be aware of and sensitive to parental attitudes. A parent's anger directed toward a teacher may sometimes be understood and tolerated when viewed from the above framework. With patience for and tolerance of distorted attitudes from professionals, a parent may ultimately come to recognize his distorted child-rearing patterns and modify his expectations for the child.

There are situations when parental attitudes may seriously interfere with a child's functioning in school and at home. A teacher may choose to discuss the problem with the school nurse or social worker, who may have the time to talk further with the parents. If necessary, and if possible, they should encourage the family to seek professional counseling. Nevertheless, the teacher can seek to foster such a child's growth and development in the time that he is in school.

The Child

There are numerous influences upon a child's reactions to an illness or handicap: the age at onset, the nature of the illness, the presence of disfigurement, the degree of parental adaptation, as well as the nature of the parent-child relationship. For example, a child who loses a limb at 6 years of age must learn to adapt to a new body image, whereas the child with a deficient limb from birth has never known normality. His attitudes will vary with age; a preschooler will react to the changes in the parents' handling or to the separation brought about by hospitalization. As he gets older, the illness or handicap will possess increasing significance for him and, by the time he reaches adolescence, it may cause considerable depression and anxiety. While the adolescent may deny his concern to others, he may be quite preoccupied with his body image and the differences he has from his peers.

Some children may consider their illness a punishment for misdeeds or forbidden thoughts while others may blame their parents for their defect. When hospitalizations are frequent, a child may be chronically anxious and may blame his mother for her lack of protection. Limitations in activity may lead to frustration and boredom. Negative reactions to his handicap may lead to self-devaluation. Thus, one may observe varying combinations of denial, rebellion, immaturity, overdependence, excessive independence, depression, anxiety, passive resignation, or mature acceptance, depending upon the many influences on the attitudes of the affected child.

It is helpful for a teacher to seek to be sensitive to a child's life situation and to communicate awareness where appropriate. Sometimes a teacher can encourage a child who has recovered to share some of his positive hospitalization experiences with his classmates, thus serving as a means of overcoming the anxiety that the hospitalization provoked. However, some children may not wish to be singled out or to have their health discussed in the class. Their privacy must be respected. Moreover, acknowledgment of feelings does not mean interpretation of them, and teachers should seek to listen rather than to explain or give suggestions.

The overdependent child who seeks to be singled out and to give excuses does indeed pose a difficult problem for teachers (and for parents). Everyone is fearful of pushing a child beyond his limit and causing harm, yet giving in to fears and excuses is not helpful either. It is best for a teacher to discuss the nature of such a child's limitations with his parents, the school nurse, and, if possible, his doctor, so that appropriate expectations can be formulated. To help a child learn that he can function well without excuses can be a major advance in his maturation. Observing such growth can bring much satisfaction to his teacher.

The Teacher

Like parents, teachers are bound to feel inadequate in handling a child with a disorder they do not understand. They may feel they were not trained to deal with physical illnesses and would prefer to see others dealing with the problem. However, with some exceptions, such a child's development is best fostered where he is not segregated. So it is through courses on handicapping conditions and books such as this that teachers may come to feel more comfortable with a different child in their classroom. The child with a chronic disability can be a challenge—a challenge to learn about a physical disorder, a challenge to utilize one's abilities in fostering a child's growth, and a challenge to develop one's skill in helping other children accept and tolerate significant individual differences.

Having a child with an illness or defect may provoke in the teacher many of the reactions described in parents. Teachers frequently feel they receive very little support from others in handling such a problem. Books may enhance their knowledge, but discussions with the school nurse, psychologist, social worker, or the physician may facilitate their coping process. In this way, a teacher can be a beneficial influence on a handicapped child's life.

COMMON CHRONIC CHILDHOOD ILLNESSES

Cystic Fibrosis

Cystic fibrosis (CF) is a chronic hereditary disease involving the lungs, the pancreas, and other organs. It is ultimately fatal, although many more children are now surviving to adolescence and adulthood. The specific cause is unknown, but it is known to be hereditary, and a biochemical defect should ultimately be found. It occurs in approximately 1 in 3,000 live births.

Children with cystic fibrosis tend to develop recurrent and progressive problems with respiratory tract infections or pneumonia. Although most children with CF have a chronic cough, they are not contagious to other children. As the disease progresses, they suffer increasingly from shortness of breath, so that physical activities, including walking, become progressively more limited. They may be hospitalized from time to time for pneumonia which requires antibiotics and other measures. Even when well, most children with CF sleep in a mist tent to keep the secretions in their lungs moist and loose, and they require physical therapy with postural drainage to remove these secretions.

The term "cystic fibrosis" was coined because of the pathologic changes seen in the pancreas, an organ which produces digestive enzymes (as well as insulin which is usually not affected in CF). As a result of the cystic fibrosis, the damaged pancreas cannot secrete certain digestive enzymes, and so these children cannot digest and absorb their food properly. This results in large bulky stools. With inadequate absorption of nutrients, these children may grow poorly. These problems can be greatly reduced by regularly providing the pancreatic digestive enzymes in a synthetic pill form.

The diagnosis of cystic fibrosis is based on a special laboratory test, known as a "sweat test," which can be done at any age, including the newborn infant who is suspected of having CF. Children with CF are born with a tendency to have very salty perspiration which can usually be distinguished from normal perspiration. This sweat defect also means that such children should be careful not to exert themselves too much on hot days. They should be provided with an adequate fluid and salt intake.

The prognosis for children with CF has improved in the last 20 years. However, modern publicity about the disease has made many children more aware of the nature of their illness. As their symptoms progress and hospitalizations are more frequent, they may become depressed. CF children and their families require much emotional support to lead lives as close to normal as possible.

Cardiac Disorders

Within the last 30 years, dramatic changes have taken place in the management of children with heart disorders. Most severe congenital heart defects become apparent early in life. Advances in technology and improved surgical techniques have greatly reduced the mortality in certain heart lesions. Acquired cardiac disorders, such as rheumatic fever, are preventable if proper medical care is instituted.

Rheumatic Fever Rheumatic fever is caused by a specific streptococcal infection, usually a sore throat. The disease is characterized by a fever, arthritis (inflamed swollen joints), and a skin rash. Sometimes the heart is affected. Precise examinations and blood tests must be conducted in order for the physician to establish a diagnosis of rheumatic fever since other disorders may show similar symptoms. In past years, children were hospitalized and bedridden for many months with rheumatic fever, while today they may be confined for only 2–6 wks. Early return to school is thus anticipated, with gradual increase in physical activities, as directed by the doctor. Once a child has had rheumatic fever, frequent medical evaluations are mandatory. In addition, the child must receive prophylactic penicillin or other antibiotics indefinitely to prevent the development of recurrent sore throats which may initiate an exacerbation of rheumatic fever. The school nurse and teacher should assist the child who has had rheumatic fever in receiving proper medical supervision. Because poor drug compliance may lead to a recurrence of the disease, careful monitoring of the frequency of drug intake may assist in the management of the child on prophylactic penicillin. By these vigorous efforts to prevent the recurrence of rheumatic fever, chronic heart abnormalities due to this disease are becoming less prevalent. Hence, rheumatic fever is becoming a less serious chronic health disorder in children.

Not all children with rheumatic fever develop heart defects, so one should be cautious, as in all medical problems, not to frighten or worry a child with unnecessary information. Many children and their parents have confused ideas about rheumatic fever and should be encouraged to discuss their questions with their physician.

Congenital Heart Defects Some children are born with defects of the heart. These are extraordinarily complex and will not be detailed. The defects occur during the first 1–3 months of embryonic development, at the time the heart is being formed. There are several known causes of such malformations. Chromosome aberrations, such as Down's syndrome (mongolism), which begin at conception, may result in heart defects as well as improper formation of other body organs. The virus of German measles (rubella), contracted by a mother during the first 3 months of pregnancy, may cross the placenta to produce heart, hearing, visual, and mental defects in the fetus. (German measles can now be prevented by immunization.) Some heart defects are hereditary. Many times, however, the cause is unknown, and the heart abnormality is the sole defect present.

Children with congenital heart disease may complain of shortness of breath, limited exercise tolerance, and occasionally, may have cyanosis (blue appearance of the skin due to poor oxygenation of the blood). The disorder is usually recognized at birth or in early childhood and may be detected by the presence of a heart murmur, although not all heart murmurs in children suggest an abnormal heart. Some heart defects are incompatible with life, and death usually occurs within the first year. Those children with congenital heart defects who have reached school age generally are less likely to have a life-threatening problem. Many have had complete surgical correction of the defect in early childhood (Figure 3).

Parents and teachers may be apprehensive about a child who has or has had a cardiac disorder. Heart defects seem mysterious and frightening. It is helpful to understand the status of a child's condition so that one can know what to expect. The child with continuing heart problems should not be pressed to the point of excessive fatigue, while the child with complete surgical correction should be encouraged to participate in all activities. Despite correction of the heart defect, a child may continue to be fearful and use many excuses to conceal his apprehension, while a significantly handicapped child may push himself to the limit. Careful discussion with the parents, school nurse, and, at times, the doctor may help the teacher to arrive at appropriate expectations of activity for each individual child.

Chronic Renal Disease

Kidney Infections   The kidneys are the organs which remove waste products from the blood and are located in the abdominal cavity close to the backbone. They are connected by tubes to the bladder, which delivers urine to the outside of the body. These passageways are susceptible to infection by bacteria in some individuals, particularly if there is some obstruction of the normal flow of urine (Figure 4).

Children with kidney infections may initially demonstrate a fever, but they may also void frequently and complain of back pain or burning during urination. Any child with these symptoms should be examined by a doctor. Of course, frequent requests to be excused may be a sign of anxiety, a small bladder, or simply an excuse to leave the classroom!

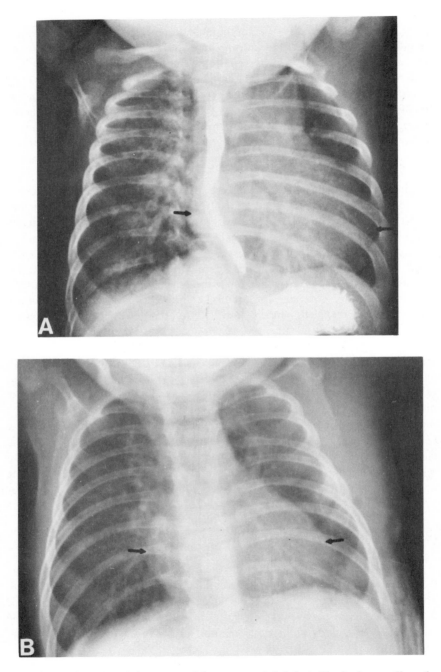

Figure 3. *A,* the enlarged heart caused by a congenital defect. The barium outlines the esophagus and stomach and assists in the evaluation of cardiac size. *B,* significant decrease in the abnormal heart size following surgical correction. Compare distance between *arrows* in both chest x-rays (presurgery and postsurgery).

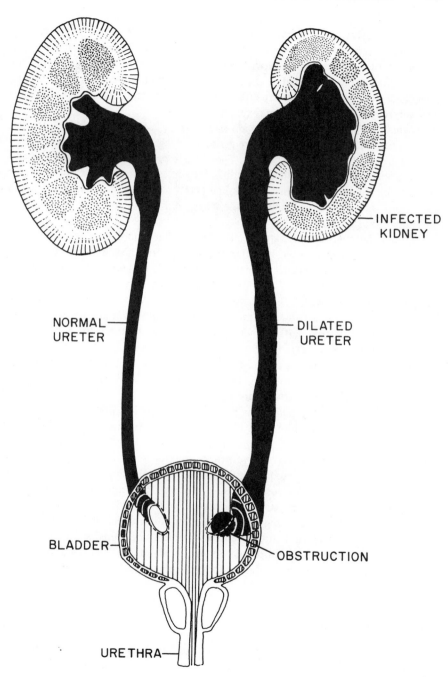

Figure 4. *Left,* normally the kidney produces urine which is delivered to the bladder via the ureter. *Right,* the obstruction as the ureter enters the bladder enlarges the ureter and damages the kidney.

Kidney infections can be detected by special studies of the urine and by radiologic examinations (x-rays) of the kidney itself. Careful diagnosis and treatment of kidney infections with antibiotics are extremely important. The school nurse should see that a child returns for regular checkups since kidney infections may recur. Recurrent infections may ultimately damage the kidneys so severely that kidney failure may result.

Kidney Failure When kidneys are damaged by infections or other diseases, such as congenital anomalies, that are gradually progressive, the kidneys may not be able to rid the body of its wastes. These waste products then accumulate and cause a number of symptoms, including fatigue, swelling of the ankles, poor growth (in children), and, in the terminal stage, clouding of consciousness and even coma. Associated problems include susceptibility to infections, convulsions, and high blood pressure.

Kidney failure will ultimately cause death unless the disease is treatable or the kidney function arrested in some manner. Several measures are utilized by the physician, but the primary means to prolong life is either through kidney dialysis or transplantation. Dialysis is a method of cleansing the blood via a machine connected with tubing to an artery and a vein. The patient's blood passes from the body through the machine which removes impurities by dialysis. In adults, this can frequently be done at home, one to three times a week. A home program is not often used with young children because of technical obstacles. Transplanting a kidney from a close relative or a person who has just died (cadaver donor) has proved a significant means of returning many persons with kidney failure to a relatively normal life.

Children with kidney failure may require frequent hospitalization for many associated problems. A child may be encouraged to return to school, but, on occasion, a home teacher may be necessary because of fatigue and other symptoms. Decisions concerning return to school require the careful consideration of the doctor and parents. Close communication with the parents may enable the teacher to comprehend and adapt her expectations, since this life-threatening illness has many associated problems. When a transplant can be performed, a child may regain much energy and interest and, thus, be able to resume a normal school life. Frequent medical checkups will continue to be necessary. Fortunately, more centers are available for dialysis and kidney transplantation so that the outlook for this once fatal condition is not as gloomy.

Leukemia and Tumors

Leukemia Leukemia is a malignancy of the bone marrow in which there is a massive overproduction or abnormal formation of white blood cells. It is usually fatal in children, although modern methods of treatment have greatly increased survival time. The cause of leukemia is still unknown, although it has been found to be related to mongolism, massive amounts of irradiation, and viruses in animals (but not in humans).

A child in whom leukemia is developing may show symptoms such as pallor, fatigue, fever, weight loss, joint pains, and excessive bruising. However, these symptoms are not specific for leukemia and can occur in other less serious illnesses. The correct diagnosis must be made after a careful examination by a physician with the performance of several blood tests, including studies of the bone marrow where the blood cells are formed.

Treatment of leukemia has increased the survival time from less than 6 months to as much as 5 years and even longer. Groups of doctors throughout the country have collaborated to share experiences and, thus, to gain more knowledge in a shorter time about the treatment of this dreaded disease. The medicine (chemotherapy) used includes cortisone derivatives (prednisone), specific chemical antagonists to metabolic processes in the blood cells (methotrexate, vincristine, and 6-mercaptopurine), and agents toxic to the malignant blood cells (cyclophosphamide). New drugs are continuously being developed. A child receives the initial treatment in the hospital and may have complete disappearance of symptoms and signs so that his parents and teachers would not recognize that he had an illness. The remission may last for months to years before the disease reappears. Medicines are frequently given even when there are no outward signs of the disease. These potent drugs may produce side effects; among those that may be observable are a moon face and truncal obesity (from cortisone), and loss of hair (alopecia). Children with leukemia may have a tendency toward infection and bleeding, but their doctors watch carefully for such complications and decide when it is safe to have the child in school. Some children may have to be hospitalized frequently, while others may be able to attend school for prolonged periods without many absences.

Tumors Tumors are the results of excessive growth of cells that may occur in any organ of the body. A benign tumor does not usually lead to death, while a malignant tumor has such uncontrolled cell growth that a fatal outcome is more likely. While less common than leukemia, some tumors are more readily cured with modern methods of management, which include surgery, radiation, and medication (chemotherapy). Common malignancies in children include tumors of bone and cartilage, central nervous system, kidney, and adrenal gland. Thus, a teacher may have a child return to class after treatment for cancer. Some discussion with his parents is in order to determine whether he may have a fatal illness or may expect prolonged survival. Regardless of the prognosis, a child may have many fears about the nature of his disorder, to which the teacher must be sensitive.

Allergy

The term allergy refers to an excessive and sometimes abnormal response of the body to foreign substances (allergens). Several allergic conditions are commonly observed in children of school age.

Hay Fever and Allergic Rhinitis Many are familiar with the stuffy nose, sneezing, and itchy eyes of hay fever which occurs in late summer as a reaction to ragweed pollen. It may also occur in spring, all year around, or sporadically in response to other allergens in the environment, such as cat hair or various dusts.

Antihistamines and related drugs are utilized to control symptoms. Some physicians use specific hyposensitization immunizations given periodically, depending upon the cause and severity of the symptoms. Some children may miss school due to these conditions, but it should not interfere greatly with the educational process apart from being a nuisance to the child.

Asthma Bronchial asthma is a disorder characterized by labored breathing or wheezing due to excessive constriction of the small air passages with overinflation of the lungs (Figure 5). Like many allergic problems, it tends to run in families and appears to be a constitutional abnormality. Those with such a defect may develop wheezing in association with colds, in response to many allergens, and sometimes as a result of emotional stress. The wheezing can become quite severe and even life threatening, requiring emergency hospitalization.

Many children with asthma attacks can be managed by various oral medications. On occasion, adrenalin must be given intramuscularly to control an acute attack. Some children are allowed to use inhalers, but these should be used under a doctor's supervision since inhalers can be abused and overutilized. Hyposensitization shots are also utilized to reduce the asthmatic attacks. Occasionally a child with severe asthma must be treated with a cortisone drug which may produce a moon face and truncal obesity. However, modern methods of administration of cortisone drugs and their usual short-term use in the treatment of asthma tend to minimize side effects.

Severe wheezing can be a frightening experience for a child. As a result, some children develop excessive dependency on their parents, particularly their mothers. Chronic asthma poses a stressful drain on families, both financially and psychologically. Optimal management of asthma includes careful attention to psychologic factors which may aggravate this chronic illness. Within the classroom, the teacher can support a child's growth toward independence and can help him function with satisfaction in this area of his life.

Eczema Children with asthma and allergic rhinitis may also have problems with a skin condition known as eczema. While it occurs more commonly in infants, school-age children and adults may suffer from the problem as well. It presents as an itchy, thickened, reddened area in the creases of the elbows, at the back of the knees and on the neck, but the skin changes may, on occasion, be more widespread. Scratching the involved areas may cause weeping sores to develop. Eczema is not a contagious disorder, but rather a chronic skin condition which, at times, may become quite severe. It is aggravated by scratching, poor hygiene, allergens, psychologic stress, and other, unknown factors. Topical agents applied to the skin (particularly those with cortisone derivatives), oral medications, and other skin care measures can usually control eczema fairly well.

A child with eczema may be embarrassed about the appearance of his skin. The educator can play an important therapeutic role through his own attitudes

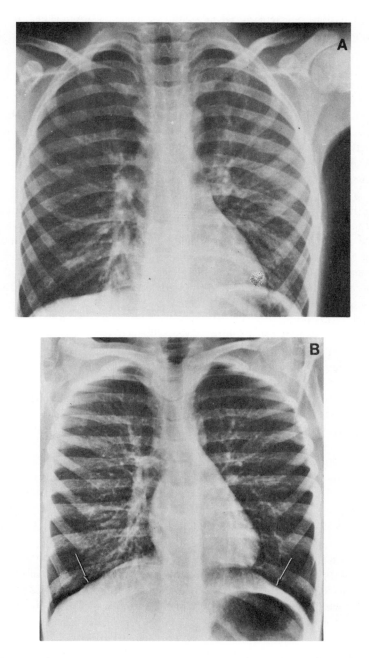

Figure 5. Two chest x-rays on one boy. *A*, the film during a period of good health. *B*, changes during an asthmatic attack. The dark areas (representing the lungs) become darker and overinflated pushing the diaphragms (*arrows*) downward.

and explanatiòns, particularly when a child's classmates are repelled by the skin condition. Support and encouragement may foster the child's feeling of acceptance.

Juvenile Rheumatoid Arthritis

Rheumatoid arthritis in children (JRA) is an uncommon disorder, with only 3 new cases per 100,000 population occurring each year. However, since the chronicity of JRA is from 1–10 years or more, a child with JRA will occasionally be encountered by the teacher in the classroom. The etiology of JRA is unknown. It occurs more often in girls and begins particularly between 1–4 years of age, and between 9–14 years of age. The outlook for a useful, productive life is excellent, and the prospect for the absence of an associated handicap is good, given excellent medical management.

The symptoms are quite variable. The arthritis or joint involvement may be sudden and severe with painful, hot, swollen joints; it may begin gradually and insidiously with joint stiffness, swelling, and limited motion, especially noticeable upon waking in the morning. Commonly only one or two joints, such as the knee or ankle, may be affected, and there is a good prognosis for recovery within 2–3 years. The more familiar diffuse involvement of knees, ankles, feet, wrists, and fingers, as well as other joints, is more likely to last longer and may lead to residual joint complications. Fever, irritability, and poor appetite are common accompanying symptoms during the active phase of the disease and may persist for weeks without associated joint complaints. Anemia and rash are common. Involvement of other organs including the heart, liver, and spleen does occur in young children and requires careful management by the physician. Inflammation of the eyes (uveitis) is a complication which must be looked for in all cases, since lack of treatment may lead to blindness.

The diagnosis of juvenile rheumatoid arthritis requires the physician's careful consideration of the history and physical findings and his use of various laboratory tests both to rule out other disorders and to support the diagnosis of JRA. Differentiating JRA from rheumatic fever can be difficult and sometimes only careful monitoring and management over several months will establish the diagnosis.

The management is demanding and time consuming since the disorder may wax and wane for several years, even though the outlook for remission is good. Medications found to be effective in reducing the symptoms include aspirin, cortisone, and gold salts. Because each of these agents, like all medications, have their dangerous side effects, the choice of their use to reduce the inflammation depends on balancing the relative anticipated benefits with the potentially harmful effects. Children on long-term aspirin should be monitored for signs of salicylate toxicity which include hyperventilation, drowsiness, and gastrointestinal upset. Physical therapy is very helpful in maintaining and improving joint movement and muscle strength. A child with JRA will determine his own activity and generally does not require bed rest. During the active phase of the disease, the child may be quite uncomfortable and irritable and, thus, voluntarily restrict painful movement. The physician's goals in the total management of a child with JRA are the reduction of the symptoms during the active period of the disease, the maintenance of as close to normal functioning as possible at home and at school, and the prevention of long-term physical and psychologic handicaps.

The teacher should be on the alert for a child with JRA who complains of bright lights (photophobia), painful eyes, or difficulties in vision. These are signs of eye involvement which require urgent treatment by an ophthalmologist to prevent serious impairment of vision.

The child with JRA who is of school age may have varying degrees of difficulties with transportation to and from school, stair climbing, and absences from school because of exacerbations of the disease. When it is possible, attendance at a regular school is preferable to homebound teachers or separate schools. Prolonged immobility in school may increase joint stiffness, and a student may prefer to get up and walk around the classroom to relieve his discomfort. A child can become demanding and cranky during the active phases of his illness, and this may persist and become a personality trait, with passive uncommunicative hostility and manipulativeness as common features seen in children with JRA. As difficult as it is to discern the differences between these states, the teacher should encourage participation in school activities to the best of the child's abilities, both physical and mental, based on guidance from the physician, school nurse, and the parents.

Peptic Ulcer

It is a common belief that peptic ulcers (or ulcers near the outlet of the stomach) are found only in adults. Peptic ulcers, however, are frequently being recognized in children as well. The causes of peptic ulcer are not clearly understood. There is a hereditary tendency that predisposes an individual, psychologic stress plays an important role, and increased acid production by the stomach contributes to the ulceration.

Symptoms from a peptic ulcer include episodic pain in the upper abdomen 1–3 hrs. following meals, which is typically relieved by milk or alkali. Vomiting can also be a common symptom. However, many children who have complaints of abdominal pain do not have a serious underlying disease. Pediatricians frequently perform careful examinations (x-rays, blood tests, etc.) in certain children with chronic stomach aches and do not uncover a cause for the pain. Some children, particularly girls, seem to experience frequent abdominal pain which may be related to constipation or some other physiologic change. For some, it is a psychologic symptom that is used in order to be excused from school or some other stressful event.

Nevertheless, the occasional child is found to have a duodenal ulcer, upon obtaining x-rays of the stomach (Figure 6). Once a diagnosis has been established, treatment includes milk or antacids, frequent bland snacks, and medica-

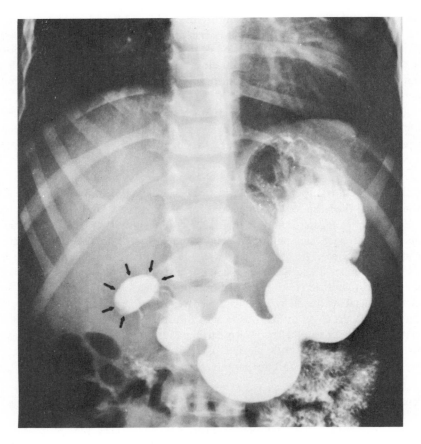

Figure 6. Barium in the stomach (large white area) empties into a C-shaped passage (duodenum). The ulcer crater (*arrows*) is in the duodenum and is outlined by barium.

tions, termed anticholinergics, which diminish stomach acid secretion. With these measures, the ulcer should heal, although recurrence is a distinct possibility given continuing stress. Treatment should, thus, also include attention to the psychologic stresses that may have contributed to the development of the ulcer. Frequently, children with ulcers are bright, conscientious, and very self demanding. They are tense and anxious, and their ulcers have developed in situations of stress or conflict. The high pressure some parents place on their children for outstanding school performance contributes to their anxieties, especially at examination time.

Teachers may help by being aware of the role of stress in the development of an ulcer, and by examining the school situation for contributing causes. Is the child capable of performing the school work? Are his classmates teasing him? Are there any situations that could be modified? Frequently, however, the stress is at home or within the mind of the child. Treatment of the latter usually requires the assistance of a child psychiatrist.

Residua of Accidents

The most common cause of death (mortality) in the United States today is accidents (see Figure 1). Yet significant numbers of children survive accidents with residual morbidity. A description of a few of these handicaps may demonstrate the seriousness of the risk of accidents to children.

Limb Deficiencies   One-half of limb deficiencies are congenital; the remainder are accidentally acquired. Cars, bicycles, snowmobiles, and farm vehicles are major sources of accidental loss of limbs. With the loss of a leg, an artificial prosthesis usually enables a child to return to normal ambulation fairly promptly. The loss of a hand or arm may or may not be successfully replaced if the child has one remaining functional hand. Artificially powered limbs are useful in some, but not all, cases. Careful and periodic assessment at regional juvenile amputee clinics is most beneficial for optimal selection and care of the prosthesis.

Brain Damage   Head injuries from such trauma as car accidents and gunshot wounds, anoxia from drownings or other asphyxiating events, and ingestion of medicines (including aspirin) and poisons may all lead to some degree of irreversible brain damage and dysfunction. The end results include mental retardation (see Chapter 11), perceptual and learning defects, motor handicaps, seizures (see Chapter 4), blindness, and hearing deficits. While a child's brain seems to have greater capacity for recovery than an adult's, significant residua occur commonly. Some children are able to return to regular classrooms with temporary periods of learning and behavioral difficulties. Common behavioral symptoms include hyperactivity or hypoactivity, short attention span, inadequate mechanisms for anger control, and discipline problems. Some children require special class placement because of these or other neurologic residua noted above. A few children are so damaged that home care, day care placement, or residential care are the only possible alternatives.

Burns   A child who survives a serious burn from fire, hot water, or other thermal agents frequently has severe residual scarring. There may be severe limb contractures and disfiguring appearances. Plastic surgeons are able to prevent or to improve some of the scars, but the impact of the terrifying event causing the burn, several prolonged painful hospitalizations, and the acquisition of a distorted and disturbing body image may lead to a variety of emotional problems with marked fears, emotional regression, nightmares, and social withdrawal. Children with facial disfigurations require considerable professional guidance along the road to physical and mental recovery.

Birth Defects

Birth defects are receiving increasing attention as research has begun to reveal some of the causes, and new techniques have become available for treatment. Birth defects may result from genetic disorders (see Chapter 10). Some drugs are well known for their ability to produce congenital abnormalities. Almost everyone is aware of thalidomide, a drug once used to counteract the nausea of the first 3 months of pregnancy. It interferes with the normal growth of the extremities during fetal development and results in an infant with absent arms and legs. This explains why physicians are very cautious about what medications are prescribed for pregnant women. There are several infections which can cause serious problems to the fetus. German measles or rubella during the first trimester may cause deafness, cataracts, mental retardation, and cerebral palsy; syphilis can lead to a miscarriage or to a baby with several deformities.

There are still many birth defects whose causes are unknown. Modern biochemical research may clarify many; careful epidemiologic studies of the influences of drugs and other chemicals may assist in explaining others. Regardless of cause, many structural defects can be cured by surgery (e.g., heart defect, club feet, intestinal defects, and cleft palate). Medications can be of help when an organ is defective in producing an essential hormone (e.g., thyroxin corrects an abnormality in a baby whose thyroid gland is deficient). Special diets may prevent severe consequences in infants with specific metabolic disorders (e.g., phenylketonuria).

Cleft Lip and Palate   One of the more frequent defects that a teacher is likely to encounter is that of cleft lip and palate. The incidence of cleft lip or palate in the population approximates 1 per 800 live births. This is an abnormality whereby the upper lip fails to fuse during the fetal life (Figure 7). It may or may not be associated with a defect in closure to the hard (bony) palate. The cause is unknown, but probably many factors are operational, including a very important hereditary role in some cases.

The lip is normally corrected surgically within the first 2 months of life, and the cosmetic result is usually quite pleasing. The baby with a cleft palate requires special feeding techniques until his palate is repaired surgically several months or years later.

Children with cleft lips and palates need long-term follow-up in a multidisciplinary clinic because they may be confronted with a large number of problems which demand careful monitoring and prompt treatment. The surgeon decides upon the necessity of revision of the lip or palate; the dentist attends to dental and orthodontic care; the audiologist looks for hearing deficits because of the tendency toward recurrent ear infections; the speech pathologist monitors the need for speech therapy; the psychologist is concerned with learning and adjustment problems; and the social worker assists the family with the demands that this handicap can produce.

A child with a cleft lip and palate is usually self-conscious about his appearance. If he is fortunate to have an accepting family, he may be able to relate readily with his peers, while others may need considerable assistance in enabling them to relate comfortably with peers and the public. A teacher can seek to include such a child within the group and should also be alert for hearing problems which may be the source of inattentiveness, poor school performance, or even social withdrawal (see Chapter 3).

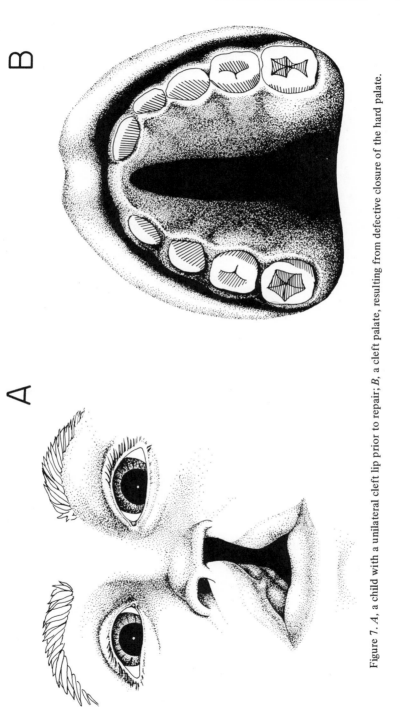

Figure 7. *A*, a child with a unilateral cleft lip prior to repair; *B*, a cleft palate, resulting from defective closure of the hard palate.

Phenylketonuria (PKU) Phenylketonuria, a hereditary condition that causes mental retardation, may now be prevented by treatment. It has been estimated that PKU occurs in approximately 1 in 20,000 live births. Phenylalanine is an amino acid (one of the building blocks of proteins) that is normally present in the diet (e.g., milk) and converted in the body to another amino acid, tyrosine. If a baby lacks the enzyme for this conversion (phenylalanine hydroxylase), the phenylalanine and other products build up in the blood and spill into the urine as phenylketones, thus resulting in phenylketonuria. These chemical abnormalities interfere with normal brain development. Thus, the baby becomes severely mentally retarded, develops seizures and eczema, and, invariably, has blond hair and blue eyes.

If a diet low in phenylalanine is given to such children from birth to 4 or 5 years of age, the incidence of mental retardation will decrease significantly. The earlier the diet is instituted, the better the result. The diet is specially prepared by artificially reducing the quantity of phenylalanine in the milk (Lo-Phenalac).

Thus, it is important to identify all such children at birth. In most states, during the first week of life, infants must, by law, be screened for phenylketonuria. A blood test for phenylalanine after a baby has begun to eat is the usual procedure (Guthrie test) and it is performed prior to discharge from the hospital. A high blood phenylalanine found by the screening test must be documented by more specific and elaborate biochemical determinations before a diagnosis is established.

After institution of the diet, regular blood checks are necessary to monitor the blood phenylalanine level. It is uncertain at this time when the diet may be safely discontinued, although most experts advocate its use until at least 5 years of age.

There is no special management for such a child in school. However, there may be some conflict with a child who must remain on the diet (which is unpalatable) and who wishes to eat other food. With mounting attention and apprehension associated with being a special child, there is an increased risk for adjustment problems.

Hemophilia Hemophilia is a birth defect even though the defect is not a visible structural abnormality nor is it always immediately obvious at birth. Hemophilia is a bleeding disorder due to a hereditary deficiency in certain coagulation factors within blood. (There are many factors essential in the clotting of blood but their deficiency is not usually hereditary.) The most common, classical hemophilia, is a hereditary deficiency of antihemophilic factor (AHF) and occurs only in boys (see Chapter 10).

A boy is usually recognized as having hemophilia in the first 2–3 years of life by easy bruising, prolonged bleeding from minor cuts, bleeding into joints, or excessive bleeding at an operation. Since there are other disorders of the blood producing similar symptoms, careful blood tests are necessary to establish the nature of the disorder.

Fortunately, a treatment controlling or preventing the bleeding tendency is available. The AHF can be obtained from blood plasma and given intravenously to treat bleeding in these children. More frequently, boys receive AHF regularly to prevent bleeding problems. Many efforts are being made to give this on an outpatient basis or even at home and, thus, reduce hospitalizations. However, bleeding into joints—the commonest problem during school age—may require hospitalization for rigorous treatment to prevent complications.

With these treatment meausres, hemophiliacs are able to lead more normal lives. Most attend regular schools. Most boys wish to be active, and this may lead to conflict with their parents and teachers. Some participate in sports. Decisions about activities depend on the severity of the disease, availability of prophylactic AHF programs, the boy's interests, and parent-child relationships.

Despite some increased risk for life, most hemophiliacs can be expected to lead full lives, which includes marriage and jobs. Hence, attitudes by the child's family and teachers which foster an excessive dependency situation may be detrimental. A hemophiliac and his family require careful guidance to avoid the extremes of isolated inactivity or self-destructuve risk taking.

Sickle Cell Anemia The biochemical defect which results in sickle cell anemia has been well described even though there is no specific treatment yet available. It is an abnormality of the hemoglobin molecule, the oxygen-carrying protein in the red blood cells. The structure of hemoglobin is known to consist of four chains of amino acids which are identical in most humans. Because *one* of the amino acids is different, the hemoglobin molecule of patients with sickle cell disease is modified, oxygen is not transported as well, and the cells are altered from a round to a sickle shape (Figure 8).

Sickle cell anemia is a hereditary problem. It takes one sickle gene (S) from each parent to produce the disease (SS) in the offspring. (See Chapter 10 for a description of autosomal recessive inheritance.) People with only one gene (SA) have *sickle cell trait* which causes no symptoms since half of their hemoglobin is normal. Sickle cell trait is found in 8% of American blacks, while sickle cell disease occurs in only 0.3%. Blood can be tested to identify the trait (SA) and the disease (SS).

Sickle cell anemia is a chronic disorder which may cause death in childhood, although many patients live for extended periods. The symptoms result from anemia (low blood count) as the sickled cells are destroyed by the body more readily than normal red blood cells. The children fatigue easily and are small for their age. When the cells sickle and clog blood vessels, hospitalization may be necessary for the treatment of crises which include fever, abdominal discomfort, or bone pain. These patients are susceptible to strokes (blood clots in the brain) and ulceration of the legs.

There is currently no available therapy which will correct the defect in the hemoglobin molecule or prevent the sickling, but there is considerable research underway to discover a more appropriate form of therapy. At the present time,

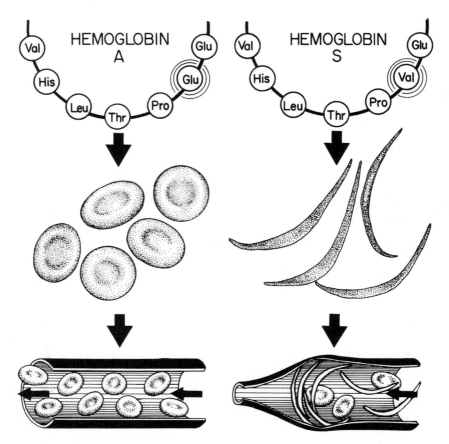

Figure 8. *Left,* the normal red blood cell and, *right,* the sickle-shaped red blood cell characteristic of sickle cell anemia. The normal round red blood cells readily flow through the blood vessel. The sickle-shaped cells become lodged within small vessels and form a clot. The sickle cell hemoglobin molecule results from an abnormal substitution by the amino acid valine (val) for glutamic acid (glu) as shown in the diagram.

multiple blood transfusions with supportive care for pain and the treatment of complications are the mainstay in the management of these patients. Treatment is not required for sickle cell trait which causes no problems in normal everyday living. With the recent emphasis on screening blacks for sickle cell disorder, many people may become unduly concerned because of the confusion between sickle cell trait and the disease.

Children with sickle cell anemia can attend school and be expected to participate in most activities except for physical exercise which may tire them. Since many children with sickle cell anemia require almost constant medical care, close cooperation between the school and the physician is essential.

Spina Bifida (Myelodysplasia) A congenital abnormality presenting at birth known as spina bifida, or myelodysplasia, poses profound medical and ethical dilemmas for our society. It is a defect occurring in approximately 3 in 1,000 live births, and because of vigorous intervention beginning at birth, more children are surviving, but with significant serious chronic handicaps. Teachers will increasingly encounter such children in the normal classroom—children who have normal intelligence but significant physical impairments.

The defect begins early in embryogenesis as the central nervous system is developing, with a failure of the spinal cord to close over at its lower end (Figure 9). The lesion at birth appears as a swelling, with or without a skin covering, at the lower part of the back (lumbosacral region). This swelling may contain only the membranes covering the spinal cord, or more often, portions of the defective spinal cord. The term myelodysplasia refers to the entire group of central nervous system malformations. It is the damage to or defect of the spinal cord that results in several handicaps in these children.

Paraplegia Disruption of the motor tracts from the brain to the muscles at the spinal cord level leads to weakness and paralysis of muscles. The extent of the weakness depends upon the level of the spinal cord damage or defect. If the defect is at the base of the spine, the weakness may be limited to the muscles of the feet and ankles and the child may only require short leg braces for normal ambulation. A midthoracic defect may give a flaccid paralysis below the waist, necessitating use of a wheelchair. Such defects rarely occur in the neck region so as to affect the arms.

Sensory Loss Disruption of the sensory tracts from skin, bone, and muscle at the spinal cord level results in absence of sensation on the skin, which is roughly but not always parallel to the areas of muscles weakness. Such anesthesia increases the risk for injuries and pressure sores, especially on the feet and buttocks.

Urinary and Bowel Incontinence The spinal cord damage interferes with normal voluntary sphincter control and may be one of the biggest obstacles to a child's existence in a regular classroom.

Kidney Infections Poor urinary drainage lowers the threshold for infections of the kidneys and ureters, which may ultimately end in kidney failure, if untreated.

Hydrocephalus A frequently associated defect is hydrocephalus, the accumulation of fluid in the ventricles of the brain (Figure 10). It is often treatable with the use of shunts, which divert the accumulated cerebrospinal fluid to some other area of the body, either to the atria of the heart or to the abdominal cavity. Treatment would appear to prevent or reduce the degree of mental retardation—a common finding in children with spina bifida and hydrocephalus.

The management of children with myelodysplasia is expensive, frustrating, and time-consuming and creates great hardship for the family. It requires the cooperation of several professionals—the neurosurgeon, neurologist, pediatrician, urologist, general surgeon, orthopedic surgeon, physical therapist, nurse, and social worker to name a few. Surgical procedures are common; medication for

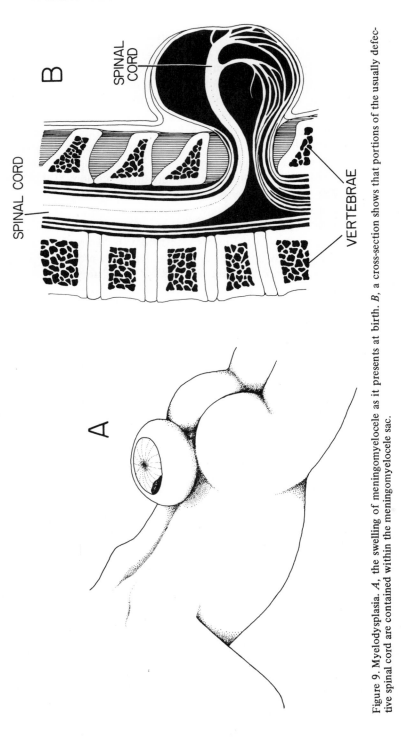

Figure 9. Myelodysplasia. *A*, the swelling of meningomyelocele as it presents at birth. *B*, a cross-section shows that portions of the usually defective spinal cord are contained within the meningomyelocele sac.

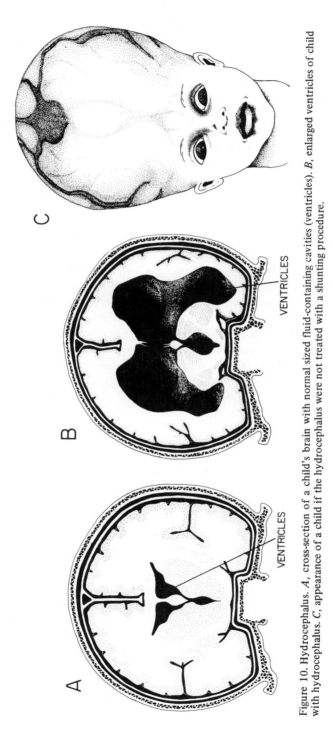

Figure 10. Hydrocephalus. *A*, cross-section of a child's brain with normal sized fluid-containing cavities (ventricles). *B*, enlarged ventricles of child with hydrocephalus. *C*, appearance of a child if the hydrocephalus were not treated with a shunting procedure.

urinary and bowel problems are often required; bracing and wheelchairs are commonly necessary; and urinary collecting devices must be utilized. The results of this enormous effort are increasing numbers of individuals who are able to become useful citizens, even though some will remain dependent and may require institutional care.

Many children with myelodysplasia present so many management problems that separate classroom placement is usually indicated. The extra personnel available to help with bowel and bladder problems and the facilities to handle wheelchairs are two reasons for such placement. Nevertheless, there are some children that can handle regular school and who do not impose excessive demands on their teachers. They can be real assets to their classrooms.

CONCLUSION

A child who has a chronic illness or handicap should have the right to grow and mature to the best of his physical and mental capabilities. His relationships with society via his family and teachers can either negatively or positively affect his ability to function as an adult. We, as professionals, can have a beneficial influence on the child and his family through the skillful use of our knowledge about a disorder and a sensitivity to the family's attitudes. Collaboration and cooperation between physicians, allied health professionals, and educators is essential in fostering optimal growth for each child.

REFERENCES

Cooke, R. (ed.). 1968. The Biological Basis of Pediatric Practice. McGraw-Hill Book Company, New York. 1,592 p.
Green, M., and R. Haggerty. 1968. Ambulatory Pediatrics. W. B. Saunders Company, Philadelphia. p. 85.
Kubler-Ross, E. 1969. On Death and Dying. The Macmillan Company, New York. 260 p.

SUGGESTED READING

Apgar, V., and J. Beck. 1972. Is My Baby All Right? A Guide to Birth Defects. Trident Press, New York. 492 p.
Bain, H. 1974. Symposium on Chronic Disease in Children. Pediatric Clinic of North America, pp. 743–1049. W. B. Saunders Company, Philadelphia.
Barker, R. G., B. A. Wright, L. Meyerson, and M. R. Gonick. 1953. Adjustment to Physical Handicap and Illness: A Survey of the Social Psychology of Physique and Disability. Social Science Research Council, New York. 440 p.
Cruickshank, W. M. 1963. Psychology of Exceptional Children and Youth. Prentice-Hall, Inc., Englewood Cliffs, N. J. 624 p.

Debuskey, M. 1970. The Chronically Ill Child and His Family. Charles C Thomas, Publisher, Springfield, Ill. 203 p.

Downey, J. A., and N. Low. 1974. The Child with a Disabling Illness: Principles of Rehabilitation. W. B. Saunders Company, Philadelphia. 627 p.

Haller, J. A. (ed.). 1967. The Hospitalized Child and His Family. Johns Hopkins Press, Baltimore. 121 p.

Harper, P. 1962. Preventive Pediatrics. Appleton-Century-Crofts, Inc., New York. p. 630.

Heisler, V. 1972. A Handicapped Child in the Family: A Guide for Parents. Grune & Stratton, Inc., New York. 160 p.

Moore, K. 1974. Before We Are Born: Basic Embryology and Birth Defects. W. B. Saunders Company, Philadelphia. 245 p.

Phibbs, B. 1971. The Human Heart: A Guide to Heart Disease. C. V. Mosby Company, St. Louis. 247 p.

Robertson, J. 1958. Young Children in Hospitals. Blakiston Company, London. 103 p.

Somekh, E. N. 1972. Parents Guide to Children's Allergies. Charles C Thomas, Publisher, Springfield, Ill. 187 p.

Somekh, E. N. 1974. Your Allergic Child. Harper & Row, Publishers, New York. 271 p.

Spock, B., and M. O. Lerrigo. 1965. Caring for Your Disabled Child. The Macmillan Company, New York. 373 p.

Weiner, F. 1973. Help for the Handicapped Child. McGraw-Hill Book Company, New York. 221 p.

7

Teacher Awareness Of Drug Abuse Problems

Thomas J. Craig, M.D.

This chapter is designed to provide the teacher with basic information regarding the recognition and management of common forms of drug abuse which may be encountered in the classroom situation. For this reason, the chapter has been divided into four sections: (1) an overview of the current status of drug abuse among student populations; (2) a brief description of the most common drugs of abuse; (3) a listing of behavioral clues which may be of use in the recognition of active drug use among students; and (4) a description of important considerations in the management of drug abuse problems among students.

OVERVIEW OF THE CURRENT STATUS OF STUDENT DRUG ABUSE

Despite the countless surveys which have proliferated in recent years, most information on the prevalence of drug abuse among students must be regarded with skepticism. However, some general trends may be identified over the past decade. The use of drugs by students has shown two distinct directions: drugs are being abused by larger and larger proportions of young people at increasingly younger ages, and the type of drug abuse is a major factor in the extent of student abuse.

By far the most widely abused drug among youths, as among adults, is alcohol. Yet the National Commission on Marijuana and Drug Abuse found that only 39% of adults and 34% of youths considered alcohol to be a drug (Second Report of the National Commission on Marijuana and Drug Abuse, 1973). After alcohol, marijuana is the most popular intoxicant among secondary school and college students. The prevalence of marijuana use escalated markedly in the late

1960's. The Gallup poll has indicated that marijuana use increased from 5% of the college student population in 1967 to 51% in 1971. Unpublished surveys reported by Pillard (1970) revealed that 20–25% of high school students had smoked marijuana on at least one occasion. Recent reports suggest that the use of marijuana may have peaked, and relatively little increase was noted among either youth or adults between 1971 and 1972.

Narcotic use, particularly heroin, has been more generally confined to certain segments of the population, especially inner-city poverty areas. However, in recent years, heroin use has gained a foothold among middle class youth as well. Use of sedatives, in particular the barbiturates and the new nonbarbiturate methaqualone (quaalude, sopor, etc.), has become a serious problem among a substantial number of adolescents and college students. In this regard, the Gallup poll indicated in 1971 that 15% of college students had experimented with barbiturates.

Amphetamines have recently been revealed to be abused by large numbers of middle class adults, particularly women, for whom the initial use is frequently via prescription for appetite suppression or as a mild antidepressant. Experimentation with lysergic acid diethylamide (LSD) and other hallucinogens has been largely limited to older high school and college students. Despite the rapid rise in use in the late 1960's, as evidenced by the Gallup poll's increase from 1% of college students in 1967 to 18% in 1971, the incidence of use of these drugs appears to have peaked. Deliriants, particularly glue sniffing, have been employed principally by younger adolescents on an experimental basis. Reliable estimation of the prevalence of this practice is unavailable, but their occasional use is probably fairly widespread, although fortunately, relatively few cases of serious physical damage have occurred.

Contrary to the popular image of the pusher (an anachronistic term) lurking around schoolyards, most youths are introduced to drugs by friends or via the family medicine chest. A myriad of reasons have been advanced to explain the current epidemic of drug use among the youth of the country. The phenomenon is far too complex to explore in this chapter.

DRUGS OF ABUSE

Before the most common drugs of abuse are described, several definitions are essential to the understanding of the drug abuse phenomenon. Drug *dependence* is a state of psychologic and/or physical reliance resulting from chronic, periodic, or continuous drug use. *Habituation* is the psychologic desire to repeat the use of a drug intermittently or continuously because of emotional reasons (such as escape from tension, dulling of reality, euphoria, etc.). *Addiction* is a physical dependence on a drug which is manifested by the development of tolerance, in which the user requires larger and larger amounts of the drug to produce the same effect and withdrawal symptoms (such as vomiting or convulsions), if the use of the drug is abruptly discontinued.

Marijuana

Marijuana is a drug derived from the Indian hemp plant. Its active ingredient is tetrahydrocannibinol, which is most prevalent in the flowering tops of the plant with smaller quantities in the leaves and little or none in the stalks and seeds. Marijuana varies considerably in strength. Hashish (hash) is the resin collected from the tops of the plant and is at least five times as potent as crude marijuana. Marijuana is not physically addicting and does not show tolerance or withdrawal effects, although sudden withdrawal may provoke restlessness and anxiety in chronic users. Marijuana use can lead to serious psychologic dependence, however, and is habituating. In addition, an amotivational state, characterized by apathy and loss of interest, has been described in long-term users.

The effect of marijuana varies with the user's prior experience and mental makeup. Thus, an individual who has experienced pleasurable "highs" in the past will be more likely to have similar experiences in subsequent trials. Marijuana is most frequently used to produce a mild sense of euphoria and relaxation. However, it may also cause sensory distortion and interfere with work and driving ability.

Sedatives

There are four general groupings of sedatives important in drug abuse: (1) barbiturates (long-acting, such as phenobarbital, and short-acting, such as nembutal); (2) nonbarbiturate sedatives, which are primarily sleeping pills (Quaalude, Doriden, and chloral hydrate); (3) minor tranquilizers, used primarily for daytime sedation (Valium, Librium, and meprobamate); and (4) alcohol.

Strictly speaking, sedatives are drugs which induce sleep. In small doses, they may reduce tension and anxiety, and even appear to stimulate, due to cerebral depression which initially produces disinhibition. This is perhaps most dramatically apparent in the use of alcohol, in which initial small doses, by reducing cerebral cortical inhibition, may appear to "loosen up" the individual, although further use will progressively diminish consciousness and could lead to coma.

All sedatives are physically addicting, to a greater or lesser degree, in that tolerance to the drug develops (as well as cross-tolerance between drugs of the same class), and severe withdrawal symptoms will appear upon abrupt cessation of the chronic use of the drug. The sudden discontinuance of sedative drugs may produce the most serious of all withdrawal symptoms and is far more dangerous than narcotic (e.g., heroin) withdrawal. A severe withdrawal state resembles the delirium tremens evident with alcohol withdrawal and includes agitation, anxiety, sleeplessness, tremulousness, hallucinations, and, in a significant number of cases, convulsions. This withdrawal syndrome is a medical emergency requiring immediate gradual detoxification in a medical setting. In addition, the sedative drugs produce marked psychologic dependence. Acute intoxication with sedatives also constitutes a medical emergency, as this can lead to coma and death.

Sedative drugs are generally used to reduce anxiety, although young persons abusing sedatives often employ them for their intoxicating effects as well. In addition, persons abusing amphetamines often utilize sedatives to counteract the stimulation produced by the amphetamine. Most sedative drugs are obtained either legally (by prescription or over the counter) or illegally through diversion of legally produced medications.

Stimulants

Stimulants are drugs which increase alertness, reduce hunger, and afford the user a euphoria or sense of well being. Two major stimulant groups are abused by students: (1) amphetamines (including methamphetamine—"speed") and (2) cocaine. The amphetamines are legally produced and prescribed for a limited number of medical conditions. When ingested in large amounts, amphetamines can be physically addicting, leading to tolerance, the use of larger doses for the desired effect, and withdrawal on abrupt cessation. Withdrawal is less serious than that following cessation of sedatives, and consists primarily of severe depression.

Cocaine is much less widely available, but has become a more serious problem in recent years. Cocaine is not physically addicting due to its short duration of action. Amphetamine and cocaine are markedly psychologically habituating. Several recent reports have linked chronic stimulant abuse with violent behavior. In addition, the "speed freak" frequently shows a deterioration in social, familial, and moral values, as well as a physical deterioration due to poor eating habits and personal hygiene.

Stimulants are used primarily for feelings of alertness, well being, and euphoria. However, as use continues and tolerance develops, their utilization may be more to prevent withdrawal depression than for any positive benefits.

Hallucinogens

Hallucinogens are drugs which can provoke changes of sensation, thinking, self-perception, and feelings in susceptible individuals. User proneness is markedly influenced by self-expectation, personality type, prior experience, and mental set. LSD was the earliest hallucinogen to gain widespread use, although other synthetic drugs (DMT, STP) and naturally occurring hallucinogens (psilocybin, mescaline) produce similar effects.

The major influence of the hallucinogens has been alteration of sensation. Users of these drugs seek pleasant images and warm emotional feelings (a "good trip"). However, the alterations in perception and sensation may be unpleasant, especially under unfavorable conditions, such as excessive anxiety, and in certain personality types. Some hallucinogen users have experienced "flashbacks" for months after the last dose. This experience may be provoked by emotional or physical stress, other drugs, or marijuana, and is more common in cronic users. "Flashbacks" can have a considerable emotional impact on the individual, often leading to a fear of losing one's mind or a suicidal depression.

The hallucinogens are not physically addicting but may lead to psychologic dependence. Their use has diminished somewhat during the recent past, perhaps due to much adverse publicity concerning "bad trips" and possible chromosomal damage.

Narcotics

Narcotics are drugs which relieve pain and induce sleep. They include opium and its derivatives, such as morphine and heroin, as well as synthetic compounds (such as Demerol) which possess morphine-like properties. A small proportion of narcotic abusers have become addicted due to employment of the drug by a physician to relieve pain. The vast majority, however, have developed their habit through illegal use. Young males from inner-city poverty areas have been the most frequent group to become addicts. However, in recent years, some middle class youths have begun to abuse narcotics as well.

Narcotics are physically addicting. On abrupt cessation, withdrawal symptoms may occur, including sweating, tremulousness, nausea and vomiting, muscle aches, abdominal pain, diarrhea, and chills. While not as dangerous as sedative withdrawal, narcotic withdrawal can be excruciating, and is best accomplished in a medical setting with gradual reduction in dosage.

Deliriants

Deliriants include a heterogeneous group of substances capable of inducing delirium, characterized by agitation, sensory disturbances, disorientation, and alterations in consciousness which can lead to coma and death. Included in this group are: (1) medications such as anticholinergics often found in over-the-counter sleeping preparations and cough mixtures; (2) volatile solvents such as airplane glue, gasoline, paint thinner, etc.; (3) nutmeg and mace in large quantities; and (4) naturally occurring substances, such as belladonna and jimson weed. These substances have been abused primarily by immature adolescents and, in a few cases, have resulted in death or irreversible physical and neurologic damage. Their use is primarily for the "high" of predelirium. They are not physically addicting, but may induce some degree of psychologic dependence. Use of volatile solvents is particularly hazardous in view of the danger of serious kidney and liver damage.

BEHAVIORAL CLUES TO ACTIVE DRUG USE

In this section, certain behavioral features will be discussed which may suggest the presence of active drug use in a student. It must be remembered, however, that no single behavioral change or set of changes is indicative of drug use. Most of the following signs and symptoms, while suggestive of drug abuse in the absence of other illness, may also be seen in a wide variety of medical and psychiatric conditions unrelated to drug use. Any of the following clues should be viewed as indicators for further diagnostic evaluation in a collaborative manner by the student, his parents, teacher, physician, and others, rather than as evidence to be used to convict the student of drug use.

Nonspecific Behavioral Clues

The following behavior, while not directly caused by the action of the drug itself, is frequently observed among student drug users.

Behavioral change can be defined as any significant change in behavior related to drug use. Thus, for example, the good student whose performance suddenly deteriorates, the quiet student who becomes outgoing and boisterous, and the congenial student who appears irritable and argumentative should all be evaluated with respect to the possibility of drug abuse.

Dissocial or antisocial behavior, defined as a tendency to disregard usual social codes and often to come into conflict with them, is frequently seen among drug users. This symptom must, of course, be evaluated in light of the counterculture developments of the past decade, in which young people generally found themselves in conflict with some of the social codes (especially with regard to dress and appearance) of their elders. However, the drug user's conflict with society may exceed the limits of adolescent rebellion and take on self-destructive aspects, such as truancy, crime, and violence. In this case, it is often argued, with considerable justification, that the antisocial behavior and the drug use are both symptoms of an underlying personality disorder, and that to focus on the drug use is to lose sight of this complex interrelationship which may severely limit the potential effects of intervention.

Seclusive, withdrawn behavior may be observed in some drug users, and again, may be either the accentuation of a long-standing underlying personality disorder or the manifestation of the chronic effect of the drug itself. In this regard, as was mentioned earlier, an amotivational syndrome consisting of a general decline in purposiveness in life, apathy, decrease in scholastic achievement, and rambling, tangential, fragmented, and disorganized thinking has been described in chronic users of marijuana, although this has not been definitively shown to be the result of the drug per se.

Association with the drug culture, including excessive use of drug terminology, may be considered indicative of some predisposition toward drug use in the involved student.

Specific Behavioral Clues

The following behavior represents a more specific indicator of physical or psychologic distress in which drug abuse may play a role. Again, as with nonspecific clues, none of these symptoms or signs are diagnostic of drug use but should be investigated, as they suggest the possibility of more serious underlying dysfunction, whether drug induced or not.

Physical Clues

General Appearance A flushed face is often seen in association with the use of hallucinogens, narcotics, and deliriants. Weight loss and emaciation may be indicators of the use of stimulants and narcotics, both of which tend to suppress appetite and lead to an attitude of carelessness and lack of concern for personal appearance and hygiene. Sleepiness may be observed as the result of the use of marijuana, sedatives, and narcotics. Tremor and shakiness may be associated with the use of stimulants, as well as in the withdrawal phases of sedative or narcotic abuse. Hunger is sometimes related to marijuana use. Abscesses, needle marks, and tracks in the veins of the arms and legs may be seen with the intravenous injection of drugs, notably stimulants and narcotics.

Eye Signs Reddening of the eyes and chronic conjunctivitis (inflammation) are complications of chronic marijuana abuse. Dilated pupils may be observed during the acute phase of hallucinogen and deliriant intoxication and, to a lesser degree, in the use of marijuana. Contracted pupils are evident with narcotic abuse. Double vision may be associated with the use of deliriants. Temporary blindness may be an outcome of the acute use of deliriants.

Cardiovascular Effects Increased heart rate and pulse may be seen with marijuana and hallucinogen use. Decreased heart rate and pulse are characteristic of narcotic abuse. Increased blood pressure and abnormal heart rhythm may be observed with stimulant abuse, especially methamphetamine ("speed").

Acute Intoxication This may be apparent with the use of sedatives and deliriants and, to a lesser extent, with narcotics and marijuana. Characteristic signs of intoxication include confusion, slurred speech (dysarthria), unsteady gait (ataxia), irritability, impaired coordination, and disorientation (inability to accurately determine time, place, or person).

Other Physical Signs Coughing and bronchitis may be seen with chronic marijuana smoking. Convulsions can be the result of stimulant intoxication or sedative withdrawal and, on rare occasions, have been associated with hallucinogen use. Tension, itching, and muscular pains are sometimes observed with stimulant use. Dryness of the mouth and throat may be seen with the use of marijuana, deliriants, and stimulants. Ringing in the ears may result from the use of certain deliriants.

Psychologic Clues As with the physical clues listed above, it must be recognized that the following psychologic symptoms or signs may result from a wide variety of physical and psychiatric conditions of which drug use represents only a portion of the total picture. Definitive diagnosis as to etiology must, of course, be left to the appropriate medical or mental health professionals.

However, inasmuch as these conditions may present in the classroom as behavioral problems and, in some instances, as genuine emergencies, their prompt recognition and immediate management by the teacher are essential to their overall treatment until appropriate medical or psychiatric attention is available.

Anxiety is a marked and continuous feeling of threat, especially of a frightening nature. It may become so severe as to lead to a panic reaction in which the individual believes himself to be in severe and immediate danger, causing an attempt to flee from this threat with possible disastrous results. Cases of death have been reported resulting from drug users leaping from windows, etc., while experiencing a panic attack. This symptom is most common with the use of hallucinogens and, to a lesser degree, marijuana, although some degree of anxiety may be associated with deliriant abuse or the withdrawal phase from narcotics and sedatives.

Clouding of consciousness and confusion, characterized by bewilderment, perplexity, and environmental disorientation, are often seen as a result of a toxic psychosis. This may be an extremely serious complication of the use of deliriants and hallucinogens, of sedatives in large doses, and, rarely, in marijuana use. Its presence constitutes a medical emergency and, although many medical conditions other than drug abuse can lead to this state, its sudden appearance in a formerly unaffected adolescent should raise the question of drug use as a cause. In this state, as with anxiety, the individual becomes uninhibited and impulsive and may engage in life-threatening behavior as the result of his skewed perception of reality. Immediate medical attention is mandatory in such a condition, both for management of the behavioral problems encountered and for definitive diagnosis.

Delusions are beliefs held in the face of evidence normally considered sufficient to destroy them. There are several specific types of delusions including delusions of grandeur, delusions of persecution (paranoia), and delusions of self-accusation. These symptoms may be observed in a wide variety of psychiatric and medical conditions. They may also be encountered with the use of hallucinogens (especially paranoid and grandiose delusions), stimulants (principally paranoid delusions), and very rarely, marijuana.

Depersonalization is a state in which the individual suffers from a loss of conviction of his own identity and loss of a sense of identification with and control over his body. Again, this may indicate the presence of a variety of psychiatric and medical conditions but may also accompany the use of hallucinogens and marijuana.

Euphoria is a prevailing elevated mood, including an optimistic mental set and a feeling of well being and confidence not justified by circumstances and experience. Mild degrees of euphoria are sought by many drug abusers and may be induced by marijuana, narcotics, sedatives (in moderate dosage), and stimulants.

Depression indicates a prevailing mood of sadness, despondency, or despair. It may be seen, especially with the use of hallucinogens, and may be profound when secondary to stimulant withdrawal.

Hallucinations are false sensory stimuli in the absence of an actual external stimulus. The principal types encountered are auditory and visual; however, less commonly, olfactory, gustatory, tactile, and kinesthetic hallucinations may occur. Again, in addition to the many medical and psychiatric conditions which may lead to these symptoms, hallucinations may be manifested in association with the use of hallucinogens (one of the desired effects), stimulants, and, rarely, marijuana. They are often an integral component of so-called "flashbacks" which are not well understood. The latter appear to be recurrent hallucinatory experiences subsequent to hallucinogen use, which may be precipitated by emotional stress, marijuana, and other drugs.

Illusions are false perceptions occurring in response to a misapprehension. They may occur in association with the use of marijuana, hallucinogens, or stimulants.

Suspicion and ideas of reference allude to the continual impression that the conversation, smiles, and behavior of other persons have reference to one's self, and may be observed with marijuana, hallucinogens, and stimulant use.

Inadequate affect, in which the student is emotionally dulled and detached and appears insensitive to stimuli, may be seen with marijuana use (especially the amotivational syndrome) and hallucinogens.

Increased psychomotor activity, or the accelerating of prevailing levels of motor behavior with a general dramatic increase in the person's usual activity level, may be seen especially with hallucinogens and stimulants, and, rarely, on abrupt cessation of marijuana use.

Loss of reality testing, seen as impairment of the person's ability to perceive and evaluate events and situations, may be observed as part of a psychotic state secondary to the use of hallucinogens, marijuana, and stimulants.

Stupor, the deadening of senses resulting in little or no appreciation of surroundings, is a serious medical emergency which may be associated with clouding of consciousness and confusion. It may be witnessed with the use of sedatives in large doses and narcotics. It is often a hallmark of an overdose of one of these drugs.

Emotional lability, in which the student exerts little control of his emotional expression and may rapidly fluctuate between laughing and crying in a giddy manner, may be evident with the use of marijuana and hallucinogens.

Violent behavior which can lead to overtly destructive outbursts, including homicide, has been reported with the use of stimulants, especially methamphetamine ("speed").

MANAGEMENT OF DRUG ABUSE IN THE SCHOOL SETTING

Immediate Management of Medical and Behavioral Complications of Drug Use

Perhaps the most common management problem encountered among drug abusers is anxiety in a panic reaction. This may occur in conjunction with hallucinations and delusions, and is most frequently the result of hallucinogen or marijuana use. While not physically life threatening, these reactions do pose psychologic emergencies to the extent that the individual may act upon his impulses, and as a result may seriously injure himself and others in an attempt to escape his fears. Most of these reactions are self-limited and will spontaneously resolve in 6–12 hrs.

Occasionally, such a reaction will trigger an underlying psychosis in a predisposed individual, and may lead to a prolonged panic state or actual psychotic decompensation. In the latter case, intensive psychiatric care may be necessary. However, in the more benign and self-limited panic states, school personnel can play a key role in assisting the student by "talking him down" from his anxiety. To do this, the student should be kept in a quiet room, with as few sensory stimuli as possible, and accompanied at all times by one or more persons whom he trusts and with whom he can communicate. Physical restraints should be avoided as they merely intensify the panic, and the student should be actively encouraged to recognize the reality of the situation and to "come out" of the fantasy world in which he finds panic. This can be accomplished by repeated reorientation (telling him who he is, where he is, and what is happening) and reassurance that his experience is drug induced and will soon be over.

This technique is generally sufficient to allay the individual's immediate anxiety, although it may need to be repeated at frequent intervals over a period of several hours. The student in such an episode should *never* be left unattended, as his anxiety may rapidly accelerate and may induce harmful reactions. In the rare case that is not manageable by the above procedure, psychiatric attention should be sought both for diagnostic purposes and for definitive medical management.

Fortunately, the incidence of true medical emergencies among drug users is relatively low. However, the occasional emergency involving a drug user often requires immediate attention and may be truly life endangering. Among the physical signs cited earlier, very few require emergency medical care, although some, such as weight loss and emaciation, may progress to such an extent as to pose serious health hazards. In addition, the intravenous injection of drugs carries with it risks of infection and hepatitis. Certain deliriants may lead to permanent liver and kidney damage. Temporary blindness, in view of the fact that it may represent a serious medical condition, should receive urgent medical evaluation; the student should be carefully observed for his own protection. Acute intoxication, which may be the result of overdoses, especially of sedatives and narcotics, constitutes a most urgent medical emergency, especially if it progresses to the level of stupor, coma, or toxic psychosis. The immediate management of convulsions has been described in another section (see Chapter 4). Extreme urgency must be given to convulsions which may be caused by sedative withdrawal, as death or serious permanent damage to the central nervous system are frequent consequences of this condition.

Problems of Referral for Further Treatment

Ideally the school has the opportunity to serve as a portal of entry into treatment for those youngsters found to be engaging in drug abuse. In this role, the teacher may act as a confidant to whom the students may turn in seeking help with their problems—help which may be initially unavailable from parents, relatives, or other adult sources. Additionally, the teacher can serve a screening function by being alert to the possibility of drug abuse and knowledgable about its signs. To be effective in this role, the educator must have the student's confidence so that efforts to obtain assistance for the student will be seen as evidence of interest in his well being rather than as an inquisition aimed at prosecution or persecution.

Once the problem is identified, however, the question arises as to what is the best method to follow thereafter. In most cases, the teacher may feel inadequate in providing intensive counseling to the drug-using student, and may serve primarily as a referral source for further more professional treatment. As will be mentioned below, the school system may deem the problem of sufficient importance to provide on-site treatment measures for drug users. If this is not available, the teacher will be forced to look to community resources for further assistance.

It should be remembered that the ultimate responsibility for dealing with the problem lies with the student and his parents, not the teacher. If their cooperation is not obtainable, then the hopes for a successful outcome, regardless of approach, are quite dim. However, even with complete cooperation and a genuine interest in helping the student, the teacher is confronted with several difficulties in making a referral.

Availability of Treatment Programs Drug treatment programs are largely developed by communities in response to perceived threats to the community, rather than purely as therapy centers. The alleged link (as yet unproved) between drug use and crime has been a major impetus for drug program development. Thus, the availability of treatment will be found to vary from city to city, depending on how aroused the citizenry has become with respect to this issue. In addition, since hard narcotics (heroin, etc.) have been the drugs most often linked to criminal activity, most of the treatment efforts to date have been focused on this problem. This produces the paradox that specific treatment of the soft drug users (e.g., barbiturates, marijuana, and amphetamines)—by far the more widespread problem, especially among students—is in most areas inadequate or even nonexistent. In fact, in making a referral for treatment, one is often faced with the absurd fact that treatment centers for narcotics stipulate that patients must have been addicted for several years before they are permitted entry to their program (the principle of "wait until the cancer has grown large before we treat it").

The teacher may find himself in the position of having recognized a student's drug problem, successfully enlisted his aid and that of his parents, and then find there is no place to refer him to for definitive treatment! Some community mental health centers are beginning to develop programs to fill this void, but it still represents one of the weakest links in the entire drug abuse picture. For this reason, it is imperative that the school obtain up-to-date information on all available treatment resources which could be made available to anyone desiring assistance.

Establishing the Diagnosis   In general, the absolute diagnosis of drug abuse should be left to medical professionals who are agents of the parents and the student. However, the teacher may be in the best position to raise the question of drug abuse with the student, especially if the student has developed confidence in the teacher. This should be approached in a tactful manner, and precaution must be taken to avoid appearing as a criminal prosecutor but rather to appear as a concerned adult who wants to be helpful. Often when approached in this fashion, the student will acknowledge the problem directly and appear eager for assistance. In other cases, he may be hostile and seek to hide his drug use. These initial reactions are frequently fairly reliable barometers of the probability of treatment success. However, if the latter situation develops, the teacher should attempt to enlist the aid of parents or others if drug abuse is strongly suspected. Thus, while it would be inappropriate to accuse the recalcitrant student of drug abuse without sufficient evidence, it is the teacher's responsibility to bring any erratic or suspicious behavior to the parents' attention.

Motivating the Student to Seek Help   If a student has been found to be abusing drugs, he is often unwilling to take steps to curb this abuse and may have a positive interest in continuing. In this case, the hopes for success of any treatment program are remote.

However, on occasion, the student may respond to attempts at motivation which include goal setting (i.e., more positive goals for which cessation of drug use may be necessary), limit setting (including nonpunitive sanctions on overt drug use), and provision of information to the drug user (concerning the problems of drug abuse, etc.). The specific program, of course, must be tailored to the specific problem. Often a modified operant approach of reward for positive behavior and limits for negative behavior may serve as a first step in motivating the student toward seeking assistance. Ultimately, however, the success of any program depends on the student's appreciation that drug use must be ceased with the appropriate substitution of alternative gratifications for the immediate pleasure of the drug.

Parental Consent and Confidentiality   Often parental cooperation is crucial to the success of any treatment program, since parents generally have control over the student's primary reinforcers and because, in some cases, parental behavior may be significant in encouraging a student's drug use. Unfortunately, during the past decade, parents and teachers have tended to disagree over the appropriate methods of handling students. Thus, the teacher who discovers a student drug abuser may find himself confronted with defiant attitudes from both the student and parents. In this situation, the antagonism between parents and teacher subtly encourages acting-out behavior, such as further drug use by the student. Thus, close cooperation among parents, teacher, and student is essential for a successful outcome.

If a teacher is approached in confidence by a student, the teacher must make known to the student his responsibility vis-à-vis the school system, since in most cases teachers are obliged to report drug use to school authorities. In many areas, drug use still carries strong legal restrictions, and the student should be made aware of these restrictions before confidence is betrayed. A compromise solution in such a situation might be to refer the student to a certified psychiatrist or psychologist, where his information would be protected by professional confidence.

Unfortunately, the issue of confidentiality is often a deterrent to the student's seeking the assistance of the teacher; however, if it is handled completely openly, the student will generally appreciate and respect the teacher's position and the question of betrayal of confidence will not become an issue.

Legal Aspects Drug abuse laws in recent years have been altered with bewildering rapidity. In general, the trend has been toward less severe penalties for drug possession and use, and more stringent ones for trafficking in drugs. In some states, it has been suggested that all penalties for use of drugs such as marijuana be removed, although it is unlikely that this will receive popular support in the near future, and the wisdom of such an approach is highly questionable. In general, the more severe the penalty for drug use, the more difficult it becomes to identify and deal with the problem, since strict penalties, rather than curbing drug use, merely drive it underground. The teacher must be doubly cautious in raising the suspicion of drug use if its identification might lead to unduly harsh punishment of the student which might have long-lasting effects upon his future. Again, if a compatible working relationship between teacher and student can be developed, much of the hazard will be avoided.

Types of Drug Abuse In general, students using illegal drugs fall into three categories: experimenters, occasional users, and abusers ("heads").

Experimenters generally use drugs for only a few brief forays, primarily out of curiosity, and usually do not exceed 10 episodes of drug use in their careers. In terms of personality, they are indistinguishable from their nondrug-using peers and, practically speaking, require no treatment for this drug use.

An occasional user may be the adolescent analog of the social drinker, who utilizes drugs primarily as a social lubricant, rather than as an end in themselves. A small proportion of these individuals will eventually become heavy users, similar to the progression to alcoholism in the adult population. Again, treatment for this group is probably unwarranted except in the case of escalation of drug use toward the abuse category. Frequently, the provision of factual information is sufficient to curtail these occasional users from significant drug intake.

Abusers ("heads") represent the severe end of the spectrum of drug use, although, fortunately, they represent a distinct minority of all adolescent drug users. Frequently, "heads" have severe underlying personality disorders for which drug use may represent an attempt at self-medication. However, relatively psychologically healthy but immature youngsters may also get caught up in the drug culture to the extent of becoming chronic abusers. These are the students who are most critically in need of treatment, and for whom early identification and intervention may literally represent a life-saving endeavor. Unfortunately, they are also the youngsters who are most likely to drop out of school and, thus, be beyond the reach of the educational system for assistance. Likewise, they are often the products of chaotic family systems where parental cooperation is least available. In many of these instances, intensive psychotherapy is indicated, although these students are generally the most poorly motivated for treatment.

Medical Intervention Strategies In general, two types of intervention—psychotherapy and chemotherapy—have been utilized in dealing with drug abuse, with mixed results.

Psychotherapy is based on the rationale that drug abusers require insight and empathic support both to understand the sources of their drug use and to develop new behavioral directions based on less destructive behavioral patterns. The experience of psychotherapy with drug abusers has been quite variable and, paradoxically, seems to be most effective with the least impaired individuals. All forms of psychotherapy have been attempted with drug users. Perhaps the most consistent success has come from the application of family therapy (where significant family pathology supports the drug abuse), and peer-centered group therapy (where drug users are confronted by peers who, in most cases, are reformed drug users).

Chemotherapy has been prescribed primarily in the treatment of narcotics users and has received considerable financial support from the federal government because of its apparent cost-benefit effectiveness. Two types of chemotherapy have been most prominently attempted.

Methadone maintenance is one type of intervention in which the abuser is addicted to methadone, a synthetic narcotic, on the rationale that legal addiction will reduce the desire for illegal drug abuse and its concomitant, crime. The latter has been a controversial subject for several years. Initial reports suggested high success rates for such programs with "hard core" addicts. However, more recent experience has been much less favorable, and serious questions have been raised about the effectiveness and even the appropriateness of such a treatment approach. Despite these questions, methadone maintenance represents this nation's principal and, in some cases, only coordinated treatment program for drug abuse to date.

Narcotic antagonists have been developed on an experimental basis in recent years on the rationale that by blocking the pleasurable effects of narcotics, they will reduce the user's desire for continued narcotic administration. The employment of these agents has been too recent for any definitive evaluation of their efficacy.

In both cases, for chemotherapy to be effective, it must be combined with intensive counseling and rehabilitative programs to assist the drug abuser in reorganizing his life around more meaningful and positive goals. Unfortunately, with the exception of detoxification programs to deal with acute withdrawal from drugs such as barbiturates, no effective chemotherapy has been developed for use in "soft drug" abuse. Thus, treatment approaches to nonnarcotic abuse center chiefly on psychotherapy and counseling.

The Role of the School in Drug Abuse Management and Prevention   The foregoing discussion, while necessarily brief in the context of the present chapter, illustrates the fact that any effective drug abuse program must be multifaceted, drawing on cooperative efforts from students and parents with a wide range of community resources including the medical and legal profession, the police, etc. In such an enterprise, the school is in a unique position to exert a positive beneficial effect in several areas. However, the role of the school in the drug abuse scene has been the subject of much controversy. This section will deal with three aspects of this controversy: the "educational" approach to drug abuse, the educational system's attitude toward drug abuse, and the school's role in dealing with the individual drug abuser.

The "Educational" Approach to Drug Abuse   With the rapid expansion of drug abuse among students from elementary school through college has come a parallel expansion of educational efforts aimed at arming the student with information which hopefully will provide some balance and/or deterrent to the inducements from peers to engage in drug use. The underlying assumption upon which many of these programs are based is analogous to the preventive medicine approach to infectious diseases of childhood; exposure to an effective dose of "vaccine" (drug abuse information, small group discussion, etc.) will provide "immunization" to the majority of students "inoculated" who have not as yet been exposed to the "infectious agent." Studies relating to the exact nature of the material to be presented, the teacher training necessary, and, most importantly, the long-range outcome are, unfortunately, not as yet available in adequate volume to arrive at a judicious determination as to the most successful approach in this highly delicate area.

However, the wisdom of mass drug abuse education efforts, especially in secondary schools, has been questioned in several recent reports. The National Commission on Marijuana and Drug Abuse, for example, had discouraging words about drug education efforts, stating that most information materials were scientifically inaccurate, and that too many programs were conducted by untrained teachers who might feel obliged to pass on their own misinformation or personal prejudice (Second Report of the National Commission on Marijuana and Drug Abuse, 1973). The Commission went further to state that it is possible to speculate that the avalanche of drug education in recent years may simply have raised interest in drugs. It recommended a reevaluation of the production and distribution of all new drug information materials until governmental standards for accuracy and concept could be developed. The Commission also suggested considering a moratorium on all drug education programs in schools, at least until those in operation had been evaluated and a coherent approach with realistic objectives had been developed.

The need for such a careful evaluation was pointed out in a recent report by Tennant, Weaver, and Lewis (1973) of several drug education programs in diverse settings. They found that there was no evidence that drug education programs in secondary schools decreased illegal use in the target population. With regard to drug education programs among elementary school students, however, they stated that there did seem to be a degree of positive influence on attitudes, and gave some measure of cautious encouragement. However, the report pointed out that the latter program was given by a specially trained teacher. The study concluded that the drug education effort in elementary schools may reach an age group that is young enough to be influenced, whereas secondary school students may be too old and may have established inflexible attitudes that cannot be significantly altered by health-related education. The foregoing evidence suggests caution in the implementation of drug education programs, but is not intended to imply that there is no place for them.

The Educational System's Attitude Toward Drug Abuse   The attitude, both overt and covert, which the school manifests may have a considerable impact on the prevalence of drug abuse among students and, more importantly, on the degree to which students with drug problems seek assistance through school channels. It is certainly legitimate for the school to expect that drug usage and dealing should not be permitted on the school grounds and to set consequences for infractions of these rules. The penalties, however, must be flexible to be effective and if possible, established with the active cooperation of the students (e.g., a student government) so that the administration does not become stereotyped into the role of a rigid, authoritarian disciplinarian. A fixed set of rules will not survive for long, but if the school clearly expresses disapproval of all drug use (this can be legitimately supported on educational and not merely moral grounds since drug use significantly impairs the student's learning capacity) and seeks cooperation of students and parents in limiting the use of drugs, an effective and responsive program may be developed in which the student's welfare is the primary consideration (*not* the school's reputation or the principal's job).

A more subtle aspect of this situation involves the teacher's attitudes toward drug use. Recent reports have revealed that teachers vary widely as to their permissiveness with regard to drug use among students and as to their *own* use of drugs (both legal and illegal). The chief variable in this wide range of attitudes appears to be the age of the teacher. Older teachers generally report negative (and in many cases punitive) attitudes toward student drug use and virtually no drug use themselves. Younger teachers increasingly demonstrate more tolerant attitudes toward drug use and more frequent reports of *personal* drug use (principally marijuana). In fact, teachers in their twenties reported virtually identical attitudes toward drug use and personal drug experience as did the reports of college upperclassmen. The impact of teachers' personal attitudes and drug experience on student drug use is obviously very difficult to ascertain since, in most cases, the effects will be covert and indirect. However, it is only logical to assume that a teacher who personally participates in drug use and condones its use among his students may well subtly encourage such use, even without his own conscious awareness of such a situation.

A third reflector of the school's attitude toward drug abuse is the extent to which the school provides remedial assistance for students who have been drug abusers. No matter how well intentioned, if the school merely establishes guidelines outlining penalties associated with being apprehended for drug use without developing a program designed to assist the drug abuser, a clear message of noninvolvement will be transmitted to the student and parents. As indicated earlier, this may drive the drug problem underground so that it will be less apparent, will fail to provide any constructive solutions, and may eliminate involved students from a most effective source of assistance.

A more positive attitude can be created by the provision of programs aimed at assisting the student who has become involved in drug abuse to deal with his problems. This may be an essential resource for many students who are unable to go to their parents for help. One or more school counselors may be designated as drug abuse advisors, providing them with adminstrative immunity with respect to confidentiality. Preferably, these personnel should receive specific training in drug abuse counseling and should have well-defined attitudes of their own toward drugs. In addition, the school might establish a "rap center" where peer groups could meet to discuss a variety of adolescent problems, including drug abuse, in an atmosphere which would promote free discussion without labeling the discussants as drug abusers. Finally, the school should establish close ties with local treatment programs whenever possible so that students with drug problems might be most efficiently channeled into such programs as soon as possible.

The School's Role in Dealing with the Individual Drug Abuser In addition to the establishment of a general climate of nonacceptance of drug use with support for the drug abuser as outlined above, the school should take specific steps which may be crucial in assisting the individual student to deal with drug abuse. First of all, nonpunitive limit setting with regard to actual drug use on the school premises is essential. To be effective, outlined consequences for specific behavior should be established in advance and published widely among students and parents so that potential drug users will be fully aware of them. If possible these consequences should be determined with the active participation of students and parents so that an open, ongoing dialogue may be established among these groups. Without active cooperation among school personnel, parents, and students, any program will be rendered ineffective.

In general, consequences should not interfere with the student's ongoing education. Unfortunately, many school officials can only think in terms of suspension from school, if a student is found to be using drugs. This usually only compounds the problem, since the drug user is often a marginal student and any interference with his education merely increases his apathy and lack of motivation. More positive alternatives might include using the "infectious disease" model of disease prevention. In this model, if drug use is seen as an "infectious desease" with high potential for contagion, the student who has been "infected" might be more effectively "treated" and the student body "protected" from infection by a "quarantine" procedure. This might take the form of isolating the student from his classmates and providing him with continuing instruction, until it is felt that the "infection" has been dealt with satisfactorily. This, of course, might necessitate the establishment of special classes for drug abusers which might also include specific remedies for the "infection," including group discussions as well as intensive instruction in drug abuse problems.

CONCLUSION

In general, the most favorable results in the management and habilitation of a youthful drug abuser accrue when the student feels enlisted as an ally by school officials rather than treated as an alien. As indicated, a multidisciplinary approach to drug abuse is essential. However, the school can often play the decisive role as a "front-line" agent of assistance, both for "first aid" in the case of a drug use casualty and for facilitating entry into a treatment program which will be truly beneficial to both student and society.

With regard to specific counseling procedures which may be utilized with drug abusers, if possible, a trained counselor should be sought for more severe problems. However, in general, the counselor should adopt a nonpunitive approach aimed at opening channels of communication and establishing mutual trust between the student and himself. The counselor should listen without judging, but must be careful not to give the impression that he condones the behavior. It is most crucial to attempt to understand the meaning of the drug to the student and then to search for nondrug alternatives. Often, group counseling sessions are quite successful in developing a positive solution when led by the counselor and students who have experienced the drug problem.

Ultimately, the success of any program depends on the motivation of the drug abuser to discontinue his habit. However, the above general guidelines often help to minimize the obstacles which society may place in the student's path, and may encourage students who are ambivalent about drug use to seek a positive course away from this problem.

REFERENCES

Pillard, R. C. 1970. Marihuana. New England J. Med. 283: 294–303.
Second Report of the National Commission on Marijuana and Drug Abuse: Drug Use in America: Problem in Perspective. 1973. United States Government Printing Office, Washington, D. C.
Tennant, F. S., Jr., S. C. Weaver, and C. E. Lewis, 1973. Outcomes of drug education: Four case studies. Pediatrics 52:246–251.

SUGGESTED READING

Cohen, S. 1969. The Drug Dilemma. McGraw-Hill Book Company, New York. 139 p.

Gottschalk, L. A., G. C. Morrison, R. B. Drury, and A. C. Barnes. 1970. The Laguna Beach experiment as a community approach to family counselling for drug abuse problems in youth. Compr. Psychiat. 11:226–234.

Nowlis, H. H. 1969. Drugs on the College Campus. Anchor Books, Doubleday and Company, Inc., Garden City, New York. 144 p.

8

Cerebral Palsy And Associated Dysfunctions

Arnold J. Capute, M.D., M.P.H.

A vast change has taken place in the overall view of cerebral palsy (CP) during the past 30 or 40 years. Cerebral palsy is no longer considered a condition with a pure motor component but rather as a multidimensional disorder in which the type and distribution of the motor disability has become a neurodevelopmental marker for underlying associated neurologic, cognitive, and perceptual impairments. Thus, when the pediatrician is confronted with such a child, he must view the problem in an interdisciplinary fashion, fully realizing that the motor involvement may not be the most disabling manifestation. While there must be close supervision and monitoring of the motor disability by the team approach, utilizing the skills of the pediatrician, orthopedist, occupational and physical therapist, and others, the teacher plays a major role during the preschool and school years, since it is during this formative period that education is most likely to make an impact on the development of the child's cognitive and perceptual abilities. If the educational program is not optimal nor suitable for a particular child, as an adolescent he will enter prevocational and vocational training academically unprepared, and, therefore, unable to be employed in a position compatible with his cognitive level. This might further compound the emotional turmoil which confronts the adolescent and adult CP, and prevent him from obtaining social and economic independence.

DEFINITION

Cerebral palsy is a developmental disability in which children have difficulty with the motor control of certain groups of muscles, frequently resulting in

This paper was supported in part through Project 917, Maternal and Child Health Service, United States Department of Health, Education, and Welfare.

functional impairment. This is the result of a cerebral defect on insult to the motor cortex (area of the brain gray matter which controls movement) occurring in the early developmental stages of brain growth during the first 5 years of life. Many physicians do not adhere strictly to the 5-year period; some consider injury during the first 3 years as the most critical for the evolvement of cerebral palsy, since the brain has attained three-quarters of adult size by that time. Others utilize the early preadolescent years (8 or 9 years) as the upper limits of early brain development, since it is known that the cortex remains somewhat plastic until this time, and that loss of a particular function resulting from an injury to one hemisphere can be accommodated by another part of the brain. This is best exemplified by the preadolescent or younger child who is struck by an automobile and, as a result, develops a transient expressive aphasia; that is, his receptive language is unaffected so that he understands what is said to him, but he is unable to expressively put his thoughts into words. If a similar cerebral accident occurs in late preadolescence (over 9 or 10 years) or thereafter when the brain is fully developed and has lost its adaptability, this particular function will not be assumed by undamaged sections of the brain and an irreversible disability will result (see Chapter 4).

Cerebral palsy has been defined as a disorder of movement and posture resulting from a permanent, nonprogressive defect or lesion of the immature brain (Bax, 1964). Regardless of the definition used, it is important for teachers to consider cerebral palsy as the motor manifestation of a much broader syndrome of brain damage which may also include intellectual, sensory, behavioral, and perceptual problems frequently found in combination. Hence, a multidiscipline approach is essential for comprehensive and successful habilitation.

PREVALENCE

Estimates of the prevalence rates of CP in children of school age (5–15 years) vary from 0.6–2.4 per thousand. Studies in Great Britain reveal the prevalence to be at 2.0 per thousand (Mair, 1961). Sex incidence determinations show cerebral palsy to be slightly more frequent in the male population, with a ratio of approximately 55:45. Thus, cerebral palsy is a common disorder, and children with this condition may be pupils in virtually any school system.

HISTORY OF CEREBRAL PALSY

An English orthopedic surgeon, William John Little, initially described the entity cerebral palsy in 1843 (Little, 1853). He not only presented the first comprehensive clinical description of this syndrome, but also suggested modalities of therapy such as manipulations, gymnastics, and braces. He emphasized birth trauma and premature delivery as etiologic factors of this condition. Subsequently, birth palsies of cerebral origin were referred to as Little's disease.

Sigmund Freud, a prominent neurologist and neuropathologist as well as a celebrated psychiatrist, was another pioneer in this field. He published a monograph in 1897 based upon his clinical experience with cerebral palsied children in both Paris and Vienna. He also devised a classification which was used during the early part of the twentieth century.

While the name "cerebral palsy" was first coined by Sir William Osler, when he described childhood neuromuscular diseases in the late nineteenth century, this term was not commonly utilized until the 1930's when Dr. Winthrop Phelps significantly contributed to its popularization. During the course of the following three decades Dr. Phelps perspicuously demonstrated that these children could be successfully habilitated (Wolf, 1969).

In the late 1950's, Dr. Eric Denhoff quite properly placed cerebral palsy in the syndromes of cerebral dysfunction, emphasizing that cerebral palsy should be viewed only as the motor manifestation of an extended syndrome of brain damage or defect which may be coupled with mental retardation, convulsions, visual, hearing, or perceptual problems, as well as speech, behavioral, and emotional disturbances (Denhoff and Robinault, 1960). At one end of this spectrum is the child with minimal cerebral dysfunction (MCD), which is usually accompanied by a learning disorder, and at the other end is cerebral palsy with or without mental retardation and associated conditions such as a learning disorder (Figure 1).

Henceforth, the 1970's will continue to place more emphasis upon the associated neurologic, cognitive, and perceptual deficiencies, with the educator playing a paramount role in the child's habilitation. If educators are to devise proper methods for teaching these children, the accompanying deficits must be remediated whenever possible.

CLASSIFICATION

In current practice, it is most common to use the clinical classification (motor and topographic) of cerebral palsy. As the early stages of brain development continue to be studied and as cerebral insults and injuries are more precisely correlated with neurologic findings, an accurate neuroanatomic classification will evolve. Unfortunately, the adult brain cannot be readily substituted as a model for an immature brain. Cerebral insults occurring in early life usually involve several anatomic sites, which makes it more difficult to accurately delineate a neuroanatomic classification.

An etiologic classification would also be most beneficial, for a clear understanding of the cause of a disorder often provides the framework for its eradication. However, at the present time, the cause of only one CP entity is definitely known, namely, bilirubin encephalopathy or kernicterus, which in its

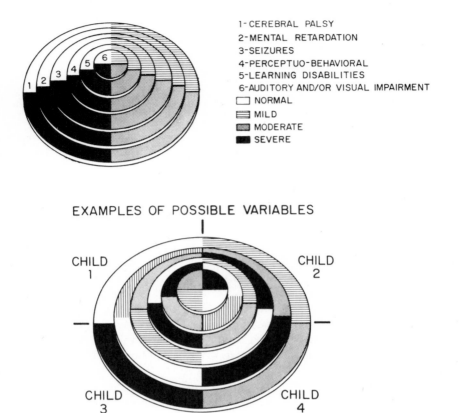

1-CEREBRAL PALSY
2-MENTAL RETARDATION
3-SEIZURES
4-PERCEPTUO-BEHAVIORAL
5-LEARNING DISABILITIES
6-AUDITORY AND/OR VISUAL IMPAIRMENT
☐ NORMAL
☰ MILD
▨ MODERATE
■ SEVERE

EXAMPLES OF POSSIBLE VARIABLES

CHILD 1

CHILD 2

CHILD 3

CHILD 4

Figure 1. The spectrum of cerebral dysfunction. A reordering of the various disorders demonstrates their complex interrelationship. (Compare children 1, 2, 3, and 4.)

chronic form can be recognized by a tetrad of clinical characteristics: a movement disorder (athetosis), supraversion gaze palsy (inability to look upward), auditory imperception (high frequency hearing loss with or without central auditory imperception, the latter frequently referred to as central deafness), and enamel hypoplasia or staining of the primary teeth (Figure 2). This type of cerebral palsy is caused by a rapid and sustained rise in serum bilirubin due to red blood cell destruction in the newborn. Since the primary cause of this type of CP is known to be rhesus (Rh) sensitization, primary prevention by the maternal injection of anti-D gamma globulin or secondary prevention by exchange transfusion of the affected newborn has significantly decreased the incidence of this entity.

The American Academy for Cerebral Palsy lists the various types of CP as spasticity (increase in muscle tone), athetosis (slow writhing movements), rigidity (extreme tenseness and stiffening of extremities), ataxia (incoordination of muscular action due to disturbance of balance sense), tremor (regular and

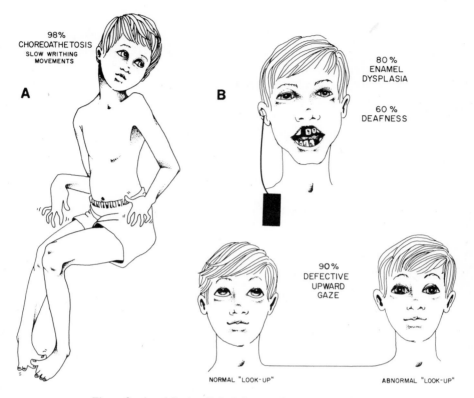

Figure 2. *A* and *B,* the clinical characteristics of kernicterus.

rhythmical involuntary shaking movements), atonia (lack of muscle tone, limp-ness, and flaccidity), and mixed, based upon tone and movement criteria observed primarily in older children and adults (Minear, 1956). The categorization utilized by Crothers and Paine (1959) appears to be more useful in dealing with the younger child in that it attempts to separate the spastics (pyramidal type) from the extrapyramidal (all types excluding spasticity), specifying the topographic distribution of the involvement (i.e., quadriplegia, hemiplegia, etc.) when possible. Thus, the clinical classification consists of two parts: (1) the type of movement disorder that is evident and (2) the topographic distribution of the motor impairment.

There are two types of movement disorders, pyramidal and extrapyramidal. Pyramidal cerebral palsy is commonly referred to as spastic CP, which is by far the most common, comprising 60% of the CP population. The spastic or pyramidal type is produced by damage sustained to the neuron (nerve cell), which is found in the motor cortex (gray matter of the brain containing nerve cells which initiate motor impulses to the muscles). The usual nerve cell involved is shaped like a pyramid, hence the name pyramidal. In addition, these nerve cells have tracts (axons) that extend from the neuron in the cortex to the spinal cord, and these cells eventually connect with nerve tracts that innervate the limb, so that muscle movement can be carried out. If these nerve cells (pyramidal cells) or tracts are injured, then spasticity results (Figure 3). The second type, extrapyramidal cerebral palsy, has its origin in the deep gray matter of the brain (basal ganglia), which consists of conglomerates of nerve cells whose interference leads to extrapyramidal movements or CP types which are classified as athetosis, rigidity, tremor, atonia, ataxia, or a mixture of both pyramidal and extrapyramidal movements (Figure 4).

The second part of the clinical classification, the topographic distribution, is usually not applied to the extrapyramidal type of cerebral palsy which involves all four extremities. The spastic cases are subdivided into monoplegia (involvement of one extremity only, either arm or leg) which is extremely rare, triplegia (impairment of three extremities) which is unusual, hemiplegia (abnormality confined to one-half of the body, either the right or left side with the arm more involved than the leg), bilateral hemiplegia or double hemiplegia (weakness or paralysis of both sides of the body with the arms compromised more than the legs), quadriplegia (involvement of all four extremities with more disability of

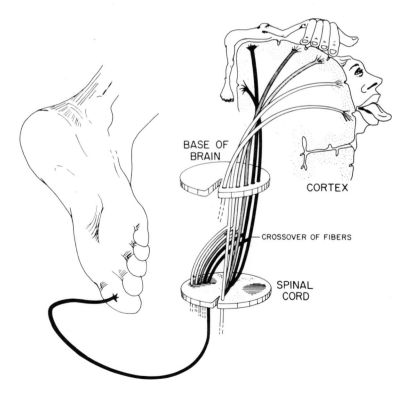

BASE OF BRAIN

CORTEX

CROSSOVER OF FIBERS

SPINAL CORD

Figure 3. The pyramidal tracts; a schematic illustration of the motor cortex. Note the disproportionate representation of the lower face, tongue, lips, and hand on the motor area of the brain. Injury to the cerebral cortex in the region of the foot (*darkest line or tract*) will result in spasticity in the opposite extremity.

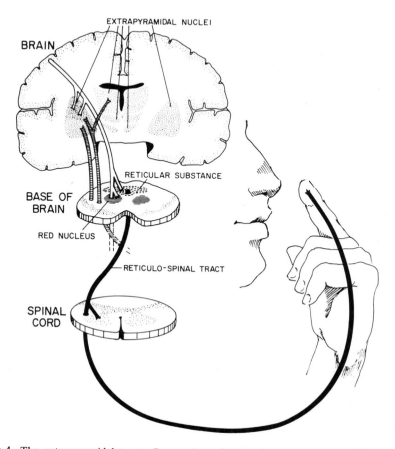

Figure 4. The extrapyramidal tracts. Destruction of the various components of the extrapyramidal nuclei may result in a movement disorder (athetosis, rigidity, tremor, atonia, and ataxia). The abnormal movements may become extremely noticeable when the patient performs certain tasks, such as pointing to his nose.

the legs than the arms), diplegia (all four extremities affected with minimal involvement of the arms), and paraplegia (neurologic dysfunction of the legs only).

It should be noted that the spastic hemiplegias are by far the most common single group, and represent 40% of the total CP population. Next in frequency are patients with cerebral palsies of the extrapyramidal group (22%), those with spastic quadriplegia (19%), and those with mixed types of cerebral palsy (13%) (Crothers and Paine, 1959).

It is essential that special educators and teachers, especially those who will be instructing the cerebral palsied child, have some understanding of the clinical classification. The peripheral manifestations (clinical classification) of cerebral palsy have been highlighted because these serve as neurodevelopmental markers for pediatricians to identify associated sensory, perceptual, and cognitive deficits. Also, peripheral involvement is clearly delineated so that orthopedists and physical and occupational therapists may administer their treatment. Hopefully, either medications or neurosurgical procedures will be available to enhance motor function once the central neuroanatomic, neurophysiologic, and neuropathologic data are studied and better understood.

The peripheral neurologic manifestations can indicate the child who is at high risk for an associated deficit. For example, the incidence of seizures is higher in the hemiplegic child (67%) than in the quadriplegic (56%) or paraplegic (31%), but the hemiplegic child is usually of better intelligence than the quadriplegic. Tizard showed that approximately 50% of hemiplegics have an associated sensory impairment of the involved side (Tizard, Paine, and Crothers, 1954). This is manifested by the child's inability to recognize an object by touch or feel (astereognosis), or diminished awareness of light touch or pain. Hemiplegics with this cortical sensory impairment may have a "blind" limb which is useless to the child and more handicapping than a motor-impaired limb. A child may commonly choose to utilize an extremity which is disabled due to motor impairment, yet which may be more functional than a limb hampered primarily by a severe sensory disturbance. Approximately 25% of hemiplegics also have loss of vision in either the left or right half of the visual fields of both eyes (homonymous hemianopsia) (Tizard, Painer, and Crothers, 1954). The presence of a visual field deficit usually correlates highly with a sensory impaired limb. The former abnormality may interfere with normal reading. Hence, it is most important for professionals to be aware of these deficiencies when a hemiplegia is diagnosed.

The athetoids are usually of higher intelligence and have a much lower incidence of convulsive disorders than the spastics. The child with the rigidity type of CP is usually quite severely retarded and has a high incidence of convulsions.

TREATMENT OF CEREBRAL PALSY

Motor and language development progress in a sequential fashion depending a great deal upon the neurologic maturation of the central nervous system. In early infancy, a motor developmental lag is evidenced by the persistence of primitive reflexes (e.g., suck and rooting reflexes and grasp and creeping movements) which are usually present at birth or soon thereafter and disappear in the early months of life. In the motor-handicapped infant, these primitive reflexes are followed by poorly developed automatic postural reflexes from which voluntary functional motor activities arise, such as rolling over, sitting, standing, and walking. It is postulated that because of the persistence of primitive reflexes which occur with brain insults, injuries, or anomalies, the postural automatic reflex reactions are delayed or even abolished so that purposeful motor activity cannot take place.

The majority of physical and occupational therapists utilize the Bobath method or a modification thereof, which consists of the inhibition of primitive reflexes and facilitation of the postural reflexes enabling the infant to progress to the next stage, with subsequent development of purposeful motor activity (Bobath and Bobath, 1972). Many therapists feel that early detection and intervention are essential for a cerebral palsied infant to progress more rapidly with both upper and lower extremity dexterity.

Physical therapists concentrate upon posture and locomotor skills, with emphasis upon ambulation, particularly walking. They work in conjunction with the orthopedist to determine what supportive measures are indicated for the child to walk to the best of his ability. With certain cases of CP, braces will be indicated for support, correction of the deformity, or prevention or reduction of extraneous movements observed in athetoid CP. Crutches or canes are frequently used for assistance. The orthopedic surgeon may perform certain operations such as lengthening or transplanting tendons and muscles to improve the function of an extremity. Bone operations are used to stabilize various joints such as the hip, wrist, or ankle, and tendon releases may be performed to lessen the degree of spasticity. In addition, physical therapy at times employs exercise programs to prevent contractures.

Occupational therapists focus upon upper extremity posturing and manipulative skills as a prelude to enhancement of self-help skills or activities of daily living. The occupational therapists also utilize methods which consist of inhibition of primitive reflexes and facilitation of postural automatic reflexes. They focus upon such self-help skills as toileting, eating, dressing, and undressing. Cerebral palsied children of the extrapyramidal type commonly have a repetitive tongue thrust which gives rise to a reversal of the normal swallowing mechanism, with most of the food pushed forward by the tongue rather than swallowed. This tongue thrust is usually accompanied by an extensor posturing (excessive stiffening) of the body. By flexing the body, the tongue thrust is reduced, and the child can more readily swallow the food. Thus, the feeding time can be significantly reduced. The occupational therapist can also assist the athetoid child in communication by having him use a special typewriter or alphabet word board.

Both the occupational and physical therapists are essential in the mangement of the adolescent CP since the skeletal deformities may progress and the skeletal-muscle ratio may change due to a spurt of bone growth, leading to loss of function at this critical time. Furthermore, these therapists can provide suggestions to the educator regarding techniques and equipment for enhancing classroom management of individual children. For example, special utensils, wheelchairs, tables, or writing aids may be available.

Since successful habilitation of the cerebral palsied adolescent is dependent upon good oral communication as well as functional upper extremity use, it is paramount that the speech therapists join in the habilitation program. The CP child must not receive undue frustration from too early an articulation program by a speech therapist when a language stimulation program at home would suffice. The CP pupil who has severe neurologic involvement of his speech-producing musculature (tongue, lips, cheeks, oral, and pharyngeal muscles) cannot be substantially improved by formal speech therapy. Those CP children who are minimally involved can be significantly assisted, especially when their mentation approaches normal.

The use of drugs for the management of the movement disorders in CP children is at present in the formative stage. Considerable attention has been directed to the treatment of athetosis with such pharmacologic agents as Artane, dopamine (drugs successfully utilized for the treatment of another movement disorder, Parkinson's disease), as well as the tranquilizer drugs. Unfortunately, at this time, a drug has not been discovered which will functionally improve the CP patient with athetosis (Capute, 1974).

Many other drugs, such as Valium and dantrolene sodium (Haslam et al., 1974), have been utilized for the management of spasticity associated with cerebral palsy. Some agents appear to provide relaxation of the involved muscles by a central nervous system sedative action. If the sedation is too great, sleepiness, lethargy, and depression may result, compromising the child's mental capabilities. Finally, those concerned with the pharmacologic management of CP students should be acquainted with the placebo effect. The administration of any medication (including sugar pills) frequently improves the patient with a disability. This finding is particularly common among children with cerebral palsy. Thus, the investigation of a new drug for the control of movement disorders in CP children should be organized in such a way as to test the true drug effect and not the placebo influence. This form of investigation is coined a double-blind crossover study.

Neurosurgical procedures have been developed which may occasionally relieve severe rigidity or spasticity in the CP child. For the most part, these include the production of lesions within the basal ganglia of the brain by the neurosurgeon in order to ablate certain groups of nerve cells which control motor function. At the present, there is considerable interest in a new experimental technique of artificial cerebellar stimulation and its possible application to CP patients with exceedingly severe movement disorders. Its use in children, however, awaits clinical trial.

Thus, the principles of management of the CP child embrace the skills and coordinated collaboration of the physical and occupational therapists, educator, speech pathologist, psychologist, orthopedic surgeon, neurosurgeon, pharmacologist, and pediatrician.

ASSOCIATED DYSFUNCTIONS

Mental Retardation

Approximately 50—60% of CP children are retarded because of an overall significant reduction of their perceptual and cognitive skills. Special educators continue to play a primary role in their management since CP children should receive special education programs comparable to their level of mental functioning (see Chapter 11). For example, the educable mentally retarded (EMR) cerebral palsied pupil requires educational programs similar to those of the nonphysically involved EMR child, and, if the motor disability is mild, the child should partake in the same program with the nonphysically involved EMR child. However, should the motor disability be extensive, and if ramps, elevators, and other special devices are required to facilitate ambulation, then CP children should be referred to schools with specially constructed facilities which include the various types of special education programs required, as well as ancillary services such as orthopedics, occupational therapy, physical therapy, and hearing and speech therapy.

The trainable and subtrainable mentally retarded children with CP have goals similar to the nonphysically involved retarded child, that is, enhancement of self-help, social, and oral communicative skills for living and working in a sheltered environment. As a teenager, the trainable retarded CP requires the availability of activity centers and sheltered workshops to allow him to maintain socialization as well as the possibility of earning some income to enhance his self-esteem and assist in financial support. He will always require close supervision of his mental as well as physical handicaps.

Learning Disabilities

Since 50–60% of CP children are retarded, the remaining 40–50% have a global intelligence score of 70 or above, which usually indicates the possibility of successful school achievement in the majority of cases within regular school programs. However, since CP is the result of brain damage, it is only logical to assume that a significant number of these children will have (and do have) an uneven psychometric profile demonstrating a variability or scattering of perceptual and cognitive abilities. This is usually indicative of a learning disability, and special teaching methods must be employed for remediation. The Wechsler Intelligence Scale for Children (WISC) and the Stanford-Binet tests of Intelligence (SB) are utilized in testing the cerebral palsied child. In certain instances, psychologists must work within the constraints of the physical disability, and this may result, at times, in an underestimation of the child's potential. In addition, other psychologic tests have been developed to assess the physically handicapped child, and include the Raven's Progressive Matrices, the Ammons Full-Range Picture Vocabulary Test, and the Columbia Test of Mental Maturity. When evaluating these children, either with psychologic or achievement tests, the usual time restrictions required in testing the normal child should be eliminated. During learning experiences teachers should allow extensive time for the cerebral palsied child to more fully comprehend the presented material.

Since these children demonstrate clear-cut motor manifestations resulting from brain injury, it is recognized that certain organic behavioral characteristics are commonly associated with CP children. These include hyperactivity, emotional lability, attentional peculiarities (short attention span or perseveration), low frustration tolerance, impulsivity, and distractibility. These organically driven behavioral patterns are frequently observed in the CP child with normal global intelligence, but an uneven perceptual-cognitive profile may result in a learning disability.

These children and their families can be helped immeasurably by professional counseling to assist in maintaining stable intrafamily dynamics. Medication may be of benefit, and usually either dextroamphetamine or methylphenidate (Ritalin) may be prescribed when hyperactivity is present. However, unlike the child with minimal cerebral dysfunction, these drugs have not been as efficacious in the patient with cerebral palsy and the more severe degree of the Strauss syndrome-like behavioral pattern associated with moderate to severe mental retardation (see Chapter 11). The latter child usually requires one of the phenothiazines (Thorazine, Mellaril, or Stelazine) or haloperidol to control his severe hyperactivity and occasional temper outbursts. Behavioral psychologists can provide considerable assistance with these children by modifying or eliminating these undesirable behaviors and, thus, facilitating school and home management.

Emotional Problems

During adolescence, the CP child frequently loses some acquired skills, particularly in the self-help, communicative, ambulative, and social areas, and, thus, appears to deteriorate. Parents, teacher, and physician should be concerned as to whether this apparent degeneration is of physical, psychogenic, or organic origin. The physical and psychogenic factors are usually the most common, since in adolescence there may be a progression of an orthopedic deformity or a spurt in bone growth which, when accompanied by insufficient muscular development, may cause the loss of a particular skill, such as walking. The role of hormonal factors is as yet unknown. Occasionally, the spastic child gains excessive weight, a most important factor in inhibiting physical performance.

The child's mental attitude may result in pseudodeterioration, since the CP child, for a number of years, has exerted a considerable amount of energy as well as mental anguish to learn and perform a certain skill and, at adolescence, may seriously question whether the effort was worth it. It is during the period of adolescence that the CP individual is particularly confronted by social isolation. His normal peers begin to date, attend dances and parties, and, perhaps, for the first time, there is a total realization of the meaning of a handicap. This can certainly lead to depression manifested by both social and communicative withdrawal as well as an unconscious desire to engage in fewer physical activities. The average or superior intelligent athetoid who has involuntary movements of all extremities is probably more prone to develop a psychologic disturbance during adolescence, with depression fairly common.

Mental health counseling should be available in early life to anticipate and prevent emotional problems which may surface during the adolescence of a CP child. Furthermore, during childhood some of these youngsters are well aware of their physical incapacity and limitations, and have developed a poor self-image which may be compounded by the parents' overprotection and unwillingness to allow them to participate in many of the social and recreational activities of other children their age. In the early years of life, most CP children are in need of continuous and ongoing mental health counseling and support, which involves a great deal of participation by the educator. The parents and siblings of CP children play an important role in rendering emotional support to the afflicted family member. It may well be possible to eliminate or at least diminish the adolescent psychologic stress that may confront these children by early periodic mental health counseling for both the child and the family.

Seizures

While seizures occur in about 0.5% of the general population, they are found in approximately 25–35% of individuals with cerebral palsy, the frequency being much greater in the spastic group than in the athetoid. (For a description of seizures, refer to Chapter 4.)

Visual Impairments

Strabismus (squinting due to imbalance of eye muscles) occurs in approximately 30–35% of the CP population, and also, there is a high incidence of refractory errors, which are twice as common in the spastics as in the athetoid group. Athetoids are more prone to have hyperopia (farsightedness) while spastics can have either myopia (nearsightedness) or hyperopia. Visual field cuts, as noted previously, occur in approximately 25% of the hemiplegics (see Chapter 2).

Auditory and Speech Impairments

High frequency hearing loss can be found in individuals with athetoid CP, especially if associated with bilirubin encephalopathy (see Chapter 3). Dysarthria (imperfect articulation in speech) of some degree is usually associated with athetoid cerebral palsy, while it is present in approximately 30–50% of children who have quadriplegia. Dysarthria of the cerebellar type (indistinct speech with variable modulation) may be associated with ataxic CP. Dysarthria in the CP child is frequently accompanied by grimacing or immobile facies and drooling. There is usually a history of poor sucking or swallowing during infancy and the early childhood years.

It is important for the teacher to note that with speech development all vowel sounds are acquired prior to consonants. While the appearance of conso-nants varies somewhat, Shank (1964) has succinctly arranged them in timetable fashion as they develop in the normal child (Table 1). The educator should become familiar with these consonant developmental milestones, for they are utilized by speech therapists when initiating formal speech therapy (articula-

Table 1. Consonant Developmental Milestones

Age (yrs.)	Consonants
3½	p, b, m, w, h
4½	t, d, n, g, k, ng, y
5½	f, v, s, z
6½	sh, zh, l, th
Up to 8	ch, r, wh

tion). Thus, speech therapists do not usually begin speech therapy until a child has reached a mental age of at least 5 or 6 years. It is at this time that the child's neurologic system is capable of coping with the neuromuscular complexities of articulation. Early referral to the speech pathologist may result in setting up a program of language and speech stimulation which is then carried out at home and school by the parents and teacher. At a later date, particularly when an appropriate mental age is attained, the pupil may be introduced to specific forms of therapy by the speech pathologist.

CONCLUSION

Cerebral palsy is a common handicap which may be manifest by abnormalities of the motor system, intellect, speech, visual, or auditory systems. As a result of the widespread distribution of CP children, many can be expected to attend school in the regular classroom. Thus, the teacher must be totally familiar with the complexities of cerebral palsy. Furthermore, the educator is in a unique position to play a vital role in the habilitation of the CP child and his family.

Although CP children may demonstrate normal intellect, as a group they are at significant risk for one of the learning disabilities, undoubtedly the result of subtle defects in the cerebral cortex. Nevertheless, early identification of such a learning disorder by the child's teacher may enhance its remediation. Still other children with cerebral palsy are severely incapacitated because of disturbances of the motor system. Braces, canes, or special shoes may be prerequisite for ambulation. Others less fortunate may be limited to wheelchairs. The teacher must familiarize herself with the student's assistive devices and encourage the school authorities to provide ramps for stairs or modifications within the classroom in order to accommodate the child with cerebral palsy.

The educator must be aware of the associated abnormalities commonly observed in the CP child, including mental retardation, seizures, visual impairment, and auditory and speech abnormalities. The teacher can provide considerable emotional support to a pupil with cerebral palsy. The student with cerebral palsy may be unable to participate in certain athletic activities. The teacher may utilize that time period to engage the child in certain other enjoyable functions which may enhance the pupil's self-esteem.

Educators have made important contributions to the habilitation of the CP child, including the development of form-boards and the innovation of various methods to improve the communication skills of severely motor-impaired CP children. Further developments will occur in behalf of the handicapped child, particularly if the interdisciplinary team can function as a unit with the singular aim of providing each involved child with the very best habilitation program.

REFERENCES

Bax, M. C. O. 1964. Terminology and classification of cerebral palsy. Develop. Med. Child. Neurol. 6:295–297.

Bobath, K., and B. Bobath, 1972. Cerebral palsy. *In* P. H. Pearson and C. E. Williams (eds.), Physical Therapy Services in the Developmental Disabilities, pp. 31–113. Charles C Thomas, Publisher, Springfield, Ill.

Capute, A. J. 1974. Developmental disabilities: An overview. *In* L. A. Fox (ed.), Symposium on Dentistry for the Handicapped Child. Dent. Clin. N. Amer. 18:557–577.

Crothers, B., and R. S. Paine. 1959. The Natural History of Cerebral Palsy. Harvard University Press, Cambridge, Mass. 299 p.

Denhoff, E., and I. P. Robinault. 1960. Cerebral Palsy and Related Disorders. McGraw-Hill Book Company, Inc., New York. 421 p.

Haslam, R. H. A., J. R. Walcher, P. S. Lietman, C. H. Kallman, and E. D. Mellits. 1974. Dantrolene sodium in children with spasticity. Arch. Phys. Med. 55: 384–388.

Little, W. J. 1853. On the Nature and Treatment of the Deformities of the Human Frame: Being a Course of Lectures Delivered at the Royal Orthopedic Hospital in 1843 with Numerous Notes and Additions. Longman, Brown, Greene, and Longmans, London.

Mair, A. 1961. Incidence, prevalence and social class. *In* J. L. Henderson (ed.), Cerebral Palsy in Children and Adolescence, pp. 15–21. E. & S. Livingstone, Ltd., Edinburgh.

Minear, W. L. 1956. A classification of cerebral palsy. Pediatrics 18:841–852.

Shank, K. H. 1964. Recognition of articulatory disorders in children. Clin. Pediat. (Phila.) 3:333–334.

Tizard, J. P., R. S. Paine, and B. Crothers. 1954. Disturbances of sensation in children with hemiplegia. J. A. M. A. 155:628–632.

Wolf, J. M. 1969. Historical perspective of cerebral palsy. *In* J. M. Wolf (ed.), The Results of Treatment in Cerebral Palsy, pp. 5–44. Charles C Thomas, Publisher, Springfield, Ill.

9

Orthopedic Problems In the Classroom

Charles E. Silberstein, M.D., M.Sc.

The field of orthopedic surgery deals with the diagnosis and treatment of injuries, diseases, and deformities that occur in the musculoskeletal and neuro-muscular systems. The picture that is conjured up in the minds of most lay people is that of the orthopedist wrapping plaster on a limb with a broken bone, or of that individual who is known as "the foot doctor." However, as is implied by the aforementioned definition, orthopedic surgery applies to and touches upon numerous aspects of medical practice. With respect to the musculoskeletal system, this field of medicine deals not only with the obvious problems of fractures and muscle disorders, ligament and joint injuries, but also contributes to the diagnosis and treatment of such neurologic disturbances as cerebral palsy and the investigation and management of metabolic disturbances, including rickets and dwarfism.

The purpose of this chapter is not to describe each and every entity that is treated by the orthopedic surgeon, but rather to point out to the teacher those problems that may present themselves in the classroom in order that the teacher may participate in their detection. Since children of school age seem to spend more hours under the watchful eye of their teacher than they do their parents, it is not surprising that the teacher frequently calls to the attention of the parents potential or existing disorders. The second objective of this chapter is to explain how and why prolonged absence from the classroom is so necessary in the management of certain orthopedic disorders.

The common signs which indicate an orthopedic problem include *pain, limp* with or without pain, and *deformity*. The areas in which pain can be a factor are any part of the spine, from the base of the skull to the tailbone (coccyx), the upper or lower extremities (usually the joints), and the hips.

COMMON ORTHOPEDIC DISORDERS OF THE SPINE

Torticollis

Specific regions of the spine will reflect different disorders, which are dependent upon the age of the child. Torticollis, or "wryneck," is most often seen in younger school children, ages 4–6 years, and is usually related to a recent or concurrent throat infection. Because of the infection, the structures in the back of the throat, or just in front of the cervical spine (vertebrae in the neck), become swollen (edematous), and this causes a laxity or stretching of the ligaments supporting the cervical vertebrae. The latter become hypermobile and susceptible to very slight twisting forces on the neck which can lead in turn to malalignment of the joints of the vertebrae. Such children present with their heads tilted to one side and the chin rotated to the opposite shoulder. The treatment of this disorder consists of immobilizing the head and neck in a soft collar for 2–4 days, analgesics, perhaps a muscle relaxant, moist heat to the neck muscles, and limited activity. Occasionally, one of these joints will actually become dislocated and require a course of traction in the hospital to reduce the disrupted joint. Twisting injuries to the neck that result from tumbling, summersaults, and wrestling will cause the same injury, present in the same way, and are treated in a similar manner. Children with a rare, progressive neurologic disorder, dystonia musculorum deformans, may also manifest torticollis. They may be differentiated from those children with acute wryneck by the chronicity of their symptoms, as well as associated neurologic signs.

There are two congenital abnormalities that mimic the appearance of torticollis. The Klippel-Feil syndrome (Figure 1) results from an actual deformity in the development of the neck vertebrae and muscles, causing the distance between the ear and the shoulder on the same side to be reduced. Congenital torticollis in the infant is due to a false tumor or scar tissue forming in the muscle tissue on the side of the neck (the sternocleidomastoid muscle). This causes the muscle to be contracted, thus rotating the chin to the opposite shoulder and drawing the ear toward the shoulder on the same side. Secondary deformities that result from congenital torticollis include flattening of the face as well as the head on the same side. Today most of these problems are recognized in infancy and, for the most part, have been corrected by the time the child enters school. Occasionally, visual and hearing problems can cause a similar torticollis appearance, as the child tilts his head to focus acutely or listen intently.

Sprengel's Deformity

Sprengel's deformity (Figure 2) is a congenital high riding or elevated scapula (shoulder blade) secondary to incomplete development. It is frequently asso-

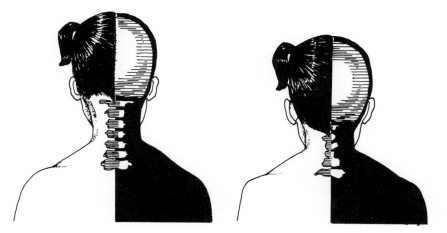

Figure 1. The Klippel-Feil syndrome. *Left,* a normal individual. *Right,* note the patient's shortened neck with malformed vertebrae.

ciated with an inability to abduct the shoulder on the same side beyond 90°—that is, the arm cannot be raised from the side of the body beyond 90°. The deformity is best treated surgically, not only to improve appearance but also to enhance function. Surgery is usually accomplished before age 10.

Juvenile Kyphosis

Juvenile kyphosis, round back deformity (Figure 3), and Scheuermann's disease are probably all one and the same, but with differing severity and variable location within the spine. Juvenile kyphosis is an acquired disorder that results from the way in which the blood vessels enter the vertebrae. Normally the major blood supply to the vertebrae is from in front, but with an increase in blood supply the bone becomes softer which leads to an anterior wedging of the vertebrae. If this process occurs in the midportion of the spine (the thoracic region), a round back deformity results. In the lower spine (the lumbar region), this pathology can create symptoms compatible with those of a herniated or ruptured intervertebral disk. Back pain, with or without leg pain, is a common complaint. Juvenile kyphosis or the round back deformity occurs in the age group 11–16 years. Many of these youngsters find that sitting in a classroom is rather uncomfortable. The treatment of this disorder consists of wearing a back corset or a brace (Milwaukee brace), heat, and limitation of strenuous physical activity if pain is present. The symptoms may linger for 1–2 years.

Scoliosis

Scoliosis (Figure 4), or a lateral curvature of the spine, is most commonly seen in the age group 12–16 years, and is more frequent in females than males (an 8:1

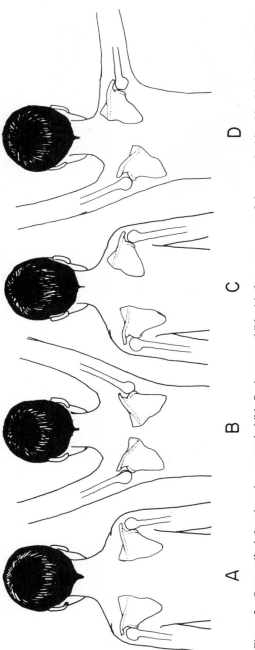

Figure 2. Sprengel's deformity. *A*, a normal child; *B*, the same child with free movement of the scapula (shoulder blade) with raising of the arms; *C*, decreased size and abnormal elevation of the right scapula in an affected patient; and *D*, limitation of shoulder movement because of the deformity.

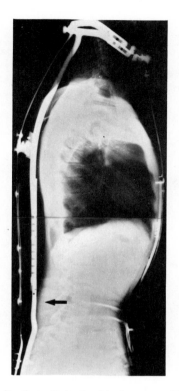

Figure 3. Roundback deformity (juvenile kyphosis). An x-ray which shows a hump formation (*arrow*) in the region of the waist. A Milwaukee brace is in place as a part of the
treatment.

ratio). These youngsters present with one scapula (shoulder blade) more prominent than the other and one shoulder or hip higher than the other. On forward
bending, the rib hump deformity is quite prominent. Pain is usually not a feature
in this disorder. The cause of scoliosis in most cases is unknown (idiopathic),
although there are instances where a congenital abnormality of one or more
vertebrae might lead to the development of scoliosis. Curvatures may also be
caused by paralytic diseases (e.g., poliomyelitis), where the muscles supporting
the spine are weakened resulting in poor support of the bony vertebral column.

The treatment of scoliosis depends upon the extent of curvature, the
location of the curve, and the age of the patient. Each curve is measured on an
x-ray of the entire spine. Curves under $20°$ usually require no treatment. Those
$20–50°$ are managed by the use of a Milwaukee brace (Figure 5), and those
$45–50°$ and above necessitate surgical correction. However, curves do progress as
long as growth of the spine is incomplete. Additionally, a 16-year-old child with a
40 to $50°$ curve who has almost completed growing is unlikely to benefit by a
brace and might require surgical correction. Ideally, a brace is applied in order to
control the scoliosis until growth of the spine is concluded.

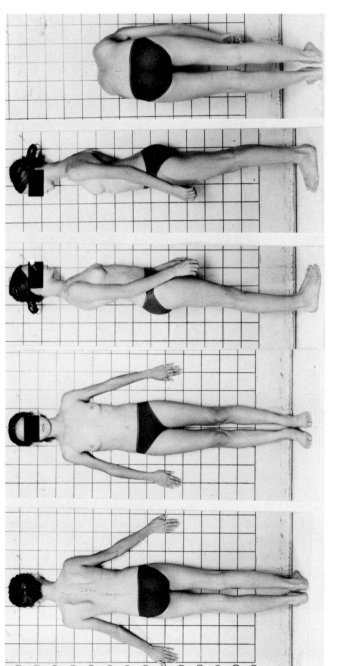

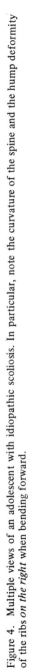

Figure 4. Multiple views of an adolescent with idiopathic scoliosis. In particular, note the curvature of the spine and the hump deformity of the ribs *on the right* when bending forward.

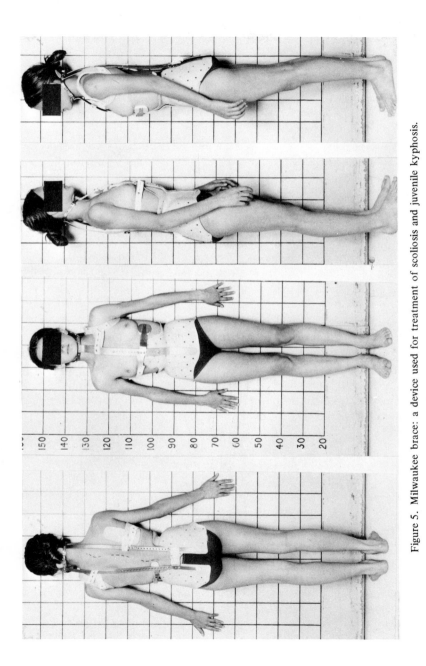

Figure 5. Milwaukee brace: a device used for treatment of scoliosis and juvenile kyphosis.

When surgery is required, it consists of inserting stainless steel (Harrington) rods along the spine to dynamically straighten the vertebral column. Further support is afforded by surgically fusing the spine. The postoperative course consists of the wearing of a plaster body jacket for 6 months, and remaining flat in bed during that entire time. Currently, attempts are being made to get some of these patients up in their casts 2–3 wks. following surgery (Figure 6).

Spondylolisthesis

Although rather rare, an occasional ruptured intervertebral disk may be seen in school age children. More common is a condition called spondylolisthesis, or a slipping forward of one vertebra on another, due to a defect in a portion of the vertebra. This defect is acquired and is felt to be secondary to an injury of the vertebra, whereby cartilage has formed as a result of the injury and has never matured to bone. This process is called spondylolysis and, if it is present on both sides of the vertebra, slippage can result. This usually occurs between the last (fifth) lumbar vertebra and the sacrum. Spondylolysis and spondylolisthesis can cause pain in the back, hip, leg, and, on occasion, unexplained abdominal pain which may be associated with low back discomfort. Frequently, these youngsters have tight hamstring muscles and are unable to touch their toes. This condition occurs after age 10. It is treated initially with a low back support and specific exercises. If the pain persists, surgery in the form of a spinal fusion to stabilize the weakened segment of the spine is indicated. This requires a period of 3–4 months at home and restricted activity for approximately 1 year.

Identical symptoms might be seen with a disk herniation (Figure 7), and the treatment is the same although, instead of a spinal fusion, the disk is surgically excised and within 6–8 wks. the patient is returned to full activity.

ABNORMALITIES OF THE UPPER EXTREMITY

Congenital and acquired conditions of the upper extremities are frequently seen. Usually these deformities have been present since birth and, in most instances, have been surgically corrected by age 5.

Brachial Plexus Injuries

Erb's palsy and Klumpke's paralysis are disorders caused by damage to the major spinal nerve trunks in the neck (brachial plexus) at the time of birth. This injury usually involves only one arm. If the injury to the brachial plexus and spinal cord has been severe, these youngsters frequently divorce themselves from their abnormal limb, even if that extremity has been operated upon to make it more functional. Most surgical procedures are designed to improve the functional capability of the extremity by appropriate muscle transfers.

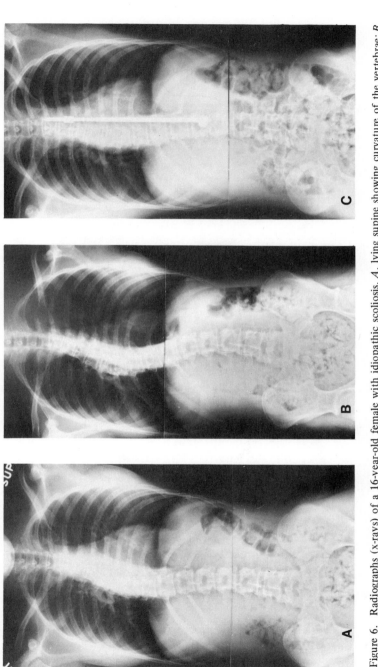

Figure 6. Radiographs (x-rays) of a 16-year-old female with idiopathic scoliosis. A, lying supine showing curvature of the vertebrae; B, standing erect; and C, following surgery and the insertion of a steel rod for stabilization.

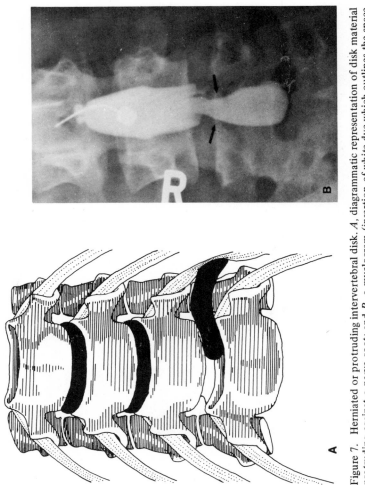

Figure 7. Herniated or protruding intervertebral disk. *A*, diagrammatic representation of disk material protruding against a nerve root; and *B*, a myelogram (insertion of white dye which outlines the space surrounding the spinal cord) showing a defect indicating a disk protrusion. The *arrows* point to the compression of the spinal column (white mass) by the disk.

Hemiplegia

Hemiplegia is usually of the spastic variety and, as the name implies, involves only one arm and one leg on the same side (see Chapter 8). Hemiplegia is the result of damage or injury to the motor center on the opposite side of the brain that has occurred before, during, or after birth. Many of these youngsters can perform in a perfectly normal fashion, while others require braces or surgery to assist or maintain ambulation. Due to diminished sensation in the affected extremity, the hands of these patients frequently do not respond to exercises or other forms of therapy.

Subluxation of the Head of the Radius

On occasion, in gym classes, teachers will notice students who are unable to completely turn their palms up or down (supination and pronation of the forearm) with the elbow flexed at 90°. Examination will show that this abnormality of rotation is due to a congenital subluxation (partial dislocation) of the head of the radius (one of two bones of the forearm) at the elbow. The bone will be prominent on the outer side of the elbow (Figure 8). Some children with this condition have bilateral subluxations of the radial head. No treatment is indicated until skeletal growth is complete, at which time the prominent upper end of the bone is removed. Congenital radioulnar synostosis is also seen and presents with the same limitation of forearm motion. It is usually bilateral and results from a congenital bony connection between the radius and ulna (the other forearm bone). Treatment varies depending on the severity of the restricted movement, but surgical correction is reserved for the most handicapped patients.

Congenital Absence of the Radius

Congenital absence of the radius causes a deformity known as congenital clubhand (talipomanus) in which the hand is deviated and the forearm shortened. Frequently the thumb is missing in combination with the absent radius. Treatment of this deformity involves stretching of the tight structures (muscles, ligaments) which are enhancing the deformity with serial plaster casts until age 2, and then surgical correction. If these youngsters get as far as the first grade in school without specific treatment, they are probably better off having no surgery. By that time, they have adapted to their deformity and have attained more function than subsequent surgery might provide.

Abnormalities of the Hand

Other hand deformities commonly seen are syndactyly (Figure 9) and Madelung's deformity. Syndactyly is a congenital abnormality in which there is an unusual connection between two or more fingers consisting of a large web

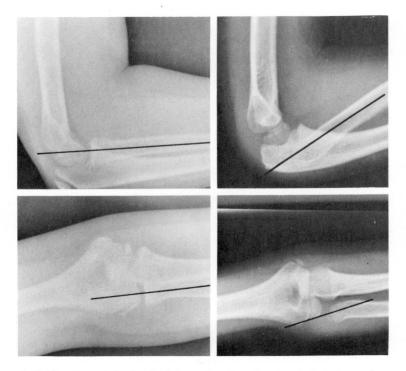

Figure 8. Subluxation of the head of the radius. Flexed and extended elbow of a normal boy in left panels. Note how a *line* drawn along the forearm (radius) of the affected patient in the right panels completely misses the elbow joint.

of skin. Most of these youngsters have had surgical correction by age 5, although it can be performed at any age. In Madelung's deformity, there is an overgrowth of the ulna at its distal end (i.e., at the wrist) with a relative shortening of the radius. No treatment is required unless function is impaired. Patients with hereditary multiple exostoses also present with a shortened bowed forearm. This deformity is associated with multiple small bony tumors (osteochondromas) at the ends of the bones adjacent to the growth plates. These painless, benign tumors are removed when they interfere with movement or function.

ORTHOPEDIC DISORDERS OF THE HIP JOINT

In the lower extremity, from the hip to the foot, abnormalities are apt to be more obvious than they are in the spine or upper extremity. Pain and limp, or limp alone, is the usual initial complaint or finding and is evident to the teacher in the classroom as well as on the playground.

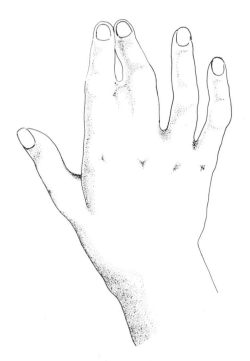

Figure 9. Syndactyly or webbing of skin between fingers.

Congenital Dislocation of the Hip

Ordinarily by age 5, youngsters born with congenital hip problems have had their condition diagnosed and treated. However, there is an occasional case of congenital hip subluxation or dislocation that slips by, particularly when both hips are involved. The reason for this is that the legs are of the same length when both are dislocated and, thus, the limp is not as noticeable. Many of these youngsters have a waddling type of gait due to the weakness of the muscles of the hip that stabilize the pelvis. Another entity which might present with the same waddling type of gait is congenital coxa vara (bending of the femur), due to a defect in the maturation of cartilage in the neck of the femur.

The treatment of a bilateral congenital hip problem in the school age child is somewhat controversial. Many orthopedic surgeons believe that these hips should remain untreated until they become symptomatic during adulthood. Others feel that reconstructive surgery with attempts to remodel the socket (acetabulum) and manually place (reduce) the ball (femoral head) within the socket is warranted. The latter techniques, which are invariably used in the older child with a unilateral dislocation, require a 6- to 8-wk. period of immobilization in a body cast and at least another 2–3 months of physical therapy and restricted activity. Thus, the recognition of a congenitally dislocated hip during infancy is of considerable importance as the treatment is nonoperative in most cases.

Legg-Calvé-Perthes Disease

During the age period from 4–8 years, a disorder known as Legg-Calvé-Perthes disease (Figure 10) is frequently observed. This condition is due to a disruption of the blood supply to the femoral capital epiphysis, or growth center for the femoral head. When the blood supply is interrupted, the bone in the growth center dies. The growth plate is then replaced by new bone and eventually the entire epiphysis remodels itself. This process goes on for approximately 2 years, proceeding in a systematic fashion through the various stages of regrowth. The younger the patient, the more expeditious the healing process and the better the prognosis. The older patients do not fare as well and frequently end up with deformed femoral heads.

The treatment of Legg-Calvé-Perthes disease seems to have been in a state of flux for the last 10 years. Up until that time, youngsters were maintained in leg traction, usually in the hospital, until their x-rays showed sufficient healing to allow weight bearing on their hips. This usually required at least 6–8 months of bed rest. During the past decade, the object of treatment has been to place the femoral head into a centralized position within the acetabulum, so that while the various stages of healing are taking place, the chances of the femoral head developing a deformed configuration are lessened. This has been accomplished by placing the legs in either a brace or a cast that allows ambulation early in the course of the disease. An alternate method of management includes surgically enclosing the head of the femur by moving the acetabulum over it or by cutting the femur so as to tilt the head deeper into the acetabulum. This latter technique has been found to hasten the healing process by 6–12 months. Use of the brace or casts permits these youngsters to go to school, whereas surgery requires a body cast for 6–8 wks. followed by 4–6 wks. of physical therapy.

Slipped Capital Femoral Epiphysis

Slipped capital femoral epiphysis (Figure 11) is most common in students between 10 and 13 years of age. It probably results from some type of hormonal effect at the growth plate of the femoral capital epiphysis which leads to a softening or weakening of the bone, allowing the head to slip off the neck of the femur. This condition is peculiar to males with the Fröhlich type body build—that is, the obese prepubertal hypogonadal individual—or the asthenic (very slender) female. All slips demand immediate surgical treatment. Those where the slip is less than one-third are stabilized with either pins or a bone graft across the growth plate to facilitate early closure and prevent further slipping. Those of greater than a one-third slip require a more major reconstructive procedure. The

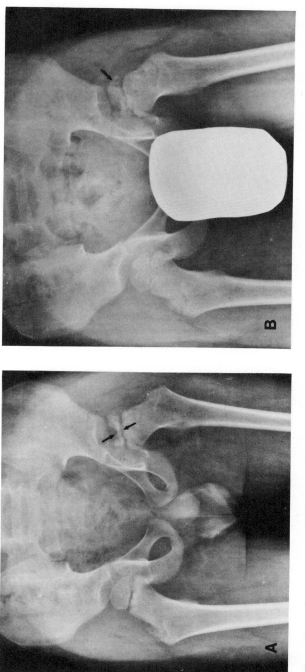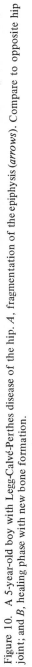

Figure 10. A 5-year-old boy with Legg-Calvé-Perthes disease of the hip. *A*, fragmentation of the epiphysis (*arrows*). Compare to opposite hip joint; and *B*, healing phase with new bone formation.

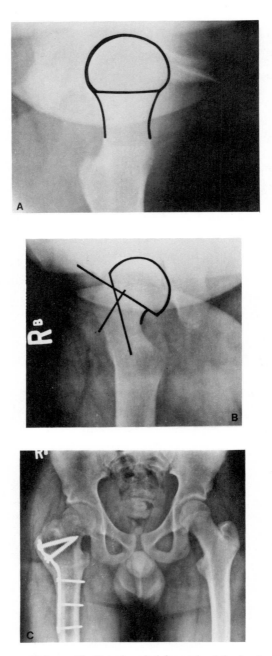

Figure 11. A 13-year-old boy with slipped capital femoral epiphysis. *A*, x-ray view of the patient's normal hip showing relationship of the head of the femur to the neck (head and neck sketched in for clarity); *B*, same view of involved hip showing bending or posterior slipping of the head on the neck; and *C*, postoperative osteotomy with a plate for support. Note the re-creation of the normal neck angle (compare to opposite side).

latter involves cutting the bone (osteotomy) just below the hip joint so as to realign the femoral head and place it in a more functional position. Whereas the pinning or bone grafting procedure necessitates only 2 wks. of hospitalization, the more extensive operation requires 2–3 wks. of traction within the hospital, or, in some instances, 6 wks., in a body cast. Slips frequently occur bilaterally and some orthopedic surgeons routinely pin the uninvolved hip at the time of surgery as a prophylactic measure.

One of the more troublesome complications of this condition, which results from the degree and acuteness of the slip as well as its subsequent treatment, is the development of avascular necrosis (bone death due to lack of an adequate blood supply) of the femoral head similar to Legg-Calvé-Perthes disease. When this occurs, an early arthritis of the involved hip is destined to occur.

The symptoms and signs of Legg-Calvé-Perthes disease and slipped capital femoral epiphysis are similar. Limp, with or without pain, is the most common finding. The pain is usually in the inner aspect of the thigh or on its anterior surface. Frequently these patients complain only of knee pain. Therefore, all youngsters who present with a limp and pain in their knee should routinely undergo x-rays of their hips. Occasionally, children with an early slip of the femoral capital epiphysis will hobble about for several months or complain of thigh or knee pain for an extended period and then, suddenly, experience a sharp pain in the groin or thigh. This usually indicates an acute traumatic slip of the epiphysis and will occasionally respond to gentle manipulation under general anesthesia to reduce the slip, followed by immediate pinning.

There is one other condition during childhood (ages 2 through 11) that mimics both of the aforementioned diseases—transient synovitis, or nontoxic synovitis, of the hip joint. It is either viral or posttraumatic in origin and causes a painful inflammation of the lining (synovium) of the joint. Usually this disorder responds to 2–5 days of nonweight bearing on the affected extremity. Occasionally, a bacterial infection in the hip joint, or pyogenic arthritis, will present with the same symptoms as transient synovitis. The correct diagnosis is made when the hip joint is aspirated with a needle and pus is obtained for culture. The latter condition requires open operative drainage of the joint and 4–6 wks. of inpatient intravenous antibiotics.

THE KNEE JOINT

Abnormalities of the knee joint in the school age child can cause some of the most trying diagnostic moments for the orthopedic surgeon.

Chondromalacia Patellae

Perhaps the most common disorder of this joint is chondromalacia patellae (softening of the cartilage under the kneecap) (Figure 12). This is seen from

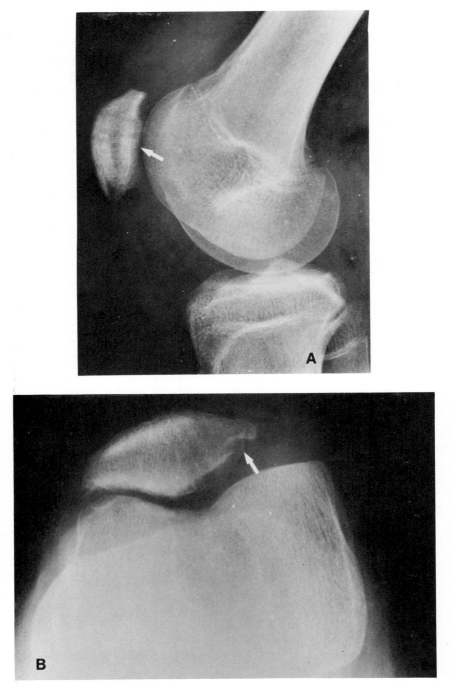

Figure 12. A 12-year-old female with chondromalacia patellae who had a 6-month history of pain and swelling of the right knee. *A*, a lateral view of the knee joint shows a ragged appearance (*arrow*) of the underside of the patella (kneecap); and *B*, a special x-ray view to show the undersurface of the affected patella.

10–17 years of age. It results from faulty mechanics involving function of the kneecap and, in many instances, is due to recurrent slippage of the patella out of position. These patients complain of a catching sensation, buckling, locking, and intermittent swelling in the region of the knee. They experience difficulty walking upstairs and running. The treatment of this condition consists of rest, aspirin, quadriceps setting exercises, and a knee support to prevent the patella from slipping. Only rarely is surgery indicated and, when performed, it is directed toward shaving down the softened areas beneath the patella or realigning the pull of the patella. Many of these youngsters go through periods of recurrent disability until growth has been completed. Females seem to be more prone to this problem than males.

Other entities which cause similar symptoms are discoid lateral menisci (abnormally formed lateral semilunar cartilage), osteochondritis dissecans, and torn menisci. Discoid lateral meniscus occurs between ages 3 and 10 and causes intermittent locking of the knee. Treatment is surgical excision of the abnormal meniscus. (Meniscus refers to the cartilage within joints that form the articulatory surface.)

Osteochondritis Dissecans

Osteochondritis dissecans occurs usually in boys ages 8–12 and results from a small fracture under the joint surface of one of the femoral condyles (articular prominence of the bone), frequently the medial one. A fragment of the articular cartilage with a small piece of attached bone may hang loosely or break off and float freely around the joint. If the disorder is recognized early, inactivity and a period in a plaster cast will allow the lesion to heal. If the symptoms of locking and swelling persist, holes can be drilled through the fragment to stimulate a new blood supply so as to heal the defect. If the fragment has fallen off, it is either surgically removed, or, if sizable, pinned back into place (Figure 13).

Torn menisci are rare under the age of 16, particularly in females. This is due to the fact that the ligaments and their attachments about the knee are stronger than the growth plates. Excessive forces that are exerted on a knee will usually cause the growth plate to slip or fracture rather than produce a tear in the ligament or cartilage. However, eleventh and twelfth grade football players frequently tear their cartilages, usually as a result of being clipped on a football field. These injuries are treated by surgical removal of the torn cartilage.

Occasionally a youngster will present with all of the signs of an internal derangement of the knee—swelling, buckling, and locking—and will turn out to have monoarticular juvenile rheumatoid arthritis. The latter is an inflammatory disorder of the synovium or lining of the joint. The diagnosis is made by performing certain blood tests and examinations of the joint fluid, and the treatment is aspirin, splinting, and physical therapy (see Chapter 6).

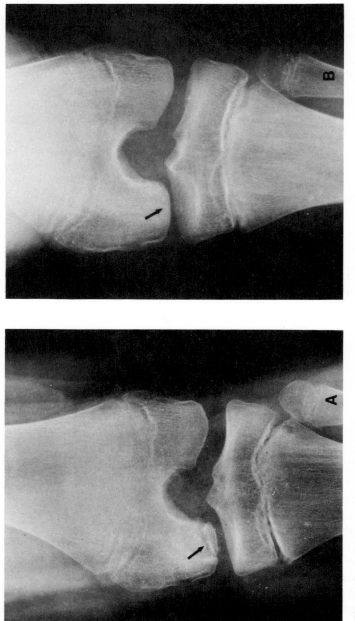

Figure 13. A 10-year-old boy with a history of locking and swelling of the left knee. Diagnosis: osteochondritis dissecans. *A*, defect on weight-bearing surface of femoral condyle (*arrow*). The fragment may break off and float within the joint. *B*, healing of the defect 6 wks. following surgical drilling through the abnormal cartilage.

Common Anomalies of the Knee Joint

Other common abnormalities affecting the knees of children include Baker's cysts, Osgood-Schlatter's disease, bowed knees (genu varum), and knocked knees (genu valgum).

Baker's cysts are located in the back of the knee and are due to a defect in the lining in the interior of the knee joint. A large sac filled with joint fluid develops. The treatment is surgical excision of the cyst.

Osgood-Schlatter's disease results from a disturbance in the blood supply to the growth center for the tibial tubercle, the bump just below the lower end of the patella, on the front of the upper end of the shin bone (tibia). This occurs between ages 10–16. The area becomes rather prominent and tender to touch. Running and climbing stairs are painful. Treatment of this disorder consists of limited physical activity, and, on occasion, casting for 6 wks. Occasionally, a local injection of steroid (cortisone-like substance) will reduce the inflammation. Rarely, if other methods of therapy are unsuccessful, the tibial tubercle is surgically removed (Figure 14).

Genu valgum or knock knee usually does not require treatment. However, if it is progressive or leads to ligamentous laxity about the knee causing instability, surgery is beneficial. The surgical procedure involves cutting through the bone (osteotomy) just below the knee so as to realign the extremity. When there has been damage to a growth plate just above or below the knee, asymmetrical growth in that plate may also cause a progressive valgus deformity. In certain cases the placing of metal staples across the growth plate, or fusing one side of the growth plate, will allow for a spontaneous correction of the deformity as the opposite side continues to grow.

Bowlegs or varus deformity occurs both at the knee (genu varum) and in the tibia (tibiovarum). The indications for correction are the same as mentioned for genu valgum deformity. However, there is one condition, Blount's disease, which requires osteotomy, and frequently repeated osteotomies (two to three times), before growth has been completed. Blount's disease is due to a defect in the inner aspect of the proximal tibial growth plate which allows for growth on one side of the plate only. It is a congenital abnormality.

Most of the surgical procedures which have been discussed require the use of a long leg cast, toes to upper thigh, for a period of approximately 6 wks. postoperatively. These are nonwalking casts but do allow the student the freedom of attending school by the use of crutches.

THE FOOT

Flatfeet (Pes Planus)

Numerous school age children have flatfeet. In most instances, this phenomenon is hereditary. For the most part, treatment is not indicated in those children over

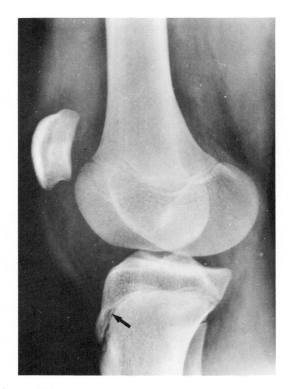

Figure 14. A 13-year-old boy with Osgood-Schlatter's disease with fragmentation of the tibial tubercle (*arrow*).

the age of 5. The use of corrective shoes and arch supports beyond the age of 5 should be restricted to those youngsters who suffer symptomatically from their flatfeet. Most flatfeet are of the relaxed type due to an inherent relaxation of the ligaments that support the arch, and, in many instances, these children will benefit from maintaining the arch with a support or sturdy oxford to facilitate running. There are operative procedures for correcting flatfeet, but these are done only on a very small number of children. The rather typical picture of the somewhat obese child who runs and walks with outturned feet associated with apparent incoordination is usually not assisted by footwear or surgery. Such youngsters should be allowed to play and participate to the best of their abilities, and, frequently, they will dramatically improve their skills with subsequent neuromuscular and musculoskeletal development.

Cavus Feet

The reverse deformity of flatfeet is cavus feet, or high arches. This, too, is usually inherited, although the progressive development of cavus feet is the result of a familial neurologic disorder. The neuromuscular imbalance that results leads to a deformity that interferes with function which may require surgical correction.

Toe Walking

Toe walking is a frequently seen phenomenon in the 5- to 7-year age group. It is caused by overactivity of the calf muscles (spasticity secondary to brain or spinal cord damage) which produces a progressive tightening of the heel cords. Muscular dystrophy (characterized by a progressive enlargement or pseudohypertrophy of the calf muscles) and cerebral palsy are the most common disorders associated with persistent tiptoeing. On occasion, toe walking is habitual. The toe walking that results from spasticity or muscular dystrophy is treated by short leg braces when the feet can be placed at a right angle to the tibia without too much resistance. When the latter is not possible, surgical lengthening of the heel cords is accomplished. The postoperative period requires 6 wks. in a long leg cast, followed by at least 3 months in a short leg brace. Night splints to maintain the correction are then necessary in most instances until skeletal maturity has been attained.

Toeing-in

Toeing-in, or pigeon-toed gait, is extremely common. This is due to any one or a combination of the following deformities: increased femoral anteversion at the hips (forward tilting of the femoral head and neck), internal tibial torsion (twisting of the shin bone), and metatarsus adductus (deviation of the foot toward the midline). Although many of these deformities are discovered and treated early in infancy, they frequently recur or remain refractory to complete correction. If toeing-in persists until these youngsters achieve school age, there is no treatment, short of surgery, that will correct the deformity. If the deformity is still present at age 8 or 9, chances are it will never be outgrown. Most orthopedic surgeons will not operate to correct these deformities unless the toeing-in is so severe as to cause the child to trip over his feet.

FRACTURES

Fractures are extremely common in school age children. Most fractures in children can be readily treated by means of a closed reduction (i.e., nonoperative) and a plaster cast. Such childhood fractures heal very rapidly and, if any malalignment remains after 6–8 wks. in a cast, remodeling of the bone secondary to normal muscle forces will correct the deformity within 1 year (Figure 15). However, the capacity for growth of a bone to correct malalignment following a fracture is dependent upon which part of the bone has been broken. The closer the fracture is to the end of a bone and its growth plate, the greater is its

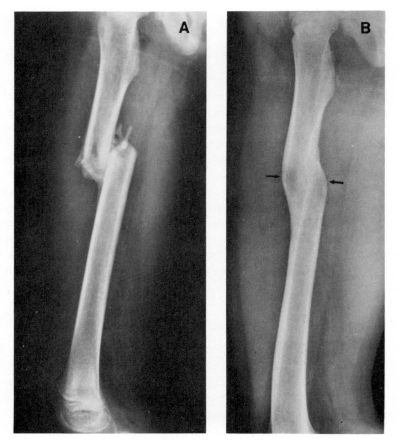

Figure 15. *A*, a 9-year-old female with a fracture of the shaft of the right femur (thigh bone); and *B*, the same patient 1 year later; note the remodeling of bone (*arrows*).

capacity for remodeling. On the other hand, fractures near the middle of a bone which heal in a bowed or angulated position lack the ability to remodel. It is, therefore, imperative that fractures which were displaced or angulated be re-evaluated by x-rays through the cast weekly for the first 3 wks. so that abnormal mending can be corrected by remanipulation before the bone has progressed too far into its healing phase.

A handful of fractures common to children require open surgery, including displaced fractures of the growth centers (condyles) on either side of the elbow, displaced fractures of the head of the femur, and malpositioned fractures about the ankle. Actually, any fracture which cannot be adequately reduced by closed manipulation or traction might require an open surgical reduction.

Additionally, there is a group of fractures that can only be treated with skeletal traction (a wire through a bone distal to the fracture). The traction is used first to reduce the fracture and then to maintain the reduction until adequate healing has taken place to allow the application of a cast to provide continued immobilization. This technique is used for displaced fractures at the upper end of the humerus, fractures in the supracondylar region of the elbow, and fractures of the femur (hip to the knee). Fractures of the femur require a body type cast that extends down the affected limb to the foot for approximately 2 months after the traction is removed. Obviously, these patients require home teaching.

While sitting immobile in a classroom for many hours with a cast on a limb, these youngsters should be encouraged to keep the limb elevated so as to prevent painful swelling of the fingers or toes. Following removal of a cast, the limb is vulnerable to reinjury for an additional 4–6 wks., so activity with that limb should be restricted.

ORTHOPEDIC POTPOURRI

Bone tumors occur frequently in children. Although many types of tumor occur which can be readily eradicated with surgical excision, there are several types of tumor peculiar to childhood which are of the malignant variety and which are ultimately fatal. The Ewing's sarcoma and osteogenic sarcoma (Figure 16) are two of the more commonly seen bone tumors, and the 5-year survival rate for each is no greater than 20%. Frequently, these two types of tumor will require radiation therapy and chemotherapy following amputation of the limb. It is the combination of amputation and radiation or chemotherapy which extends the survival time of these patients.

Children of school age are prone to the development of infections in their bones (osteomyelitis) and in their joints (septic arthritis) (Figure 17). These infections are usually hematogenous (blood born) in that they are spread from a focus of infection elsewhere—frequently the upper respiratory system. The child presents with fever, irritability, and bone or joint pain. Following the establishment of the diagnosis, intravenous antibiotics are begun and open surgical drainage of the bone or joint is undertaken. The course of treatment requires 4–6 wks. of inpatient intravenous antibiotics and rest of the extremity. Antibiotics are used for an additional 3–6 months, depending upon the nature of the infection. A cast might be required until the involved bone is completely healed.

SUMMARY

The medical specialty of orthopedics encompasses the diagnosis and management of disorders of the musculoskeletal system. Oftentimes, the condition is the result of an accident; the injury such as a sprain or fracture is self-limited and should not interfere with the normal educational process.

However, there are certain abnormalities of the muscles, joints, and bones peculiar to children which, if neglected or untreated, may result in a crippling deformity, severe loss of function, and marked emotional conflict. These ortho-

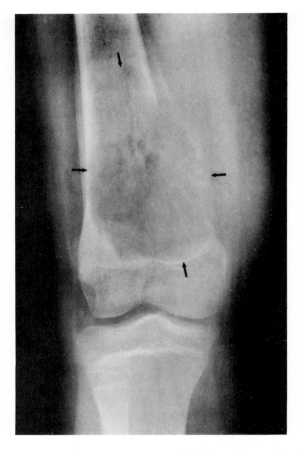

Figure 16. Example of an osteogenic sarcoma (slightly darker and expanding area) replacing the distal one-third of the femur in a 15-year-old girl (*arrows*). Despite appropriate radiation therapy and amputation of the involved limb, the patient died within 16 months after discovery of the tumor. The 5-year survival rate for this tumor is extremely poor and approximates 10–20% of patients.

pedic conditions often require a prolonged period of therapy utilizing surgical procedures, physical therapy, casting, and bracing. Extended cycles of school absenteeism may result.

This chapter reviews the orthopedic diseases common to the school-aged child. The primary symptoms of musculoskeletal dysfunction are discussed. Abnormalities of the spine, upper extremity, hip, knee, and foot are treated separately, as specific diseases of the skeletal axis tend to seek precise locations.

The teacher is in an unequaled position to detect early signs of an orthopedic disorder and, thereby, initiate appropriate and timely referral prior to the development of irreversible disability. Furthermore, the appreciation of certain musculoskeletal diseases by the educator will enhance her relationship as she interacts with the pupil during the period of rehabilitation.

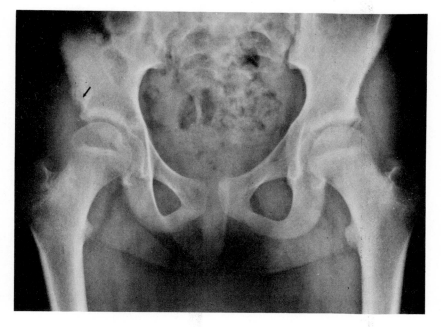

Figure 17. A 14-year-old girl with a 2-wk. history of fever and pain in the right hip. The x-ray shows erosion of the bone characteristic of osteomyelitis (*arrow*). Compare to the opposite side.

SUGGESTED READING

Blount, W. P. 1955. Fractures in Children. The Williams & Wilkins Company, Baltimore. 279 p.

Crenshaw, A. H. (ed.). 1971. Campbell's Operative Orthopaedics. 5th Ed. C. V. Mosby Company, St. Louis. 2,044 p.

Tachdjian, M. O. 1972. Pediatric Orthopedics. W. B. Saunders Company. Philadelphia. 1,767 p.

Turek, S. L. 1959. Orthopaedics: Principles and Their Applications. J. B. Lippincott Company, Philadelphia. 906 p.

10

The Role of Genetic Mechanisms In Childhood Handicaps

Thaddeus E. Kelly, M.D., Ph.D.

The aim of programs for handicapped children is to minimize the restrictions placed on a child's full participation in activities. Success in this endeavor is dependent upon understanding those handicaps and related problems as they modify a child's potential. Many handicaps are the direct result of a genetic disorder. An understanding of genetic mechanisms and disorders is helpful in fully appreciating the functional result of a handicap.

A *genetic disorder* is defined as an alteration in a child's genetic endowment which produces a physical, mental, and/or emotional alteration that may vary from a minor cosmetic blemish to a severe abnormality incompatible with life. The alteration in the genetic endowment may occur as a result of one of three general mechanisms: inheritance of an altered gene or group of genes from one parent that produces an abnormal effect in the child which is also present to some degree in the parent; inheritance of abnormal genes from each parent which have produced no abnormality in either parent, but which, in combination in the child, produce an abnormal effect; and thirdly, a change, called a mutation, that occurs in a gene or group of genes as it is being transmitted to the child through the process of fertilization of an ovum by a sperm. In the latter mechanism, neither parent has an abnormality in their own genetic composition. As there is a relationship between the nature of the abnormal effect, or handicap, and the mechanism involved, understanding of these concepts as they apply to a given child facilitates a better appreciation of the handicap.

This paper was supported in part through Project 917, Maternal and Child Health Service, United States Department of Health, Education, and Welfare.

GENES AND CHROMOSOMES

A *gene* is a linear sequence of special chemical substances called deoxyribonucleic acid (DNA). The particular sequence of the components of the DNA acts as a code to provide information to a cell enabling that cell to carry out its function. This is analogous to the manner in which a sequence of dots and dashes through the Morse code spells out a message. In the same way in which an alteration in the sequence of dots and dashes may change the meaning of a message, a modification in the sequence of the DNA of a gene may alter the function of the cell.

A change in the structure of a gene is not always detrimental. In fact, most changes are not only innocuous, but are responsible for the physical variation between individuals. The effects of these changes over a prolonged period of time are responsible for the process of evolution. A recognizable result of the effect of a gene or group of genes is called a *trait*. A trait may be a normal variation such as eye color, height, or intelligence. A trait may also be a physical defect, such as a cleft lip.

When a cell divides, a new copy of each gene results, providing the two newly formed cells with a full complement of genetic information. Multiplying cells copy genes in this process with an amazing degree of accuracy. However, rare errors may be made in the copying process that alter the sequence of DNA in a single gene or affect an entire group of genes. Such an error is called a *mutation*.

As there are thousands of genes, their physical transfer from a dividing cell to two new cells is facilitated by the arrangement of genes in packages. These packages are called *chromosomes*. Chromosomes can be seen in the dividing cell under the microscope. Each human cell contains 46 chromosomes representing all the genetic information for that individual. Different species of plants and animals have varying numbers of chromosomes that are specific for that life form. Not all the genes in every cell are functional; only those that provide information for the specific requirements of that cell are operational.

The 46 chromosomes of humans consist of 23 pairs (Figure 1). The figure shows the chromosomes as seen under the microscope and arranged in a *karyotype*. By their size and shape, the chromosomes are arranged in numerical order as pairs, numbered 1–22, with the twenty-third pair called the sex chromosomes. Techniques currently allow for identification of each pair. If the twenty-third pair consists of two large X chromosomes, the genetic sex of that individual is a female. If the pair consists of one large X and one small Y, the sex is that of a male. As a sperm and an ovum mature, they reduce their chromosomal number from 46 to 23. Thus, the fusion of the sperm and ovum at fertilization results in a cell with a new combination of 46 chromosomes. Each parent contributes equally to the genetic endowment of the child. The sperm determines the sex of the developing fetus. Because an ovum contains two X's,

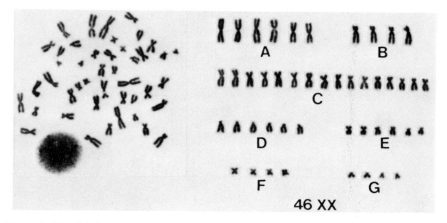

Figure 1. The 46 chromosomes of humans. *Left,* the chromosomes of one cell as seen under the microscope. *Right,* the chromosomes are arranged in a karyotype of a normal female.

when it reduces its chromosomal number from 46 to 23, it contains one of each pair of numbers one to 22 plus an X. A sperm may contain an X or a Y with the 22 chromosomes. Thus, a boy receives his father's Y and one of his mother's two X's. A girl receives her father's X and one of her mother's two X's (Figure 2).

Each pair of chromosomes contains genes for like functions, although the genes need not be identical in their DNA sequence. It is the combined action of a pair of genes operating in the forefront of the entire complement of genes and the environment that determines the exact expression of a given trait. The presence or absence of a trait may be determined by a single pair of genes, but the characteristics of the trait are influenced by the remaining genes and the environment. The same biochemical trait may have quite a different effect on a Polynesian in a warm climate and particular diet than on an Eskimo with his milieu and dietary habits.

This knowledge of genes and chromosomes can now be applied to genetic disorders. *Syndrome* is a term commonly used in referring to such disorders. Syndrome literally means a "running together." In medicine, the term is used to define a constellation of features which collectively represents a recognizable entity. A syndrome need not have a genetic causation, but many genetic disorders are referred to as syndromes. When a group of features is described in medical literature and is considered to represent a recognizable disorder, it is referred to as a syndrome often having an eponymic prefix using the name of the physician that provided the original description of the disorder. Thus, Down's syndrome is a well-defined genetic disorder owing its name to the fact that Langdon Down provided an early description of the condition. The general term "disorder" rather than "disease" is often used as these processes are inherently lifelong, are usually considered nonacute, and they may be correctable, although not curable.

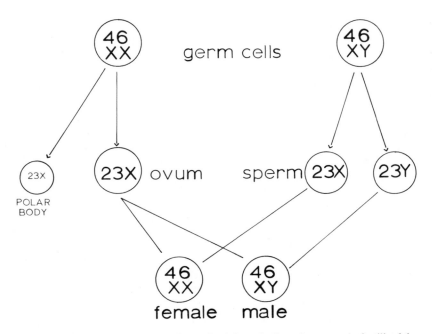

Figure 2. The sex of the fetus is determined by whether the ovum is fertilized by an X-bearing or Y-bearing sperm.

MENDELIAN INHERITANCE

A genetic disorder may result from a single defective gene or pair of genes. Such a mechanism is called Mendelian inheritance, as it obeys the two laws of inheritance described by the monk Gregor Mendel in the 1860's. While his work was done with sweet peas, the principles he defined are applicable to human genetics. Single genes may be involved in one of three patterns of inheritance as they produce recognizable traits. These are referred to as dominant, recessive, and X-linked or sex-linked. Disorders arising from the effect of groups of genes are described later.

The term *dominant* refers to a single gene producing a trait without regard to the nature of its pair member (remember that each gene is present in a double dose, one member of the pair supplied by the mother and the other by the father). Brown eyes are a dominant trait, i.e., if one of the pair of eye color genes codes for brown eyes, the individual will have brown eyes, regardless of whether the second gene codes for blue or brown. In this case, the child demonstrates a trait that is present in at least one of his parents. An individual with a dominantly inherited trait has one gene of a pair which is altered and responsible for that trait. When such an individual reproduces, he may give either member of the gene pair to his offspring. There is an equal probability of either gene being transmitted to the child. While a single individual may give the normal gene to all his children, among a large group of such people, approximately one-half of the children will have received the normal gene and one-half the abnormal gene. It also follows that this probability is dependent on the individual with such a dominant trait and not related to the spouse.

Many genetic disorders that are dominantly inherited have certain features in common. If the disorder is to be transmitted from parent to child, the effect of the disorder on the parent must be such that it does not preclude that individual's reaching adulthood and reproducing. Dominantly inherited disorders are, therefore, usually milder than recessive or X-linked disorders. Furthermore, they result in structural defects rather than abnormalities in metabolism. Structural defects include cleft lip, club foot, congenital heart disease, and others that result from abnormal development of a part of the body. As such, they are usually recognizable in infancy and the defects are congenital as opposed to developing later in life. The severity of the physical defects may vary widely between parent and child with the same disorder. Mental retardation is an uncommon feature of dominantly inherited disorders. These generalizations hold for dominantly inherited disorders as a group, but there are specific disorders which represent exceptions. Several examples will illustrate some of these points.

Achondroplasia is a dominantly inherited disorder of skeletal growth. Individuals with this disorder present a highly reproducible picture. They are dwarfed, the legs and arms are short in relation to the trunk, the head tends to be large, they are of stout build, and the base of the nose is depressed. The defective gene exerts its effect only upon growing cartilage and bone. Thus, the general health and intelligence of these people are unimpaired. Their propensity for such diseases as diabetes, heart disease, tuberculosis or others is the same as unaffected individuals. Their major handicap is short stature, with the attendant social problems which may develop. An infant with this disorder is clearly recognizable at birth, and the disorder is fully manifest at this early age. Achondroplasia demonstrates one exception to the generalizations cited in dominantly inherited disorders. That is, there is little variation in the degree of severity of similarly affected individuals. This feature has made it possible to understand an area of confusion among several dominantly inherited disorders.

A child is born with a clearly established genetic disorder inherited as a dominant. Neither parent has any of the features of that disorder. That child grows to adulthood and has children, some of whom may have the same dominant disorder. It is readily apparent that this person transmitted the gene for the disorder to his child who was similarly affected, but if he received both of his genes from his ostensibly normal parents, where did his defective gene come from? As sperm and ova mature and reduce their chromosomal number, the genes are copied one time. In that copying process an error may occur, a mutation, which will subsequently be present in all the cells of the resulting child. If that mutation leads to a defective gene producing a dominantly inherited disorder, then the disorder will be present in the child in its typical form while being present in neither parent. That affected individual may pass the disorder to his children. There is a genetic principle known as the Hardy-Weinberg law that states that the frequency of a particular gene in the population as a whole remains the same from generation to generation. If a defective gene, when present in an individual, reduces that individual's likelihood of reproduction, then with time we would expect that mutation to disappear, much as did certain now extinct animals. The frequency of the particular gene remains much the same, however, by defective genes which are lost through failure to be passed on being replaced by new mutations arising in ova and sperm.

The structural effects of a dominant disorder, when unrecognized, may be incorrectly considered to be associated with mental retardation. The Treacher-Collins syndrome results in an unattractive alteration of facial appearance. The ears may be altered to such an extent that a severe hearing loss occurs. A child with this disorder may be incorrectly institutionalized because his appearance and lack of speech are felt to be part of a problem associated with mental retardation. Later a proper diagnosis in such a child would lead to a hearing aid and cosmetic surgery which may return the child to a more normal life. This bias of attitude toward children with dominant disorders where their general appearance is quite altered, but intelligence is normal, is not uncommon.

When mental retardation occurs as part of a dominantly inherited disorder, it is usually of a mild degree. The retardation is the result of a structural alteration of the brain. The development of such children is at a slower rate, but there is no deterioration of mental function with time, and seizures are uncommon. Therefore, it is simpler to prepare long-range programs for such children as the child's status is rather stable. The mental retardation associated with chromosomal abnormalities is quite similar except that it is of a more profound degree.

A *recessive* gene is one whose presence, as only one member of a gene pair, does not result in a recognizable trait. If, however, both members of the gene pair are of a similar mutation, then a recessively inherited trait, or disorder, results. If each parent has one gene of the pair which is abnormal and a child received the defective gene from both parents, a recessive disorder would occur. Such parents are called "carriers" as they carry a mutation which produces no ill effect on themselves but may result in a genetic disorder in their child. It is estimated that each person carries five to eight recessive genes among their thousands of genes. It is only when both members of a couple have a mutation of the same gene that a disorder may occur in their child.

Tay-Sachs disease is a recessive disorder that occurs almost entirely among Jewish children. Approximately 1 in every 30 normal Jewish individuals has one of a gene pair as a defective gene which in double dose results in Tay-Sachs disease. Such individuals are referred to as carriers of the Tay-Sachs gene. When such a person marries, if the spouse is also Jewish, there is a 1 in 30 chance that the spouse is a carrier. Thus, among Jewish couples, 1 in 900 (1 in 30 $\times$ 1 in 30) have the possibility of producing a child with Tay-Sachs disease. Dominant disorders tend to occur rather uniformly among different races, whereas recessive disorders tend to occur with disproportionate frequency among certain ethnic groups. Cystic fibrosis among northern Europeans and sickle cell disease among blacks are similar to Tay-Sachs disease among Jews.

As shown in the illustration (Figure 3), if both man and wife are carriers of the same recessive gene, then any pregnancy has a 25% chance of a normal child with both genes normal, a 50% chance of a normal child who is a carrier like his parents, and a 25% chance of a child with both genes defective, thus having the disorder. A parent may give either member of a gene pair to his child with equal probability and this is independent of the gene given by the other parent. This is best illustrated by tossing two coins simultaneously. One soon realizes the results are similar to recessive genes; i.e., 25% two heads, 50% head and tail, or tail and head, and 25% two tails. It is also apparent that each toss of the coins is an independent event. Thus, among couples where both members are carriers, some may have several children with a recessive disorder, while others have none. However, the 25:50:25% ratio holds true for the collective experience of a large number of such couples.

Some generalizations can be made about the features of genetic disorders that are recessively inherited. Usually the disorder is the result of the absence or alteration of a protein, particularly an enzyme. An *enzyme* is a specialized protein which acts as a catalyst in the conversion of a chemical compound to a different form; the process is called metabolism. If both genes directing the production of that enzyme are abnormal, an inadequate amount or altered form

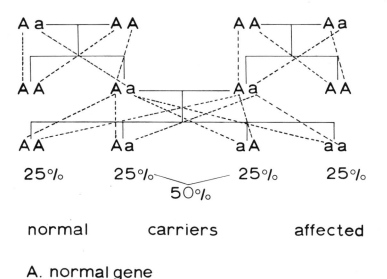

Figure 3. A recessive disorder occurs when both parents are carriers (Aa). Such a couple may have normal children (AA), carriers like themselves (Aa), and affected children (aa) with the probabilities shown.

of that enzyme is made. The resulting disorder, therefore, depends on the nature of the chemical process that requires that enzyme. Because the effect of the altered chemical process is cumulative, the disorder is often progressive. While pregnant with the child, the mother may be able to correct for the chemical defect for some disorders in the unborn child by transfer of chemical compounds across the placenta. Thus, at birth such children appear entirely normal. Without the maternal assistance, however, the effects of the chemical derangement become apparent with time.

Phenylketonuria (PKU), the disorder for which babies are tested by a heel stick blood test in the newborn nursery, illustrates these features. The effect of the metabolic defect on normal growth of the brain can be corrected by the mother's blood while she carries the child. After birth, because of a missing enzyme, the child is unable to properly handle certain metabolic products and subsequent development of the brain is impaired. These children show no structural defects, such as cleft lip or club foot, because the abnormality is restricted to a biochemical process which becomes apparent after birth. PKU is one of the few such disorders where early diagnosis and dietary management allow the biochemical error to be circumvented and brain development with dietary treatment to proceed normally.

For most such disorders, there is no effective therapy and an affected child who appeared normal at birth is subject to the constant effects of a deranged metabolic system. Such children may experience acute illnesses when their limited tolerance to certain biochemical processes is stressed. Profound mental retardation, seizures, aberrant behavior, and stunted growth often accompany the metabolic abnormality. Such defects are collectively known as *inborn errors of metabolism.*

Once such a disorder has been diagnosed, the parents are counseled that any future pregnancy carries a 25% (or one in four) risk of a recurrence, as these conditions result from a defective gene inherited from normal parents. Some of these disorders can be detected by the absence of the critical enzyme in cells grown from an affected individual. This makes possible the test known as *amniocentesis.* The term amniocentesis refers to the removal from the pregnant uterus of a small amount of the amniotic fluid which bathes and cushions the developing fetus. Within this fluid are living skin cells, washed from the fetus, which can be grown in tissue culture. These living cells are tested for the enzyme in question and make possible a prenatal diagnosis. Given the diagnosis of a specific disorder in the fetus, the couple has the option of an abortion. It should be emphasized that such programs seek to allow a couple to take advantage of the 75% probability of a normal child without the possibility of a recurrence of the severe disorder.

There are exceptions to the generalizations given for recessively inherited disorders. While most involve biochemical errors without structural defects, some do result in developmental anomalies of a structural nature and may or may not be accompanied by mental retardation. These are presumably the result of the absence of necessary chemical agents at a crucial time in fetal development.

Sex-linked or *X-linked* patterns of inheritance are so designated because the defective gene is carried on the X chromosome. This results in a unique inheritance pattern. Because a father gives his X chromosome to daughters, and his Y to sons (as noted earlier under sex determination), an X chromosome with a defective gene is given to all daughters and no sons of such a man. This lack of male to male transmission is the cardinal feature of the X-linked pattern of inheritance. As a mother gives one of her two X's to both sons and daughters, it follows that a 50% probability exists for a child of either sex to receive a defective X chromosome from the mother. Most X-linked traits are recessive, but the above features are best illustrated by a pedigree of an X-linked dominant trait, such as one form of dwarfism called hypophosphatemic rickets. In Figure 4, the pedigree shows one-half of Mrs. A.'s sons and daughters are affected, while all of Mr. B.'s daughters and none of his sons are affected.

An X-linked recessively inherited disorder is one in which one of two of a female's X chromosomes carries a defective gene, but the female does not demonstrate that trait. Males with this X chromosome demonstrate the trait, however, as their one and only X is affected. Thus, females are carriers, their sons may be affected, their daughters may be carriers, and no male to male transmission occurs. Probably the best known example of an X-linked disease is hemophilia because of its entry into royal families of Europe via Queen Victoria's offspring. Alexandra, wife of Czar Nicholas of Russia, was a carrier of hemophilia like her grandmother, Victoria. Her son, Nicholas, had hemophilia, and it was Rasputin's false claim of controlling the bleeding disorder that gave him such influence over the royal family. The bleeding disorder in males is due to a lack of protein coded by a gene on the X chromosome that is required in the clotting process. Hemophilia is now treatable by administration of the clotting protein, called factor VIII, prepared from human blood.

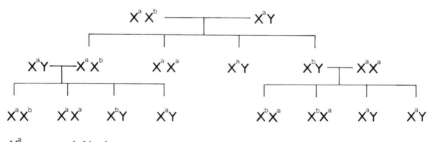

X^a normal X chromosome
X^b mutation-bearing X chromosome

Figure 4. If a man carries the mutant X (X^b), all his daughters and none of his sons will receive the mutant X. When a woman carries the mutant X, half her sons and daughters are expected to receive the mutant X.

Epidemiologic studies of mental retardation have shown a slightly greater number of retarded males than females. This difference has been ascribed to X-linked recessive disorders causing mental retardation. The only genetic disorders present in females that do not occur in males are those in which the defect is manifest only as an abnormality of female genitalia or very rare disorders which cause death in the unborn male and a milder disorder in females.

There are about 150 disorders and traits which result from altered genes on the X chromosome. Among the less severe are both forms of color blindness, while on the other extreme is a form of profound mental retardation in males associated with bizarre behavior of a self-mutilative type (Lesch-Nyhan syndrome).

MULTIFACTORIAL INHERITANCE

Groups of genes can result in recognizable traits by two mechanisms, multifactorial inheritance and chromosomal aberrations. *Multifactorial inheritance* emphasizes the fact that any gene exerts its influence in concert with the total genetic endowment, the environment within the uterus during the development of the fetus, and the environment in general postnatally. Under this mechanism, a trait appears as a result of the combined influence of a number of genes and environmental factors, and is, therefore, multifactorial. A threshold model demonstrates the input of the various components (Figure 5). As shown in the illustration, each factor contributes variously to the total and no one factor is sufficient alone to result in a specific trait. The example used in Figure 5 is pyloric stenosis (a narrowing of the duodenal lumen which interferes with the normal passage of food from the stomach to the small intestine). If the total of a combination of factors surpasses a certain level or threshold, it exerts an effect in which the defect is manifest. There is evidence to suggest that a viral infection during pregnancy is one such factor in causing pyloric stenosis. It has been clearly established that the sex of the child is another factor. The threshold required to produce the defect in a male is lower than in a female. This is an example of a sex-influenced, not a sex-linked, disorder.

Most traits which vary over a range of normal values are under multifactorial inheritance. This is best illustrated by height. A number of genes prenatally and environmental factors postnatally account for the ultimate adult height of an individual. There is a predictable cluster of heights that a child might attain based on the height of his parents (Figure 6). This cluster has wide extremes which account for the possibility of a man and woman each 60 in. tall having a son 72 in. tall. Mental retardation is not generally considered as a multifactorial trait. The distribution of intelligence is such that a couple with IQ's of 90 may have a child with an IQ of 60–70 on the basis of the combination of genes that were received from the parents. Thus, many individuals with intelligence in the

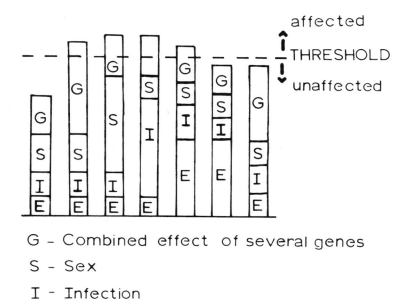

G - Combined effect of several genes

S - Sex

I - Infection

E - Other environmental factors

Figure 5. Many factors act collectively to determine if a multifactorial trait is expressed. No one factor acting alone is sufficient to determine expression.

dull range may have an intellectual handicap on a multifactorial basis rather than as a result of a specific genetic disorder or birth trauma.

Traits normally under multifactorial control may be determined almost entirely by a single defective gene. The trait is then inherited in a Mendelian fashion as previously discussed. Single genes producing dwarfism will lead to an adult height which does not seem to be influenced by the groups of genes which determined parental height. Single genes resulting in mental retardation reduce a child's intelligence to a degree unrelated to parental intelligence.

Certain birth defects are recognized to occur as a result of multifactorial inheritance. This is especially true when these defects occur as single events. Cleft lip and/or cleft palate is a common birth defect. When it occurs as part of a syndrome, that is, associated with other birth defects, it is usually caused by a single mutated gene or chromosomal abnormality. When it occurs as a single event with no other birth defect, then multifactorial inheritance is the likely causation. The cleft lip and/or cleft palate is physically the same regardless of the causation. In the same way, club foot and spina bifida (meningomyelocele) may occur as single birth defects as the result of multifactorial causation or they may occur in combination with other defects as a syndrome with a different type of causation.

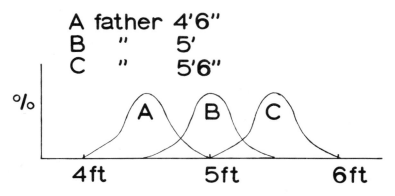

Figure 6. Based on the height of the father, an estimate can be made of the likely height of any son. The mother's height is also important in any such estimate. The *curves* represent distributions of son's height for a man with a given height.

CHROMOSOMAL ABNORMALITIES

Obvious chromosomal abnormalities visible under the microscope are the result of either a group of genes occurring as an excess of genetic material (the genes are present in a triple dose) or a deficit of genetic materials (the genes are present in a single dose). Down's syndrome (mongolism) is the result of a chromosomal abnormality when an entire chromosome (number 21) is present in triplicate rather than as a pair. Therefore, the chromosomal number in cells from an individual with Down's syndrome is 47, rather than the normal 46. A number of well-established syndromes are recognizable because of the deletion or addition of a particular chromosome. These abnormalities of chromosomal number are called *aneuploidies*. The mechanism by which such an abnormality arises is illustrated in Figure 7. The term *trisomy* refers to the presence in cells of three given chromosomes rather than the usual two. Trisomy 21 refers to the presence of three number 21 chromosomes, the mechanism for the great majority of Down's syndrome cases. *Monosomy* refers to a single member of a chromosome pair.

There are certain generalities that can be made about patients with chromosomal abnormalities. However, a distinction must be established between abnormalities involving the pairs numbered 1–22 called *autosomes* and the X and Y chromosomes (sex chromosomes). Most significant is the invariable association between excess or deficient genetic material involving the autosomes and mental retardation. Mental retardation, particularly of more than a mild degree, is not a constant feature of syndromes involving absent or extra X and Y chromosomes. When a visible imbalance of genetic material involving an autosome occurs, there are several predictable results. These consequences are illustrated for Down's syndrome, but are generally applicable to all such disorders. The defects of these syndromes are structural rather than metabolic or chemical. The genetic imbalance exerts its detrimental influence on the development of physical structures

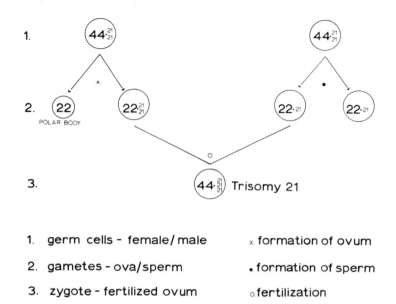

1. germ cells - female/male   x formation of ovum

2. gametes - ova/sperm   • formation of sperm

3. zygote - fertilized ovum   ₒ fertilization

Figure 7. In the germ cell *on the left,* an error in chromosome distribution during cell division called meiotic nondisjunction results in 47 chromosomes with three number 21's after fertilization.

of the early embryo and fetus. Down's syndrome is visually recognizable because of characteristic facial features consisting of an abnormal slant of the eyes, prominent epicanthal fold at the inner eye, pug nose, large tongue, flattening of the back of the skull, and microcephaly (small head). Of themselves, these are minor variations in physical appearance, but, in this case, they collectively denote a more widespread abnormality of development which can be confirmed by chromosome studies. Mental retardation occurs in all cases and is usually of at least a moderate degree. Many of these children die in infancy because of associated serious defects, such as congenital heart disease. Those who are free of severe associated defects enjoy reasonably good health. Viral respiratory infections seem to occur slightly more frequently and persist longer in children with Down's syndrome. Physical growth is restricted to some degree in all, but the shortness of stature may be minimal. Seizures are uncommon and behavior does not present a serious disciplinary problem. In fact, such children are often quite pleasant and easy to deal with.

DISORDERS OF SEX CHROMOSOMES

Aneuploidies involving the X and Y chromosomes are among the most common chromosomal abnormalities. They are significantly different in their consequences from abnormalities involving pairs 1—22. A brief summary of each is given.

Turner's Syndrome

This disorder occurs among females who possess only one X chromosome (rather than two). There may be alternative arrangements of the chromosomal material other than the usual finding in this syndrome of 45 chromosomes with one X, but, in essence, these other arrangements produce the condition by the loss of material from an X chromosome.

There is considerable variation in the expression of this chromosomal abnormality, but there are certain features that are present in most. The girls have inconstant degrees of altered development of the ovaries. As a result of the gonadal dysgenesis, they do not undergo menarche (onset of menstrual periods) or acquire the secondary feminine sexual characteristics at the normal time of puberty. This hormonal deficiency is also partially responsible for shortness of stature. Appropriate and timely administration of hormones in such girls will induce normal menstrual periods, secondary sexual development, and allow some increase in adult height. Because the dysplastic ovary is deficient in the production of estrogens as well as germ cells, these girls are sterile. They are, however, quite capable of participating in sexual intercourse and many lead happy married lives. There are developmental abnormalities which occur as part of this syndrome. Some have no significant impact on such an individual while others may have serious consequences. These include abnormalities of kidney structure, a narrowing of the major blood vessel from the heart known as coarctation of the aorta, low posterior hairline, and an excessive fold of tissue about the neck producing a webbed appearance. Additionally, some exhibit difficulty in mathematics and spatial orientation, despite normal intelligence.

Klinefelter's Syndrome

This chromosomal disorder of males is the result of an extra X chromosome. Thus, the cells contain 47 chromosomes with two X's and one Y (males normally have 46 chromosomes with one X and one Y). As in Turner's syndrome, one of the central features of this disorder is abnormal development of the gonads, in this case, the testes. There is a similar result of inadequate hormonal production with failure to attain secondary sexual characteristics at the proper age and inability to produce normal sperm. There are fewer physical clues to this diagnosis than in the Turner's syndrome, and so the disorder is recognized on the average at an older age. At an age when peers are undergoing puberty, these boys exhibit wide hips and slender shoulders, longer legs relative to total height, variable degrees of breast development (called gynecomastia), failure to grow facial, pubic, and axillary hair, and small testes and penis. The range of IQ scores of a large number of such individuals shows a wide distribution from superior to subnormal, but the average score is below 100. Hormonal therapy (testosterone) and cosmetic surgery of the breasts will largely correct the physical stigmata of Klinefelter's syndrome.

Individuals with the Turner or Klinefelter syndromes are subject to emotional and social problems which often overshadow any of the physical limitations of their disorder. However, these problems primarily seem to be secondary consequences of altered sexual development and physical appearance rather than an integral part of the chromosomal abnormality. Therefore, the complications are largely preventable given an early diagnosis and appropriate management.

XYY Chromosomal Pattern

During a survey, researchers in Scotland performed chromosomal analyses on a large group of men in penal institutions. An unexpected result was the finding of a number of tall men with deviant behavior resulting in criminality whose chromosomal number was 47 with an XYY pattern. Following this initial report, other studies among juvenile delinquents and sociopathic adult criminals disclosed further XYY cases. Further reports attempted to define physical features which were distinctive for such individuals.

Following this initial evidence suggesting a relationship between criminality and the XYY pattern, additional studies questioned the earlier assumption. Individuals with the XYY pattern were found who led highly successful lives in a number of demanding professions. Further studies failed to demonstrate any unequivocal physical features of the XYY pattern except possibly increased height. Closer evaluation of the families in several studies showed many of the individuals with the XYY pattern and criminal behavior came from family settings that were highly unstable, and, therefore, conducive to antisocial behavior.

Figure 8 shows a theoretic distribution of emotional stability for men with XY and XYY chromosomes which could explain any deviant behavior on a genetic basis. Each individual has a certain tolerance to withstand a stressful environment and maintain his emotional stability. An individual with an XYY pattern may have a lower tolerance threshold so that, when exposed to the same environmental stress, he is less well prepared to cope with it. Exceeding such a tolerance might manifest deviant behavior leading to criminality. Any conclusions on a firm relationship of the XYY pattern and criminality must await further study.

Triple X

This pattern of 47 chromosomes with three X's is more a variation than an abnormality as there are no apparent sexual, mental, or emotional changes which accompany this alteration of chromosomal number.

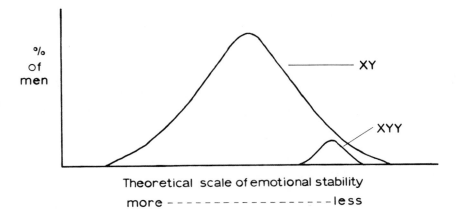

Figure 8. In this theoretic model, more men with XY chromosomes are less emotionally stable, but if a man has XYY chromosomes, he is more likely to be less stable.

Other Sex Chromosome Aneuploidies

Several other alterations of the normal chromosomal number of 46 involving sex chromosomes occur. These include 48 chromosomes with XXXX, 48 with XXYY, 49 with XXXXX, and 49 with XXXYY. These disorders result in abnormal physical, sexual, and mental development, but occur rarely when compared to the four detailed above.

PARTIAL CHROMOSOMAL DELETIONS AND DUPLICATIONS

Thus far, all the chromosomal abnormalities discussed involve either the addition or absence of an entire chromosome. A similar imbalance of the total chromosomal material can occur with cells containing the normal number of 46 chromosomes. This imbalance is the result of the absence of a portion of a chromosome, called a *deletion*, or the addition to a normal chromosome of extra chromosomal material called a *duplication*. Such alterations are shown in Figure 9. Some of these deletions occur with sufficient frequency to result in recognizable syndromes. This is particularly true of chromosomes 4, 5, and 18. These duplications and deletions may arise as a new event in the maturation of a single sperm or ovum and, thus, the resulting abnormality is restricted to a single child. Such events are very unlikely to recur in a subsequent child of the same couple, as this situation is somewhat analogous to the previously mentioned new dominant mutations. A parent may have a rearrangement of his or her chromosomes in such a way that, although the proper amount of genetic material required is present, an imbalance could recur in several children. Such a situation is shown in Figure 10. In this illustration, the mother has one of her number 21 chromosomes translocated to a number 15. She has only 45 chromosomes, but

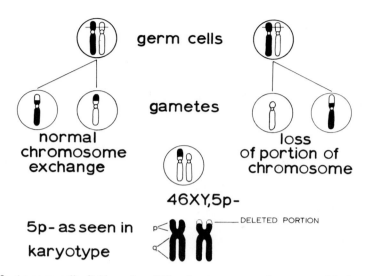

Figure 9. As germ cells divide, pairs of like chromosomes exchange material. An unequal exchange can result in an incomplete chromosome (a deletion). Severe consequences occur in the offspring.

one chromosome is composed of all the essential material from a number 15 and 21. Such an individual is called a translocation carrier. This does not produce an abnormal effect in such an individual because she possesses a full complement of genetic material. However, as shown in the diagram, as the ovum matures and reduces the chromosome number from 45 to 22 or 23 (normally from 46 to 23), an imbalance may occur when fertilization takes place. A pregnancy in such an individual may result in one of four possibilities: a normal child with 46 normal chromosomes, a normal child with 45 chromosomes who is a translocation carrier like the mother, an abnormal child with an imbalance of the chromosomes, or an abortion as a result of such serious derangement of fetal development that the pregnancy could not continue. Such possibilities hold for any pregnancy of a translocation carrier regardless of whether the carrier is a man or a woman.

CHROMOSOMAL MOSAICISM

The origin of the previously described chromosomal abnormalities is present prior to fertilization. Following fertilization, an imbalance may arise from one further mechanism. As the fertilized cell divides in the process of embryogenesis, loss or addition of an entire chromosome or deletion or duplication of a portion of a chromosome may result with any cellular division. If this occurs sufficiently early in the process of embryonic growth, the resulting imbalance can have a detrimental effect on subsequent development. This mechanism is shown in

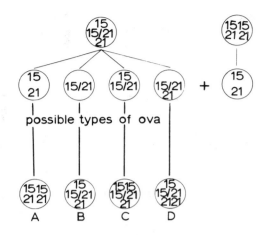

Figure 10. A number 21 chromosome is attached to a 15. This interferes with segregation of the chromosomes in division of the germ cells. After fertilization as shown in example *D*, the fetus has two number 21's and a third 21 attached to a 15.

Figure 11. Chromosomal analysis on such an individual after birth might disclose three different types of cells. Such a finding is called *mosaicism*. In the example shown, the error in chromosomal separation involved the number 21 chromosomes, and such an individual would demonstrate Down's syndrome. The effect on a patient with mosaicism may be less severe than is the case when all the cells contain three number 21's as usually seen in Down's syndrome. About 2.5% of children with Down's syndrome are secondary to a mosaicism. These children may have more intellectual potential than the usual trisomy 21 Down's syndrome.

AMNIOCENTESIS

Amniocentesis, as previously described for certain biochemical defects, can also be utilized to diagnose intrauterine chromosomal abnormalities in the fetus. As the occurrence of a genetic disorder which can be diagnosed prenatally by amniocentesis is an uncommon event, it is not presently practical to test all pregnancies. Selection must be made for those pregnancies which are at high risk for a chromosomal abnormality. The selection for amniocentesis is based on a high risk for a particular disorder that can be specifically tested for. As noted

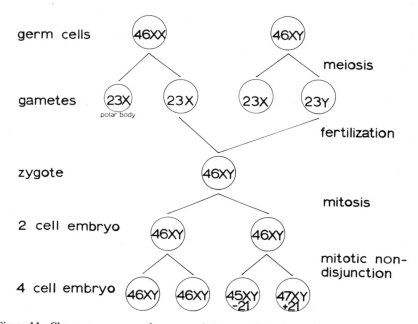

Figure 11. Chromosome separation proceeded normally in the germ cells but after fertilization an error occurred. Mosaicism refers to an individual with two or more populations of cells with different numbers of chromosomes.

earlier for the recessively inherited biochemical disorders, amniocentesis may be employed for the identification of a particular condition in a fetus among couples who have produced an affected child during a previous pregnancy, or more specifically, when both parents are known carriers for a lethal disorder, with a 25% risk of every pregnancy resulting in the disease in question. The carrier state for certain genetic disorders can be confirmed by reliable laboratory tests; however, there are serious limitations to carrier detection by testing programs. An example of a successful program for carrier detection and subsequent amniocentesis for couples at risk is that dealing with Tay-Sachs disease. Tay-Sachs disease is a rare (ultimately lethal) disorder that occurs much more frequently among Jewish infants than non-Jewish. The condition meets certain criteria that have made carrier detection and amniocentesis a practical reality:

1. The disorder is serious enough to warrant an abortion if diagnosis can be made prenatally. There is no effective treatment for infants born with this disorder.

2. There is a reliable blood test that will detect couples at risk. The testing can be performed economically enough to warrant large scale population screening. The cost of widespread screening programs is far less than the cost of providing care for the affected children.

3. The people to be tested have been partially selected by the high occurrence rate of the disorder among Ashkenazic Jews. Therefore, testing programs are directed at Jewish couples of child-bearing age.
4. The disorder can be accurately diagnosed prenatally.

There are many genetic disorders that meet some of these criteria, but because Tay-Sachs disease fulfills all the criteria, it is the only one at the present time for which a successful program has been established. Cystic fibrosis is a serious disease for which only partially effective treatment exists. People of northern European extraction have the highest frequency of the disorder. However, at the present time, techniques for carrier detection are on an experimental basis only, and prenatal diagnosis is not yet a practical reality. Sickle cell disease meets most of the criteria except that prenatal diagnosis has not yet been accomplished. Couples who are found through screening programs to have a 25% risk of having a child with sickle cell disease do not have the option of amniocentesis for prenatal diagnosis. This fact is partially responsible for some of the dissatisfaction with the results of sickle cell screening programs.

Among the chromosomal disorders, there are currently two types of criteria for the selection of pregnancies for which amniocentesis would be recommended. First, the progeny of individuals who are carriers of chromosomal translocations, regardless of whether the carrier is male or female, are tested. Couples are aware of this possibility by having had a child with an imbalanced translocation which might recur; a family member has a translocation and the rest of the family has been tested for other translocation carriers; or thirdly, the translocation may have been an incidental finding during a population chromosomal survey. Secondly, as the risk for Down's syndrome secondary to trisomy 21 increases with a woman's age, amniocentesis is currently recommended for any pregnant woman over the age of 40. At 20 years of age a woman has about one chance in 2,500 of having a child with Down's syndrome, but by the age of 45 the risk has risen to one in 40. This is true regardless of the husband's age.

It should be emphasized that while the alternative available to a couple as a result of an amniocentesis which discloses an affected fetus is an abortion, the purpose of such a program is to allow couples to have normal children when their risk of an affected child is so high as to preclude in their minds their having any children at all. At the present time, many couples who are found with a risk for which amniocentesis is recommended are identified by their having had a previously affected child, and knowledge of such weighs heavily on their future family planning.

SOCIAL AND EDUCATIONAL CONSIDERATIONS OF GENETIC DISORDERS

Genetic counseling provides information to a couple regarding their risks of having a child with a genetic disorder. As every couple faces some risk with any pregnancy they undertake (about 3% of all liveborn infants have a significant birth defect), counseling is provided to those couples who for one reason or another perceive their risk as greater than the population in general. Counseling is, therefore, directed at particular disorders or situations about which some factual information can be provided. It is the role of the counselor to provide this information in such a way that it will be usable by a couple as they consider their future family planning. Such counseling will not only involve risk figures, but interpretation of the alternatives that are available to couples. Such alternatives might include amniocentesis for a particular disorder, assistance with adoption, artificial insemination, or understanding and acceptance of a situation for which no action can be taken. It is, thus, apparent that such counseling is effective only when it provides couples with practical information and alternatives that are ethically and religiously acceptable to them.

A major problem confronting genetic counselors is a communication gap with those seeking counseling. Human biology as a subject in public school systems is sorely lacking. In the past, human biology has only been taught in medical schools. This has tended to create communication problems for all medical personnel in their exchange of information with the lay public. Human genetics has only recently been included in the curricula of most medical schools. Thus, a situation exists where geneticists are making great strides in technology and understanding of genetic influences in human disease, but lack of understanding of basic genetics by physicians outside the field of genetics, and by lay people in general, has restricted the application of this new information. When a couple present themselves for genetic counseling, the counselor often finds it necessary to spend a great deal of time providing them some basic knowledge of genetics. This is required for their better understanding of their child's disorder, but is of even greater importance if they are to appreciate the implications of such counseling in their family planning. Counseling, as the name implies, seeks to provide information on which others may make intelligent decisions. Proper use of this information and even the awareness of its availability require a better understanding of genetics by the public.

A further problem has been created by advances in genetic technology. As genetic information is put into practical use, it may raise questions of social and ethical concern. Proper answers require some sophistication of genetic knowledge by society. As an example of this issue, one need only remember the legal and ethical debates that followed the first heart transplants. The debate often involved governmental and religious leaders who were ill prepared for such problems. The capacity for mass testing of blacks for carriers of the sickle cell gene gave rise to legislation and programs which were poorly conceived and had to be rescinded.

Amniocentesis makes possible sex determination of the fetus at a time in pregnancy when abortion is legal. Whether this capability should be used to allow couples to abort a female if they desired a male has not been satisfactorily answered. Couples are making such requests, and there is no uniformity of response from medical institutions. Sterilization of individuals who might have defective offspring has been a topic of public debate. It seems appropriate for society to determine the proper use of genetic technology rather than have such technology applied simply because the capability exists. Such a realization makes readily apparent the need for improved methods of public education.

Each individual possesses a unique combination of genes. While each person prizes his singular constellation of features and attributes, he also finds consolation and reassurance through association with like persons. A great deal of individual variation may be present without interfering with one's social acceptance and respect of his personal dignity. These may, however, be unwittingly, yet cruelly, denied to persons whose variation from "normal" is such as to separate them from their peers. Misunderstanding about the cause and effect of genetic disorders has, in the past, tended to place unwarranted handicaps on persons with little more than cosmetic blemishes. Recognition that a cleft lip is no more of an indicator of one's potential than freckles has freed many such afflicted persons of unfair social stigmatization. Many dwarfs in the United States are members of Little People of America. One purpose of their organization is to assist one another with social problems they have in common. Despite their short stature, they refer to the height of taller individuals as "average." To consider taller persons as "normal" must mean that they are "abnormal." In truth, they are "less than average."

Until recently, the study of genetic disorders in man was almost a purely descriptive endeavor. As a result, there arose a terminology used in defining syndromes that was likewise purely descriptive. The same was true for all of medicine, so that a pathologist might describe a liver as having a nutmeg appearance and assume that his colleagues would find such a description helpful. The use of certain terminology, however, when applied to children, may have an unnecessarily demeaning effect. The term "mongolism" or "mongoloid" has been used for many years for children with Down's syndrome by lay and medical people alike. Compare the two following statements. "Johnny has Down's syndrome." "Johnny is a mongoloid." The former names a condition that Johnny has while the latter dehumanizes in suggesting that Johnny is a member of some subhuman species. Appropriate terms exist for genetic disorders, and their proper usage and understanding by physicians, teachers, and the general public will help insure each individual the dignity due his person.

SUGGESTED READING

Apgar, V., and J. Beck. 1972. Is My Baby All Right? A Guide To Birth Defects. Trident Press, New York. 492 p.
Bergsma, D. (ed.). 1972. Advances in Human Genetics and Their Impact on Society. Birth Defects: Original Article Series, The National Foundation— March of Dimes. Vol. VIII, No. 4. July, 1972.
Egg, M. 1964. When a Child is Different. The John Day Co., New York. 155 p.

Hunt, N. 1967. The World of Nigel Hunt. The Diary of a Mongoloid Youth. Garrett Publications, New York. 126 p.

McKusick, V. A. 1969. Human Genetics. 2nd Ed. Prentice-Hall, Inc., Englewood Cliffs, New Jersey. 221 p.

Slater, E., and V. Cowie. 1971. The Genetics of Mental Disorders. Oxford University Press, London. 413 p.

Smith, D. W., and A. A. Wilson. 1973. The Child With Down's Syndrome (Mongolism). W. B. Saunders Company, Philadelphia. 106 p.

The National Foundation—March of Dimes has pamphlets available for public education: The National Foundation—March of Dimes, 800 Second Avenue, New York, N. Y. 10017.

Pamphlets dealing with some specific genetic disorders are available from: National Institute of Child Health and Human Development, Landow Building, Room C-708, 7910 Woodmont Ave., Bethesda, Md. 20014.

11

Mental Retardation

Arnold J. Capute, M.D., M.P.H.

With the philosophy "rights of education for all children" about to be introduced on a national basis, it becomes mandatory that special educators and teachers develop sophisticated levels of awareness of the developmental disabilities. Special educators must acquire expertise in formulating and implementing programs to teach children with various types and degrees of physical and mental handicaps. Teachers in the regular classroom, especially in kindergarten and early elementary school, must become knowledgable about developmental deviations, since, as it will be shown later, the majority of children possessing mild mental retardation or a learning disability are usually not detected until confronted with kindergarten or first grade material. Children who are severely retarded, on the other hand, do not develop a mental age equivalent to the kindergarten or first grade level until adolescence. Teachers should also be aware that the presence of an educational handicap places the child at a high risk for possessing another handicap. If all handicaps are undiscovered, optimal educational programs cannot be implemented. For example, a child who is mildly retarded and has an associated significant hearing impairment will not receive maximum educational habilitation unless he is placed in a program which is devised to teach the deaf-retarded child.

Following World War II, the parents of the retarded organized associations on a national, state, and community basis (e.g., National Association for Retarded Children, NARC). These parents were most influential in persuading the school system to accept the responsibility for educating the retarded, focusing at that time upon the trainable (moderately) retarded child. Prior to this time, a significant number of these children were placed in residential care or given baby-sitting services, both of which were devoid of significant educational

This paper was supported in part through Project 917, Maternal and Child Health, United States Department of Health, Education, and Welfare.

programs. On the other hand, the educable (mildly) mentally retarded child was accepted as the school's responsibility, since these children could be taught basic subjects such as reading, writing, arithmetic, and spelling. Thus, the ultimate goal of social and economic independence was realistic and readily attainable. An optimal special educational program followed by a vocational training period could, subsequently, lead to a satisfactory placement in an occupation suitable to the mildly retarded child's abilities.

The 1970's will witness the extension of education to children with all levels of retardation. Traditionally, educators have focused upon preacademic and academic skills at the level of kindergarten or early elementary years. To meet future goals, they must become more knowledgable about the language, social, and adaptive potentials as well as the behavioral characteristics of children with various degrees of mental retardation, thus necessitating a furtherance of the training and an increase in the number of special educators for teaching these children.

This chapter will present an overview of mental retardation since it is a most important developmental disability not infrequently coupled with related disorders. Emphasis will be directed to children with variable degrees of retardation, with a description of their behavioral characteristics and mannerisms, as well as their future potential. While intelligence quotient (IQ) figures will be cited to indicate to the teacher the accepted classification of the mentally retarded, it should be pointed out that children will frequently cross over from one level to another depending upon motivation, sociocultural influences, parental attitudes, and the various community resources and activities that are available (i.e., day care centers, special education or resource classes, prevocational and vocational training programs, and social and recreational programs).

Other disciplines which may significantly contribute to the education and habilitation of the retarded will be referred to. This *interdisciplinary approach* is important, since retardation is commonly associated with other disabilities, such as hard-of-hearing, deafness, visual impairment, emotional instability, and other sensory or motor impairments.

The Developmental Disabilities Services and Facilities Construction Act of 1970 (P.L. 91-517) defines a developmental disability as a disorder "attributable to mental retardation, cerebral palsy, epilepsy, or other neurological handicapping conditions of an individual found to be closely related to mental retardation or to require treatment similar to that required by mentally retarded individuals. . . ." These conditions might well be placed along the spectrum of cognitive, perceptual, motor, and sensory abnormalities, frequently found in combination with one another. Teachers should be aware that of all the developmentally disabled children, approximately one-third have one handicap, another one-third have two, and the remainder have three or more handicaps. It is, therefore, essential for professionals and paraprofessionals to manage the handicaps in a *multidiscipline* fashion in order to render a wholesome educational program. In addition to education, the various disciplines which play an integral role in the developmental disability field include physicians (pediatricians, neurologists, orthopedists, and psychiatrists), pedodontics, genetics, psychology (including behavioral therapy and psychologic testing), audiology and speech, public health nursing, social service, physical therapy, occupational therapy, and nutrition.

It is important for members of each discipline to fully appreciate what the other may offer the patient and family in the way of diagnosis, evaluation, and management of therapy. For example, the educator should know that there are medications available to modify the hyperactive behavior frequently observed in the retarded child. In addition, there are reliable psychologic tests which correlate highly with prediction of school achievement and can provide assistance in implementing realistic educational programs to enhance the development of the limited perceptual cognitive abilities that the mentally retarded child possesses. Another example may be an understanding by the teacher of the limited value of the electroencephalogram (EEG), unless the child had a questionable convulsive disorder which the physician wishes to confirm. Educators should be aware that at least 10% of the population have an unusual EEG and that only the clinical manifestations are treated and not the EEG findings. This is an important point, as EEG's are expensive and often do not significantly contribute to the well being of a child unless there is a specific abnormality which the physician wishes to investigate, such as a convulsive disorder (see Chapter 4).

Thus, in the management, care, and habilitation of a retarded child, while education is a prime major discipline, suitable teaching programs cannot be offered unless the educator is appreciative of and engages in a *multidisciplinary or interdisciplinary* approach.

HISTORY

While mental retardation was known during biblical times and has been frequently noted in Greek and Roman literature, educators and physicians did not develop an interest in this area until the first half of the nineteenth century. This activity was initiated in France and Sweden, then spread to other civilized parts of Europe and, subsequently, to the United States.

J. E. Belhomme (1800–1880) was one of the first to advocate education for "idiocy" according to the degree of retardation. Others who contributed during the early years to the retardates' education were Johann Jacob Guggenbühl (1816–1863), who attempted to cure cretins (individuals with severe underactivity of the thyroid gland), Jean Marc Gaspard Itard (1774–1838), who spent 5 years striving to educate Victor, "the wild boy of Aveyron," at the turn of the eighteenth century, Jacob Rodriguez Pererie (1715–1780), who had limited success in an endeavor to educate a congenitally deaf mute, and Edouard Onesimus Seguin (1812–1880), a student of Itard, who dedicated his life to the investigation and education of the retarded.

Guggenbühl was the originator of the idea of institutional care for the retarded, and, thus, founded the first residential training center, Abendberg, with aspirations for the development of sensory perceptions in children afflicted with cretinism. This residential care center was located near Berne, Switzerland. Many current institutions throughout the world are direct descendants of Abendberg. Thus, Guggenbühl may be considered the father of institutional care and training for the mentally retarded (Kanner, 1964).

An American physician, Samuel Gridley Howe (1801–1876), was instrumental in establishing the philosophy that the public was responsible for training and educating the retarded. He devoted his life to developing methodologies for the education of blind and deaf mutes, as well as assisting others in working with the mentally retarded. He was responsible for establishing the Perkins Institution for the Blind which later included some retarded children. This led to the establishment of the Massachusetts School for Idiotic and Feeble-Minded Youth, which subsequently became the Walter F. Fernald State School at Waltham, Massachusetts. In a similar fashion to Guggenbühl's endeavor in Europe, Howe introduced residential training institutions for the mentally retarded in the United States.

While these residential institutions increased in number in this country during the late nineteenth and early twentieth centuries, it soon became evident that little success was being made in habilitating retarded children. It appears that the primary reasons for this failure were a lack of an interdisciplinary evaluation and management concept (since the majority of these children have more than one handicap), and the establishment of unrealistic goals for these individuals. An example of this might well have been Victor, "the wild boy of Aveyron," whom Itard treated as an educable child since it was assumed that the boy had been environmentally deprived by having lived in the wilderness throughout his life. In retrospect, many authorities suggested that Victor was retarded, abandoned by his family and that the more realistic goal would have been to educate him at the trainable level. If the child was indeed trainable, Itard was successful, for the boy's self-help, communicative, and social skills were enhanced (i.e., modern goals for habilitating the trainable mentally retarded were attained).

An important philosophy that currently exists for the retarded is the *habilitation in the community* movement (normalization principle). The national spearhead for this philosophy was the President's Committee on Mental Retardation during the administration of President John F. Kennedy. In addition to being adjacent to the family, the retardate has accessibility to the entire spectrum of education which is the preamble to successful habilitation. The latter includes the enhancement of self-help, communicative, and social skills, the fostering of perceptual development, special education programs according to the child's abilities, and prevocational and vocational training with proper job assignment. This accomplishment necessitates input from the various aforementioned biomedical and behavioral science disciplines. Thus, legislation evolved supporting the concept of habilitation in the community, and one act in particular, The Mental Retardation Facilities and Community Mental Health Centers Construction Act of 1963 (P.L. 88-164), led to the establishment of a limited number of university-affiliated facilities. The latter were to be established in close affiliation with universities so that behavioral and biomedical expertise would be available to support their primary mission—the training of professionals and supportive personnel who would render care to the handicapped child and family, particularly at the community level.

DEFINITION OF MENTAL RETARDATION

Prior to the late nineteenth and early twentieth centuries, children were classified as being retarded by an unusual physiognomy (facial appearance) and other peculiar physical features. Subsequently, there was the idea of one IQ for each person. Today it is fully recognized that there is no one IQ for any person, and that mental capacity is comprised of a number of cognitive and perceptual skills which can be tested by administering formal psychologic tests. Many take issue with using the IQ test as the sole criterion for depicting mental retardation. However, these tests do serve the purpose for which they were formulated, that is, prediction of school achievement.

A commission was appointed in 1904 by the Minister of Public Instruction in Paris to search for methods of differentiating between the normal child who could be educated in regular classrooms and those who would require special instruction. The French government was interested in devising unique educational methods and inaugurating special classes for instructing children who were unable to reach normal standards of educability. Alfred Binet, acting as a member of this commission, and Theodore Simon published a formal scale for the measurement of human intelligence in 1905. The Binet-Simon scales were translated into English in 1910 by Goddard. They were standardized on a population of mentally defective children in Vineland, New Jersey as well as normal children in nearby schools. These scales have undergone various modifications, and the current edition entitled the Stanford-Binet test has been in use since 1960. It forms an integral part of the psychometric battery employed in the evaluation of mentally retarded in many centers.

In 1973, the American Association on Mental Deficiency (AAMD) altered its definition of mental retardation deleting the borderline category. The current definition states: *"Mental retardation refers to significantly subaverage general intellectual functioning existing concurrently with deficits in adaptive behavior, and manifested during the developmental period"* (Grossman, 1973). It is most important for teachers to have a complete understanding of what this definition implies in order to understand the criteria for retardation in the preschool, school, and adult years.

"Significantly subaverage general intellectual functioning" refers to a developmental and intelligence quotient which is below 70 and represents two or more standard deviations (one standard deviation=15–16 IQ points) from the

mean or average of the population tested. The most frequently utilized techniques for determining the developmental quotient during the first 3 years of life include the Cattell, Gesell, and the Bayley tests. Even though these tests primarily focus upon sensorimotor skills, they are reliable predictors of the degree and eventual level of mental retardation (Illingworth, 1972). However, these infant developmental tests are not sensitive enough to prognosticate as to whether a child may be above normal or even superior in intellect. Their primary value in subnormal development is to ascertain levels of mental functioning as a prelude to proper educational program placement so that children may not be under- or over-challenged.

In older children, the standard tests employed are the Stanford-Binet (SB) and the Wechsler Intelligence Scale for Children (WISC), which are composed of a number of subtests quantitating various aspects of mental functioning. The WISC is reported with full scale, verbal, and performance IQ scores. This profile is a summation of 10 subscores, 5 verbal and 5 performance items (Table 1). If this profile is homogeneous, having average or above average scores, and does not show a variability in mental functioning, it is fair to assume that the child has the intellectual capacity for school achievement. Other nonmeasured factors, of course, must be considered, and include motivation, opportunity, emotional lability, social and economic elements. If there is a significant variability or scattering of the performance versus the verbal skills or within the subscores themselves, the child is at a high risk of having a *learning disability*. It should be stressed that the learning disability in the retardate refers to an overall significant depression of his cognitive and perceptual skills (global retardation), whereas the pupil with a learning disability shows a normal global intelligence but has specific perceptual-cognitive deficits which may preclude school achievement at his anticipated full scale IQ level.

The WAIS is the psychologic test for determining the intellectual capacities of the adolescent and adult (16 years and above).

The second portion of the definition, *"existing concurrently with deficits in adaptive behavior,"* implies that the individual lacks the personal independence and social responsibility expected for his age and cultural group. During infancy (1–2 years) and the preschool period (3–5 years), these deficits are measured by

Table 1. Wechsler Intelligence Scale

Verbal	Performance
General information	Picture completion
General comprehension	Picture arrangement
Arithmetic	Block design
Similarities	Object assembly
Vocabulary	Coding
Digit span (supplementary or alternate test)	Mazes (supplementary or alternate test)

developmental milestones in adaptive, language, and sensorimotor skills. Examples of the latter include the age at which infants and preschool children babble, use gesture language (wave "bye-bye" or play "pat-a-cake"), assist in dressing and undressing, button clothing, eat with a fork, utilize a table knife for spreading, or join in group play. In the school years, adaptive behavior is measured by academic achievement. In adulthood, it is gauged by social and economic adjustment, such as the ability to earn a livable wage at a competitive job and the ability to care for one's self or manage a family independently.

The third part of the definition, *"during the developmental period,"* defines the developmental upper age limit as 18 years.

Thus, for an individual to be considered as functionally mentally retarded, he should possess all three characteristics: (1) an IQ score of below 70 (two or more standard deviations from the mean), (2) manifested prior to 18 years of age, and (3) accompanied by impairments in adaptive behavior.

INCIDENCE OF MENTAL RETARDATION

Approximately 3% of the total population have IQ values below 70, according to the distribution of scores based on the normal probability curve of intelligence (Figure 1).

In the United States, there are approximately 6 million people functioning below an IQ level of 70. Of these, 89% or 5.5 million are mildly or educable mentally retarded, and tend to be found within the lower socioeconomic strata. The remaining 11% or 0.5 million comprise the trainable, severe, and profound mentally retarded groups. The latter are found in all socioeconomic levels and include most of the retarded population who have associated biochemical and chromosomal aberrations and other pathologic entities.

CLASSIFICATION AND PLANNING FOR THE RETARDED

The AAMD divides the retardate into four categories using two standard deviations below the mean or an IQ of less than 70 as significantly subaverage general intellectual functioning. Each category represents one standard deviation below this level. The mild or educable mentally retarded child has an IQ score of 69–55; the moderate or trainable mentally retarded (TMR), 54–40; the severe mentally retarded (SMR), 39–25; and the profound mentally retarded (PMR), less than 25 (Grossman, 1973).

The Educable Mentally Retarded

The prototype for the EMR group might well be the psychosocially or culturally deprived individual. The ultimate goal for the EMR is *social and economic*

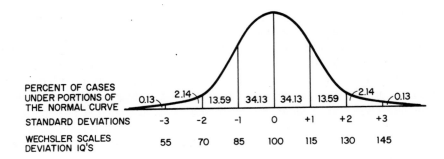

Figure 1. Normal probability curve for distribution of mental retardation.

independence, with special educators playing the dominant role in habilitation. A major problem is the early recognition of these children during infancy and the preschool years, since at this time they are not that far behind the average child. They are developing at a rate approximately one-half to three-quarters of normal, and are usually not identified until kindergarten or the first grade when confronted with academics or given IQ tests. Thus, teachers should be "tuned in" to early detection so these children may be channeled into proper educational resources.

The special educator plays a prominent role in the formative years of the EMR, preparing the child with the important academic and behavioral skills prerequisite for job training. At a later date, vocational habilitation intervenes to ready him for a suitable and profitable vocation with a smooth and comfortable integration into society. Successful vocational programming and placement depends a great deal upon the outcome of the educational program utilized in the EMR's habilitation. An unfortunate circumstance may occur when an EMR child is born into a professional family, for the parents may be unrealistic and reluctant to accept the child's educational handicap. The educator is pressured into giving social promotions within the regular class channel. The child cannot maintain the academic pace, falls behind, and does not reach his potential. In addition, this over-challenge becomes frustrating and, soon, unusual behavioral mannerisms develop which further compound his inadequate academic progression and, occasionally, may lead to inappropriate residential care placement.

One can readily agree that the EMR child should be transported in the same school bus as normally intelligent children and attend the same school, with special instructional resources being utilized for the EMR's education. It is most important that the educable child maintain social and recreational peer relations during auditorium, playground, and lunchroom activities with other children. This type of peer relationship is essential, for, with suitable habilitation, the EMR will later participate in social functions and job affairs along with the general population.

The EMR child will develop at a rate between one-half to three-quarters of normal, reaching a mental age of 8–12 years by the chronologic age of 16 years. By using the "rule of five" (subtracting 5 years from the mental age), one can convert the mental age (MA) into grade capacity (GC) or level at which the child will competently function. This may be represented by: GC=MA–5 (Dunn, 1963). Hence, educables are usually able to function ultimately at the third to sixth grade level. The majority will become literate (reading comprehension at fourth to fifth grade levels), and the educational goal, reading for information but not enjoyment, can be accomplished. Thus, the overall curriculum is aimed at the fourth grade, with few EMR's reaching higher levels. This is important, for, as adults in a competitive world, they must read the want ads for job seeking, which also requires filling out application forms, talking with employment counselors and future supervisors, getting to and from work, and developing and maintaining social activities. With adequate habilitation, approximately 80% marry, and they usually marry spouses with higher IQ's and have normal children (Charles, 1957).

When jobs are plentiful, the rate of employment for the EMR is fairly high. However, when there is a business recession, the reverse is true, and the incidence of unemployment increases (Dunn, 1963). Approximately 80% of the mildly retarded obtain employment primarily in semiskilled, unskilled, and domestic occupations. Males are readily employed as laborers, while female adults tend to obtain domestic pursuits. It has been reported that as many as 15–20% of educables are employed in skilled occupations (Johnson, 1968).

The EMR is entitled to the same rights that are extended to the population at large. They are in dire need of family planning, counseling, and guidance. For example, when married, the socioeconomic circumstances may be such that they are readily able to manage one or two children, while a third could lead to social or economic disaster. Thus, family planning should be conveniently available, so that they may avail themselves of this information and put into practice an appropriate regimen. The most applicable method is reversible contraception. The birth control pill has little or no place for the retarded female since it requires close supervision. The most suitable means of reversible contraception is the intrauterine device (IUD), which can be inserted in a nulliparous uterus (uterus never having had a pregnancy) and be retained.

With the integration of the retardate, it would be unwise and contraindicated to apply irreversible contraception or permanent sterilization to the educable group. It is possible that a divorce or death may ensue and, should irreversible procedures be employed, this might well be detrimental to the future matrimonial plans of the individual. The rights of the mildly retarded child have been infringed upon when the parents consent to an irreversible procedure, since there is a good possibility that he or she will eventually marry and want to conceive. Society has an obligation to the mildly retarded, to protect their rights and withhold sterilization until an age is reached at which they are capable of making this decision for themselves.

The Trainable Mentally Retarded

The trainable mentally retarded child develops at a rate between one-third to one-half of normal, reaching a mental age of 4–8 years by adulthood, hence precluding formal academic studies. While the educable child is frequently not discovered until confronted with academic work, the trainable youngster is readily identified by the parent or pediatrician during infancy or early childhood because of a severe developmental lag. Deviation of the normal language milestones is fundamental to detecting a child developing this slowly. Since development is sequential, the milestones lag at least one-half behind the normal rate. Thus, expected accomplishments that usually occur at age 2, such as 2-word sentences and a 50-word vocabulary, may not take place until 4 years of age. Motor and adaptive milestones, however, are more variable in their appearance because of environmental influence.

Since the TMR eventually attains a mental age of no better than 7 or 8 years, he remains illiterate as an adult. He is unable to read for information. However, the majority do possess the potential for developing functional reading and writing skills as additional means of communication. The latter provides a medium for protection from hazardous situations by heightening comprehension for stop-go signs, danger-men-at-work posters, beware-of-falling-objects warnings, the significance of a six-sided sign, and the meaning of red, green, and yellow. The goal for the TMR is enhancement of self-help, social, and oral communicative skills for living and working in a sheltered environment. While the EMR can function independently, the TMR will always require a supervisor (big brother or father figure) for assistance in activities of daily living.

Thus, it is difficult to envision the TMR child being transported on the same bus with the average child. The majority of children with moderate mental retardation are incapable of performing at the primary school level until they have reached their chronologic adolescent years. Therefore, these children cannot establish peer relationships with normal children, and their attendance in a regular school, whose classroom materials are geared to the average student, is totally inappropriate. These children, in addition, frequently have associated disruptive behavioral patterns. Their teachers must have some knowledge of behavioral modifying techniques or the assitance of a skilled psychologist to employ operant conditioning methods for successful management (see Chapter 12). Frequently, medication management can be successfully employed to extinguish untoward behavior.

Educators, once assuming the responsibility of teaching at all levels of retardation, must seek guidance from other disciplines so that instructional methods can be optimally employed. Since the goal set forth for the trainable and subtrainable child is enhancement of self-help, communicative, and social skills, the educational milieu must cross over into other disciplines such as occupational and behavioral therapy. Occupational therapy focuses primarily upon the amelioration of upper extremity function so that self-help skills may be maximized. This discipline possesses methods for improving dressing, undressing, toileting, and eating skills. The occupational therapists are also capable of testing the child's visuomotor abilities and, at times, are able to improve these skills, taking into consideration the overall mental functioning of the child as well as motivational and parental attitudes. A word of caution: there is to date no reliable data which indicate that an intensive visual or visuomotor perceptual training program can remediate or correct preexisting deficiencies. Two important questions must be answered before children are subjected to intensive perceptual training programs. Can perceptual deficiencies be significantly remediated, and, if so, can this improvement be carried over to the learning situation? At the present time, we do not know which auditory and visual perceptual abilities are required to learn to read, write, spell, or perform computational mathematics. This vital issue is not only applicable to the child with mental retardation but also to those with normal intelligence who have learning disabilities with a severe perceptual-cognitive dissociation with the perceptual abilities being much more deficient.

For personal hygienic reasons, a significant number of TMR females are unable to cope with menstruation, and, since the overwhelming majority of this group do not marry, irreversible contraception or permanent sterilization is available. For the female, a hysterectomy is the method of choice, since the menses are abolished but necessary hormonal activities are maintained, as the ovaries are not removed. While some gynecologists perform the operation in the premenstrual years, the majority wait until the onset of menstruation to be sure that the hormonal system is functioning properly. The male may undergo a vasectomy as a form of permanent sterilization.

The Autistic Child

Another group possessing severe perceptual and integrative disabilities consists of autistic children, who represent a type of mental retardation in which severe auditory perceptual deficiencies, particularly with receptive language (central auditory imperception), are primarily involved. These children are severely retarded in their ability to interpret auditory symbolization, and, thus, are unable to use language functionally. This inability to communicate and relate with others results in the child's living in a world of his own and developing self-stimulatory activities, such as head banging, rocking, finger play, and the twirling of various objects. The child's relation to environmental activities is modified, depending upon his other perceptual abilities, which are relatively much better. Other stereotype behavior patterns may arise. For example, a child functioning below the 30-month level of receptive language will frequently be echolalic. Since the autistic child is commonly below this language level, this parroting ability, if coupled with a relatively good auditory rote memory, enables the child to reiterate things said to him or to retain what was said and repeat it several days later. How unfortunate it is to observe such a child who hears an examiner state, "It's a beautiful day today, isn't it?", store this and several days later repeat the same sentence while it is raining. The latter demonstrates that the child was merely parroting and not comprehending what was said.

Some examiners mistakenly may judge these children to be normally intelligent because of their relatively better fine and gross motor skills, as well as isolated auditory or perceptual abilities, neither of which in themselves correlate with intelligence. As will be shown in this chapter, motor milestones are inferior to language skills as predictors of future intelligence. These children have what might be coined a "perversion of communication," for they do not utilize language for the reason it was established.

There is much to be learned about infantile autism, but it is pointless to use a label or special marker to segregate an entity or syndrome when therapeutic regimes or specific forms of preventive measures are unavailable. This entity has been known for over 30 years, and, thus far, there is no form of therapy that has been successful. The prognosis for the autistic child is compatible with his overall intellectual functioning; thus, one should recognize these children as displaying a type of mental retardation which exemplifies the most profound of all communicative disorders. Parents should be prevented from seeking a cure, and rather be given some assistance with behavior modification and other management techniques which are offered to the mentally retarded population.

These children appear to be part of a spectrum of cerebral dysfunctions, with the major disability a severe communicative disorder, coupled with Strauss syndrome-like mannerisms (Strauss and Lehtinen, 1947). These also occur in children with trainable, severe, and profound mental retardation who demonstrate communication problems which are compatible with their overall level of mental functioning (global IQ). This behavioral profile is also observed in children with minimal cerebral dysfunction (MCD), with or without a learning disability, but to a lesser degree, since their overall or global intelligence is normal.

The Strauss syndrome (Strauss-Lehtinen syndrome) is a behavioral profile manifested by children who have cerebral dysfunction on an organic basis. This disorder consists of hyperactivity, a spectrum of attentional peculiarities with short attention span on one side and perseverance on the other, emotional lability, low frustration tolerance, and distractibility. The syndrome is characteristic of children with MCD, which is frequently (50–65% of the time) associated with perceptual disabilities resulting in a learning disorder. A significant number of TMR children have organic brain damage and develop stereotype behavior which is an exaggerated or expanded form of the Strauss-Lehtinen syndrome. While MCD children are of normal intelligence and trainables are moderately retarded, both can be placed in sequence, with MCD pupils demonstrating major perceptual difficulties and mild cognitive deficiencies, while the TMR children have both major perceptual and cognitive discrepancies.

In addition, because of their relatively poorer communicative skills, a significant number of trainables and subtrainables develop certain behavioral characteristics which may be mistakenly interpreted as psychiatric in origin by professionals who are unfamiliar with the deviant behavioral patterns (head banging, biting, self-stimulation, etc.) found in this group. Thus, hope for a cure may be transferred unwittingly to the parents who then develop unrealistic, overly optimistic goals.

The behavioral psychologists can assist these children by modifying or eliminating the undesirable behaviors, thereby, facilitating home management as well as maximizing habilitation in day care centers, formal trainable classes, vocational training centers, sheltered workshops, and residential care facilities. At the present time, almost all of the TMR group are institutionalized by 45 years of age (Johnson, 1968).

The Severe and Profound Mentally Retarded

The severe (SMR) and profound mentally retarded (PMR) are more limited than the TMR in their abilities. It is important that their self-help, communicative, and social skills be enhanced and their social interactions remain optimal while at home, at the community day care center, or in a residential care facility.

The majority of biochemical and genetic disorders are discovered within the trainable, severe, and profound mentally retarded groups. These children tend to have certain physical characteristics in common, which consist of hirsutism (excessive amount of hair over the body), delayed bone growth, microcephaly (abnormal smallness of the head), malformed or dysplastic teeth, clinodactyly (medial or lateral curving of the finger or toe), and brachydactyly (abnormal shortness of the finger or toe).

ETIOLOGY OF MENTAL RETARDATION

The extent to which psychosociocultural and biologic (genetic, biochemical, and other deficits) factors act as a cause of mild mental retardation requires much more study, although there is some evidence which suggests the environment ultimately influences intelligence. This is important since educable retarded children might well be remediated by early intervention, if, in fact, their retardation is directly related to environmental deprivation. In all probability, day care centers will become readily available on a nationwide basis to assist mothers in obtaining employment to avoid being placed on welfare. Their preschool children may attend teaching day care centers which may emphasize preacademic skills and highlight visual and auditory perceptual training. The limit to which this nonspecific form of sensory-oriented training can be advantageous must be carefully scrutinized, so that these children are not overperceptualized from morning to night.

Approximately one-third of trainable and subtrainable individuals are retarded due to organic factors, the result of chromosomal and biochemical aberrations, certain infections in the pregnant mother (e.g., rubella or syphilis), brain anomalies, premature or small-for-date infants, and birth injuries. Birth injury appears to be a less important factor, since a number of studies have indicated that a malformation of the brain may give rise to an unusual gestational period as well as an abnormal labor, birth, delivery, and neonatal course.

Individuals with Down's anomaly or mongolism account for another one-third of the trainable and lower levels of intelligence. They are usually depicted as the prototype for the trainable group and are the most common clinical syndrome of mental retardation, explaining the significant numbers of children with Down's syndrome in trainable classes. The stigmata of these children include a short anteroposterior skull diameter along with a flattened occiput, a short neck with a low hairline, protruding tongue, broad nasion (upper portion of nose and forehead quite flat), mongoloid slant (upward slant) to the eyes with epicanthal folds, short stature, broad hands and feet with decreased muscle tone, and hyperextensibility of the joints. These children look like brothers and sisters due to their similar stature and facial characteristics. These distinctive features are caused by an increased amount of chromosomal material (see Chapter 10).

While children with Down's syndrome are regarded as amicable, fun-loving youngsters with a placid personality, studies suggest that from birth there is an ongoing degenerative process in some of these children, quite similar to Alzheimer's disease or presenile dementia, a form of brain atrophy which produces remarkable psychiatric and neurologic changes in afflicted adults. This process causes the Down's syndrome adolescent or adult to appear much older than his chronologic age and also to manifest changes in personality.

The remaining one-third of the TMR, SMR, and PMR individuals have unknown etiologic factors as a cause for their retardation. Continued research will undoubtedly discover additional causes of mental retardation within this group.

FUNCTIONAL DEVELOPMENTAL EVALUATION

In order for teachers to fully appreciate atypical, abnormal, retarded, or deviant development, they must become acquainted with recognized and pertinent developmental milestones in the motor, language, adaptive, social, and language areas. Growth and development take place in a sequential fashion, and, thus, the child at particular age periods performs certain tasks which have been standardized within the normal population. If development is followed in its various parameters, one notes that it occurs in an orderly fashion with simple, less integrated tasks taking place prior to more complex ones. For example, in the language area, normal infants will develop a social smile at 4–6 wks., coo by 2 or 3 months, babble before 6 months, use gesture language at 7–8 months, recite "mama" and "dada" appropriately by 9 months, say the first word before 1 year, and possess a vocabulary of a minimum of 50 words by 2 years of age, at which time the infant will utilize a 2-word sentence with a pronoun or noun accompanied by a verb (Table 2). Thereafter, the vocabulary repertoire increases tremendously, with psycholinguistic skills playing an important factor in language development.

If the child or infant is retarded in the language area, then sequential development will be altered proportionally. A child who is trainably mentally retarded and functioning at approximately 50% of normal (IQ 40–55), will have milestones progressing at a rate approximately one-half behind the norm, and, thus, will babble at 6 months, use "mama" and "dada" appropriately at 22 months, and not utter a 3-word sentence until 6 years of age. The adaptive, social, and motor milestones also follow a fairly predictable course; however, the motor milestones are less valuable in establishing the current developmental status as well as prognosticating future development, since there is some variability of the developmental age at which motor milestones appear, and two developmental milestones in particular, sitting and walking, not uncommonly appear at the average expected age in the retarded child.

Parents of retarded youngsters have a common tendency to overprotect their children, anticipating their wants and needs and disallowing them an opportunity to fend for themselves. This behavior prevents the child from attaining his highest functional level, particularly in the self-help, language, and social skills.

Table 2. Language Developmental Milestones

Age	Developmental Milestones
1 mo	Alerting response to sound (sound recognition)
4–6 wk	Social smile
4–5 mo	Orienting response to sound, voice, or noise (turns toward source of sound)
6–7 mo	Mature babbling ("ma-ma" and "da-da" inappropriately)
7–8 mo	Gesture language (waves bye-bye, plays pat-a-cake)
9–11 mo	Says "ma-ma" or "da-da" appropriately
11 mo	First word
12 mo	2-word vocabulary
14 mo	3-word vocabulary
15 mo	2–6 words; immature jargon
18 mo	2–20 words; mature jargon (with several intelligible words)
21 mo	2-word phrases
2 yr	50 plus word vocabulary; 2-word sentences using pronoun (inappropriately) or noun and verb
30 mo	Uses pronouns and prepositions appropriately
3 yr	250 plus word vocabulary; 3-word sentences; forms plurals
42 mo	Understands and will follow at least 3 prepositional commands
5 yr	Able to follow 3-step commands in correct order; asks questions about the meaning of words

Significant strides can be made in these areas by working with the child and the family.

It is recommended that the educator not only become acquainted with the language milestones which are found in Table 2, but also with the social, gross motor, and manipulative skills which are necessary for self-care development (Capute and Biehl, 1973).

The language milestones listed in Table 2 are utilized at the John F. Kennedy Institute during parent interviews and have been found to be most useful in ascertaining the mental age level. These milestones have been well standardized and are an overall compilation of ones proposed by Cattell (1940), Gesell and Amatruda (1941), Illingworth (1972), Sheridan (1960), and others notable in the field of developmental pediatrics. They can be readily transferred into an appropriate question for the parents to answer, and careful evaluation of the sequence at which various components of language developed will be useful as one important indicator of the level of intellectual potential.

CONCLUSION

This chapter has presented an overall view of mental retardation to provide teachers and special educators with some guidelines as to the importance of the educator's role in the total habilitation programming of children with mild, moderate, and severe intellectual disabilities. The educational goal of children with mental retardation is to allow the child to reach his potential in the academic skills, so that his vocational achievement and job placement will be most appropriate for his abilities. In habilitating the trainable child, educators must become knowledgable with the techniques of other disciplines and utilize them in maximizing the self-help, oral communication, and social skills of their pupils.

REFERENCES

Capute, A. J., and R. F. Biehl. 1973. Functional developmental evaluation: Prerequisite to habilitation. Pediat. Clin. N. Am. 20:No. 1, 3–26.

Cattell, P. 1940. The Measurement of Intelligence of Infants and Young Children. The Psychological Corporation, New York. 274 p.

Charles, D. C. 1957. Adult adjustment of some deficient American children. Am. J. Ment. Deficiency, 62:300–304.

Dunn, L. M. 1963. Educable mentally retarded children. In L. M. Dunn (ed.), Exceptional Children in the Schools, pp. 53–127. Holt, Rinehart and Winston, Inc., New York.

Gesell, A. L., and C. S. Amatruda. 1941. Developmental Diagnosis. Paul B. Hoeber, Inc., New York. 447 p.

Grossman, H. J. 1973. Manual on Terminology and Classification in Mental Retardation. Garamond/Pridemark Press, Baltimore. 180 p.

Illingworth, R. S. 1972. Development of the Infant and Young Child, Normal and Abnormal. 5th Ed. The Williams & Wilkins Company, Baltimore. 377 p.

Johnson, G. O. 1968. Special education for the mentally retarded. Pediat. Clin. N. Am. 15:No. 4, 1005–1016.

Kanner, L. 1964. A History of the Care and Study of the Mentally Retarded. Charles C Thomas, Publisher, Springfield, Ill. 150 p.

Sheridan, M. D. 1960. Developmental Progress of Infants and Young Children. Her Majesty's Stationary Office, London. 11 p.

Strauss, A. A., and L. E. Lehtinen. 1947. Psychopathology and Education of the Brain-Injured Child. Grune & Stratton, Inc., New York. 206 p.

12

Classroom Evaluation, Management, and Organization For the Mentally Retarded

Michael Bender, Ed.D.

The traditional role of the special educator has long been a multidimensional one. Included among the many responsibilities of the teacher has been the necessity for acting as the evaluator, behavior manager, and classroom organizer. While many educators have relied on commercially prepared curriculum material, programmed instruction, and prepared courses of study, many have developed their own materials and have utilized them quite effectively. The theory that retarded children can be educated in terms of treating them as groups and planning lessons accordingly has tended to confuse many beginning teachers and educators who quickly lose sight of children's individual differences. The time-honored cliché that it is not what is taught but how it is taught has also undergone close scrutiny in most recent years, as educators will strongly agree and as vehemently disagree with the way educational objectives are being implemented.

Most often, it is assumed that the individual working with a handicapped population is well qualified, but this is not always the case. Certification requirements for teaching the mentally retarded vary from state to state (Balow, 1971), and, as of now, only a few states have any certification requirements at all for teachers of the severely or profoundly handicapped.

Another assumption is that the educational material being presented to the mentally retarded population has been piloted, tested, and proved to be effec-

This paper was supported in part through the United States Office of Education Grant for Special Education Programs in University Affiliated Facilities and the Joseph P. Kennedy, Jr. Foundation.

tive. Again, this has not always been substantiated. A more common practice is the finding that commercially prepared programs are being used in school systems without prior thorough testing based on objective standards, including monitoring and close follow-up studies.

The teacher who assumes the responsibility for teaching a class of children does so knowing that she will strive to do her best. Despite this dedication there are many teacher failures in all areas of education. In analyzing these failures, it has been found that unsuccessful teachers do not really know enough about the individual children with whom they are working. Attempts at gaining information often have been hindered by bureaucratic and administrative paper work, and, on many occasions, there appears to be insufficient time to investigate all available data on a particular child.

Educational theories also impede and obstruct the success of teachers. One hypothesis suggests that the more that is known about the individual and the more information assembled and effectively utilized, the greater the ultimate understanding of that child. This especially appears to be true when dealing with the severely handicapped child where it might be imperative that specific learning rates and past accomplishments are recognized. Another theory is based on the assumption that the child will tell the teacher all she needs to know about him in due time. People believing the latter suggest that prior knowledge of a child may bias the teaching process and act as a self-fulfilling prophecy. The fallacy of this criticism is especially obvious in teaching the more severely handicapped population. Many times this group will be unable to communicate with their teachers as freely as would a population of higher functioning individuals, and in essence, previous records may be a very valuable resource.

One method of gaining information is to utilize educational tests (Ashlock and Stephens, 1967). While most teachers are able to review psychologic test scores, hearing and speech reports, and other relevant information concerning their students, they tend to rely most heavily on educational assessments which might help them plan their program. However, it has become increasingly difficult for the classroom special teacher to depend on yearly educational assessments before she refines her program. The educator realizes that this must be done on a continual basis so that programs may be restructured and behavioral objectives restated. Teachers of the severely or profoundly retarded may have to rely on their own informal testing to establish baselines and develop appropriate curriculum material.

EDUCATIONAL ASSESSMENT

Most lay people tend to interpret how a child is progressing in relation to a continuum of grades (see Table 1). While this is a reasonable chronology for the normal student, it is quite different for the child who is mentally retarded. The rate of development of the mentally retarded child is critical, and curricula must

Table 1. Continuum of Grades

Age (yrs.)	Grade	Activities
3	Nursery	Pre-readiness, play
4	Nursery	Pre-readiness
5	Kindergarten	Readiness
6	First	Reading, arithmetic, social skills, etc.
7	Second	Reading, arithmetic, word discrimination, problem solving, etc.

be adaptive and flexible enough to allow for educational lags and developmental rate plateaus, as well as for academic growth spurts. The child who has been classified as educably mentally retarded (EMR) or mildly retarded demands a curriculum quite different from that of a child who has previously been called the slow learner or the student who is experiencing some difficulty in school. In the same manner, the pupil who has been classified as trainable or moderately retarded (TMR) requires a totally different curriculum than the educably mentally retarded child. The severely (SMR) and profoundly retarded (PMR) are in need of curriculum and method changes which have not yet been totally developed. Many educators are still hesitant to accept the retarded population as an integral part of the regular spectrum of education.

What type of testing then is effective for children whom the teacher suspects as being in need of help? Is she capable of administering these particular measures? If so, what can she derive from the results of these tests for her curriculum planning? All of these questions are critical ones for the teacher who is working with a mentally retarded population. Initially, a teacher will look toward a formal measure as a means of accurately assessing how a particular student is functioning. While there are many tests commercially available, few offer the teacher suggestions as to how to alleviate the weaknesses the test has documented. It is the educator's responsibility to chart the strengths and weaknesses as evidenced by test results and plan a corresponding program of remediation. Table 2 will offer the teacher some suggestions as to the type of formal tests she may wish to investigate for future information.

For example, the assessment of a 10-year-old child in a class for educably mentally retarded may involve testing in readiness areas. Readiness refers to those areas which give an indication as to how the child might educationally function were he required to perform first grade academic work. Included on this particular test would be an evaluation of a child's listening skills. He would be required to listen to statements which would vary in complexity and length, and then be asked to select an appropriate response. He may also be given a picture vocabulary test which may check on the extent of his oral vocabulary. Readiness testing has been used extensively in kindergarten classes where formal

Table 2. Suggested Areas in Formal Testing

Area	Test
Early development	Minnesota Pre-school Scale
	SRA Pre-primary Profile
	Bayley Scales of Infant Development
	Denver Developmental Screening Test
Readiness	Metropolitan Readiness Test
	Lee-Clark Reading Readiness
	Murphy-Durrell Diagnostic Reading Readiness Test
	Harrison-Stroud Reading Readiness Tests
Achievement	Metropolitan Achievement Test
	Stanford Achievement Test
	Iowa Test of Basic Skills
	Wide Range Achievement Test
	California Diagnostic Test

group readiness tests are administered and used as one source of predicting success in first grade. Other areas to be included on a formal battery would include the matching and copying proficiency of a child, which encompasses his visual perceptual skills as well as his motor control utilized in handwriting. Two of the major readiness areas the teacher should be familiar with include those of numbers or arithmetic skills and knowledge of the alphabet. These two skill areas have been suggested as being very important indicators of success in first grade.

For the child who cannot be tested formally or who is not at the stage of readiness, other problems are posed. This child may very well be functioning at a 2-, 3- or 4-year level educationally. While there are many psychologic tests, such as the Binet, Wechsler Intelligence Scale for Children (WISC), Cattell, and the Gesell, to test children's intelligence levels, the teacher is usually unable to interpret the results or functionally use them. The teacher may opt to informally test these students. Informal testing has undergone considerable criticism during the past years. The argument has long been that informal testing is based on subjective measures which can be different from evaluator to evaluator and that few standards are utilized. Advocates of informal testing suggest that these evaluations can be beneficial if they are obtained by first setting out educational guidelines based on standardized developmental levels. As an example, the educational milestones of a child functioning at a 4-year level may include the ability to count two objects out of a number of objects or select the biggest or smallest from a number of items. A 4-year-old child should be able to tell his age, know the difference between morning and afternoon, name at least three or more colors, and point to his major body parts. These children are expected to button and unbutton, zip and unzip, and lace their shoes. A student who is functioning at this age level should also be able to hold a pencil in his hand and copy a circle. He may very well imitate and copy a cross and crudely draw a man on request. In administering an informal measure, the evaluator must be particularly careful to be as objective as possible. Before indicating that a child's drawing of a man is immature, the examiner must make certain that he is considering keys or samples which offer accurate comparisons of similar age groups.

If a teacher realizes that her student is not progressing in these developmental areas, she should refer him for professional diagnostic testing as soon as possible. It is equally important for the teacher who is assessing children who are in the severely and profoundly retarded range to be aware that many of these individuals possess skills which are encompassed on infant tests (Alpern and Kimberlin, 1970). It is, therefore, no longer appropriate to state that a child who may be functioning in this profoundly or severely retarded range is untestable.

In presenting this very brief overview of the educational assessment of a child, it is important that priority areas in need of remediation be incorporated within the curriculum. The fact has been stressed that information obtained from many formal and informal evaluations may be functional and can be incorporated into an educational program, making it more meaningful and relevant.

CURRICULUM OBJECTIVES AND MATERIALS

In analyzing the curriculum objectives for a specific population of exceptional children, it is important that one considers the functional value of such objectives. While it may be possible to teach alphabet and letter recognition skills to a child who has been classified as moderately or severely retarded, one would wonder about the functional value of such a skill when the vast majority of these children will not be able to formally read. Curricula for the trainably mentally retarded have often been developed by persons who have been prepared to teach the educably mentally retarded. The idea that an EMR curriculum can be "watered down" and made appropriate for trainable children is not only a fallacy but may very well be harmful to the trainable student who must suffer through the frustration of not understanding what is being required of him. The educably mentally retarded population has received the most emphasis curriculum-wise over the last several decades and is summarized as follows.

Educably Mentally Retarded

As has been previously noted, any curriculum should be based upon the interests, capabilities, and needs of those individuals who will be receiving the instruction. As much as possible, the educational setting should promote personal and social growth and help a child become ready for society. A major goal for the EMR child has been toward developing social and economic independence.

In most school systems, there are classes for the educably mentally retarded which may be subdivided into three groups. These would include the primary group consisting of children ranging in age from 6–9 years; the intermediate group, 9–13 years; and an advanced group, 13 years and older. The curricula which would be relevant for these types of children have been documented in many publications and resource guides throughout the years (Kirk, 1972). As an example, in the area of reading, children in the younger grades would be offered a pre-reading program, including pre-readiness and readiness skills of listening, observing, talking, and imitating. They may be exposed to some very simple sight vocabulary words and introduced to word attack skills. They also would study a protective vocabulary based on words they would functionally need to know. The ultimate goal for reading achievement of the EMR may be at a fourth to sixth grade reading level. While this educational goal may appear quite advanced for this population of children, many never attain these goals but still manage to blend into society and become very productive members. Therefore, academic emphasis for this population is placed on functional reading. This would include the ability to read the newspaper, write and read letters, read simple books, magazines, or catalogs. These reading skills would hopefully be incorporated into future job activities such as the ability to read employment forms, work memoranda, or work schedules.

In the area of arithmetic, the educably mentally retarded may be expected to learn and utilize number concepts ranging from the number recognition stages to number concepts employing three-place digits. These students are usually able to sequence numbers and count by twos and threes and functionally use these skills in society.

The educable child is able to use and understand most coins and money concepts. He may master the ability to tell time and use measurement information functionally. The children who advance through arithmetic processes are able to start with very basic addition facts and work up to simple multiplication tables and division problems. The EMR with reading and arithmetic skills at the fifth or sixth grade level is, of course, much more likely to maintain employment.

Thus, the educably mentally retarded child may, with appropriate education, achieve vocational and social skills which would contribute to his support. At present, this has become increasingly more difficult due to the current economic problems of our country. The jobs previously available to the EMR are now being filled by the worker who has been terminated from his regular employment. The EMR requires considerable guidance and assistance in arriving at critical decisions and will need to know that advice and supervision will be available.

The EMR has been defined as functioning at one-half to three-fourths that of normal (Kirk, 1972). It is important that the overzealous educator does not lose sight of this fact. Many times the child will, with apparent ease, achieve goals in select areas, and this is taken as a sign that he is really normal and not of educable intelligence. These children must be closely monitored as behavior problems tend to be created when they are placed in stress situations or become frustrated by academics above their level.

Research studies have indicated that many of today's EMR programs are not successful (Guskin and Spicker, 1968). Many children appear to benefit from placement in a regular class with additional educational support. This has been referred to as mainstreaming an EMR child. There is still, however, a great need for EMR classes. It is imperative, therefore, that, if educable classes are to exist, the information presented in these classes be relevant, practical, and of functional value for this particular population.

Trainably Mentally Retarded

The objectives of the curricula for the trainably mentally retarded or moderately retarded have undergone close scrutiny over the past several years. Courses of study have recently been initiated in many colleges and universities specifically in the area of teacher education for the trainably mentally retarded. In analyzing the objectives of a curriculum for trainable children, they can best be divided into several key areas. These are as follows: (1) developing self-care and self-help; (2) developing communication; (3) developing gross motor skills; (4) developing fine motor skills; (5) social adjustment in society, home, and neighborhood; and (6) functional academics.

For each of the above areas, the child who is functioning as trainable is basically performing at a rate of one-third to one-half that of normal. Therefore, a child who is chronologically 8 or 9 years of age may be performing educationally at a 3- to 4-year level. Formal measures have defined trainables as having IQ's ranging from 30–35 to 50–55. In adulthood, the trainably mentally retarded child develops at the same rate and, thus, educationally may function as a normal child of 5–8 years of age. In all likelihood, the child who is trainable will not acquire sufficient skills in the academic areas associated with traditional schooling. TMR's are individuals who usually will be unable to meet any standards for literacy (reading at a fourth to fifth grade level), and are not educable in the academic sense in that they are unable to profit from an academically oriented school program. In adulthood, the trainably mentally retarded require continual supervision. Many will assume job responsibilities as part of a sheltered workshop program or be a participant in a work study program which may originate in the school. Specific examples of objectives for the TMR may be found in Table 3.

Severely and Profoundly Retarded

The severely and profoundly retarded tend to develop at a rate which is below one-third normal. This population of individuals usually has poor motor development, speech is minimal, and they are generally unable to profit from many

Table 3. Examples of Educational Areas for the Trainably Mentally Retarded

Self-Care	Gross Motor	Fine Motor	Communication	Socialization	Functional Academics
Toilet skills	Rolling	Picking up objects	Gestures	Community helpers	Labels on clothing
Cleanliness	Pulling to stand	Grasping	Facial expressions	Eating in a restaurant	Printing name
Grooming	Walking	Buttoning/unbuttoning	Expressive oral language	Safeguarding self	Survival words
Eating and drinking	Avoiding obstacles	Snapping/unsnapping	Receptive oral language	Working with peers	Concepts of first, next, last
Health habits	Closing doors and windows	Tracing	Vocal-tone patterns	Behavior in community	Counting objects

objectives and activities which are outlined in a curriculum for the trainably retarded (Geddes, 1974). While, in the past, this population has been relegated to institutional care, this is no longer true. Recent legislation and class action suits have utilized this population as test cases in demanding rights to education. Many of these children are now being admitted to public school programs throughout the country in classes for subtrainables. For this population, education is not the typical reading, writing, and arithmetic, but includes areas such as self-care, ambulation, toilet training, and modifying inappropriate behaviors. The severely and profoundly retarded appear to be especially adaptable to the use of behavior modification techniques, and many such programs have been incorporated both in private and public facilities. Many severely and profoundly retarded children demonstrate characteristics which make their curriculum a difficult one to develop and implement. Bradtke, Kirkpatrick, and Rosenblatt (1972) have stated that the profoundly retarded exhibit a diminished awareness of themselves, others, and their environment, as well as a lack of response or an inability to cope with tactile, auditory, or visual stimuli.

Of necessity, many parts of the curriculum for the severely or profoundly retarded must begin at infant activity stages. Thus, the procedures of learning to roll, walk, and stand, as well as creeping and crawling, may be important skills to be taught over a prolonged period of time. Webb (1969) has stated that profoundly retarded individuals present gross underdevelopment in four general areas of behavior: (1) level of awareness, (2) movement, (3) manipulation of the environment, and (4) posture and locomotion. It, therefore, becomes increasingly difficult for the teacher to plan appropriate activities for this population if she has not been specifically trained in the management and education of these children.

Suggestions have been offered concerning the curriculum for the severely and profoundly retarded which would encompass all those skills which are essential for communication, ambulation, and self-care (Webb, 1969). For example, in planning the program for the severely and profoundly retarded to raise their level of awareness, the classroom teacher may wish to stimulate their senses of taste, vision, and touch. This can be done with such activities as drying faces or hands with a towel, hair brushing, following a flashlight, or gesturing and uttering sounds. In essence, the teacher attempts to alert the children to external stimuli. They can also be exposed to extreme odors or temperatures, and they appear to be receptive to mirror and water play activities. In the area of improving movement, the child may be assisted in rolling over or raising his head. Many of these activities work well with music, which tends to interest the child as well as motivate the teacher. Many fine motor skills such as reaching, grasping, and developing holding techniques are required to improve manipulation of the environment.

While much of the curriculum currently utilized in institutions or residential facilities for this population has focused upon vast numbers of students, educators today find themselves in the position of teaching available objectives based upon a 1:3 or 1:5 teacher to pupil ratio. No longer can it be said that education cannot or should not be offered to a severely retarded child because he is unable to profit from the regular educational program. However, innovative educational programs for this population must be developed which will allow a retarded child to develop to his greatest potential.

In summary, some of the curriculum considerations for the three major types of mentally retarded children have been examined. It must be emphasized that, while many of these activities are geared to the ambulatory mentally retarded, many are also available for use with the child who is nonambulatory and nonverbal and who may very well constitute a significant population increase in public schools during the coming years.

CLASSROOM MANAGEMENT AND ORGANIZATION

It has long been thought by some educators that the teacher of the special class has a strong advantage in being able to work with fewer numbers of students than the traditional elementary or secondary school teacher. The pupil to teacher ratio has continually been the source of many pedagogic arguments and has in itself acted as a barrier between the special teacher and the regular teacher. Those who have taught in special classes find it difficult to believe that the need for a lower teacher to pupil ratio is not obvious. The lament of many special educators has been that they receive the students who are unable to profit from the regular grades. These students may not only be academic failures but behavioral failures as well. While many tend to think of special education in terms of the trainable and, perhaps most recently, the severely retarded, the majority of special educators are associated with children of educable intelligence whose inability to cope with peers may add to the pupils' reasons for unsuccessful classroom performance.

Physically, the special classroom in itself can take many forms. There have been periods of tightly structured physical settings, open spaced settings, and a combination of both. The approaches employed in these classrooms have also run the gamut from very traditional in nature to very free ones. Whether or not recent eclectic attempts at combining methods and physical settings are effective is still under considerable scrutiny and discussion.

The physical structure of the room for educably mentally retarded may differ in space considerations, but many times appears to be organized according to the nature of academic work expected of this population. EMR classes may be self-contained, used as resource classes, or function as part of an open space program. Maximum use of instructional aids and materials and the level of curriculum dictates the type of apparatus and equipment used. Today it is not unusual to find many EMR classes employing methods typically utilized in the regular grades. An example of this is individual learning stations which have recently become quite popular within the EMR class. The classrooms for these children are usually decorated with the thought of reducing stimuli. The physical surroundings of the EMR classroom tend to allow freedom for the child and yet, at the same time, provide structure. The academic areas require a variety of audiovisual aids and support devices.

In the physical arrangement of the class for the trainable child, once again it is noted that structure tends to be the key word. Many classes have prearranged areas in which to undertake self-care of dressing skills, toileting independence, and related activities. Much use is made of various sized tables in addition to the more traditional classroom desks. Again, it is important to note that the curricula for the TMR child in essence dictates the type of physical arrangement of the classroom. Chairs and desks would not be lined up in the customary rows if the major objective for the morning was to teach feeding and dressing skills.

In the area of classroom arrangement for the severely and profoundly retarded, major renovations of the physical setting are imperative. Such examples would include handbars by drinking fountains, ramps by steps for wheelchairs or children on crutches, modification of furniture which would allow children with braces to sit, and the addition of many nonskid floor coverings for children who are just beginning to learn to ambulate. In most states, a child can no longer be omitted from a public school program for the handicapped or retarded because he or she is not toilet trained. Toilet training has now become an integral part of the curriculum and, therefore, the physical arrangement and organization of the classroom must reflect this.

There are many behavior intervening techniques which are in existence today. There are several traditional ones, however, which have been most effectively used by teachers for many years. Rather than interpret each of the terms found in behavior modification literature, it is important that the teacher understand what he or she can implement in a classroom setting. Three major premises have dictated the need for a flexible but realistic behavior modification program. These are as follows. (1) Many schools are not physically equipped to handle the procedures employed in implementing behavior modification techniques. As an example, few classes have time-out booths, charting materials, or equipment for recording the frequency of occurrence of behaviors. (2) Teachers may not be knowledgeable enough in the techniques of behavior modification, and qualified approaches may be less effective. (3) Many methods which today are labeled under the umbrella heading of behavior modification have been successfully utilized for many years in the classroom. Many teachers have effectively used reward and punishment, as well as ignoring techniques, in formulating their classroom management plans.

It is important to emphasize once more that many school discipline problems in regular classes, as well as special education classes, are the direct result of an inappropriate curriculum. If the teaching levels are beyond the comprehension of the students, or, in some cases, on too low a level, frustration and poor motivation may add to the management problem (Van Til, 1956).

Swanson and Jenkins (1969) charted sentiments which were typical of children in the classroom. These responses continue to constitute a major framework of many classroom management programs and are especially relevant today. Examples are included in Table 4. As can be seen in the table, the likes and dislikes of children are important considerations when developing any type of classroom management program. With new populations of special students gradually being assimilated into the school system, the teacher needs more and more skill in the organization and systematization of her classroom. A major learning assumption which often goes unnoticed is that children who are introduced into a classroom learn to *misbehave* as well as to *behave* in this setting. The teacher must be cognizant of all her actions and responses for they are quickly imitated and easily distorted.

What then are the major approaches which can be used to help manage the classroom? Techniques utilizing praise, ignoring, reinforcement, and punishment all have been quoted in behavior modification literature and have long been a standard part of the repertoire of the good classroom teacher. In analyzing the actions of children, the teacher often may not witness what immediately precedes or follows an unacceptable behavior. Punishment or reinforcement is sometimes introduced at the inappropriate time and for the incorrect act. It is important, therefore, that the teacher becomes an accurate observer of behaviors. While it is more difficult when class size is large, the teacher must make herself acutely aware of the student's actions. When a child performs a behavior which is unacceptable to the teacher, she must immediately analyze what followed that behavior. As an example, when a very small baby begins to cry and puts his arms out for his mother, the mother picks up the child. In essence, she is rewarding the child for crying by making the consequence immediately following the crying a very positive one. When a consequence immediately follows a behavior and the behavior then occurs more frequently, it is defined as an accelerating consequence (Sheppard, 1973). A classroom example of this would include the child who is doing well in an activity and receives praise from the teacher. The child will usually continue or increase what he is doing well for a variable period following the commendation. Praise, therefore, can be a very effective method of controlling a child, particularly when it is appropriate that the child continue in the same activity. It does, however, soon loose its effectiveness if it is offered on a continuing basis. It is, therefore, incumbent

Table 4. Likes and Dislikes of Children

What Children Like	What Children Don't Like
The teacher who is for the child	Hollering
Loyalty	Being ridiculed
Honesty	Ridicule of the family
Frankness	Having too much expected of them
Willingness to listen	Grudges
Protection of property	Threatening
Strictness	Continually talking
An outgoing teacher	Criticism of other teachers

upon the teacher to decide how often she shall praise a child for participating in an appropriate act or for exhibiting suitable behavior.

The classroom teacher may wish to utilize a *preferred activity* in helping to manage her class. For instance, the teacher might offer a child who refuses to follow her directions something he would like to participate in if he will adhere to her wishes. This has been quoted in the literature as the *if-then* technique, where "if" you do something, "then" you may take part in a preferred activity. Preferred activities are those which a child will participate in when he has free time. It is, therefore, important that the teacher carefully observe how a child behaves or what toys he plays with during free time and then make note of these activities as possibly representing his favorite or most cherished.

One effective technique a teacher might use in aiding the control of a classroom is ignoring. As has been mentioned, when the teacher wishes to accelerate a consequence she may praise it or offer the student preferable activities. When the educator wishes to decrease a behavior, she may employ the reverse and totally ignore it. An illustration might include several children in the room raising their hands and shouting out answers. In this situation the teacher should disregard those pupils who may be shouting at her and direct attention to a child whose behavior she may want the other children to model. *Ignoring techniques are very important in the special education classroom.* They cease to be effective when they are overused or applied to behavior that is so extreme it is unaffected by the ignoring method. Knowing when to ignore as well as recognizing when to praise becomes an art that the teacher develops with experience. Its use depends highly upon timing, the situation, and teacher confidence.

One of the best methods to slow down or eliminate a behavior which the teacher finds unproductive is to diminish or exclude its accelerating consequence. Such an example is the child who, in striving for attention, behaves like the classroom clown. While it takes a concerted effort on the part of the teacher and the class, the behavior will tend to gradually decrease and may eventually be eliminated if the child is not laughed at or reinforced for his actions. It is important to remember that children seek variety in the type of reinforcement they receive; thus, it is advisable to diversify accelerating consequences for effective behavior control.

A major technique for modifying the behavior of a disruptive child is the time-out procedure. This form of intervention is basically a social isolation which is accomplished for a very short period of time in which the uncooperative child is removed from his setting. Time-out procedures may be less effective than other methods of behavior shaping if the student is uninformed as to why he is being removed from the situation. Effective social isolation is executed by telling the student why he is being removed from the class. The actual location for the isolation process should be well conceived and devoid of dangerous materials or objects. When the child is returned to the classroom, he should be treated as though he is a new child in the class. A significant failure of educators who employ social isolation is that they tend to return the child to the exact milieu that created the initial disturbing condition. It is suggested that such items as toys, school supplies, or other distractive objects be eliminated from the immediate environment of the child. Rearrangement of the desks when he returns may reduce or deter many of the forces which have acted as accelerating consequences for his behavior. As with other techniques, time-out should only be used when necessary if it is to be repeatedly effective.

The final area to be considered in the management of children with behavioral problems is *punishment*. Punishment, however, is not strongly advocated for many reasons. While it may succeed temporarily, it tends to be ineffective as long-term approach for handling behavior problems. Punishment, even over an extended period of time, is not as effective as presenting a desirable behavior to a child and reinforcing it, rather than punishing him for an undesirable one. Children also react negatively to, or dislike, people who punish them. The teacher who continually chastises her students encourages absenteeism in the class as children begin to dislike coming to school.

One major reason to avoid the use of punishment in dealing with the mentally retarded child is that he tends to mimic these acts with his peers. It is a common experience to witness a trainable child imitating an activity (Bender, 1971) or some form of punishment he has received with children on the playground. The degree of punishment may also be very harmful for certain populations of handicapped children who might not fully appreciate the significance for this type of treatment.

Punishment should be considered separately from the use of *reprimands*. The reprimands of "no," "hands down," and "sit down" are very effective tools in the behavior training of the mentally retarded child and may play an important part in a structured teaching program. They may be employed effectively providing they are not used constantly.

If the teacher can remember to reinforce appropriate behavior spontaneously, utilize accelerating consequences appropriately, incorporate ignoring measures when necessary, and use social isolation only in predetermined cases, she will be in a position to avoid many behavioral problems. The teacher who initially establishes firm guidelines will find it simple to relax the structure as the year progresses. It is extremely difficult, however, for the teacher to be an effective class manager if structure is loose and behavior has gone unchecked for any length of time.

MAINSTREAMING

The practice of mainstreaming has taken on new dimensions in recent years. Mainstreaming is based on the principle of educating the educably mentally retarded in the same classroom as other children. It provides special education on the grounds of learning needs rather than on the categories of the particular handicap (Birch, 1974). One of the main advantages for mainstreaming is that children with various learning problems can receive assistance from well-qualified personnel, such as special education teachers or resource teachers, without having to be excluded from regular activities which are open to their peers. It also avoids the labeling stigma so often associated with special education. Proponents for mainstreaming have argued in favor of such a program in terms of its ability to share skills and knowledge with the regular classroom teachers. Ideally, the special educators who work within the mainstreaming program can offer their resources to the entire school instead of restricting them to the special students. There have been many explanations for the plethora of mainstreaming programs and their popularity. One of these reasons has been the scarcity of special classes or programs for the educably mentally retarded. As early as 1955, Birch and Stevens (1955) suggested a mainstreaming approach as a service that may be provided for the EMR child within the school system.

The provision of quality special education for educably retarded students while they remain in regular classes received its impetus from several sources (Birch, 1974). One justification for mainstreaming in this country grew out of the movement to label various children with handicaps. Many local school districts have refused to respond to state education agency questionnaires requiring that they label the retarded children they serve. An obvious stimulus for mainstreaming has been the parental reaction to segregating certain students in special classes. Parental concern has long been on the side of educating retarded children in classes with normal children so that they may benefit from the socialization experiences of the regular school program.

Recent consent decrees and court actions have also accelerated remarkable changes in the provision of special education services. The Right To Education Acts such as those in effect in the states of Pennsylvania and Maryland dramatically point out the parents' responsibility and role in ensuring that their children receive an appropriate program. The Right To Education Acts, while initially mandated for severely and profoundly retarded children who were excluded from existing school programs, also affected those children who were educably retarded. Consent agreements were formulated which affirmed the right for all children to receive a free education, regardless of the type or degree of their handicap. More specifically, the courts followed the recommendations of many leaders in special education who testified that one of the most desirable settings for special education is in the regular classroom. This expert testimony by special education leaders provided momentum for the proponents of mainstreaming.

Mainstreaming has also been advocated on the basis that many children are psychologically classified as mentally retarded when in fact they are not. Those that support mainstreaming continually stress that it is unfair for nonhandicapped children to be socially and educationally segregated from handicapped children. They argue that it is very difficult for normal children to accept the differences of others, be they physical or mental, when they have had little or no experience with them. Many regular class students who were questioned as to whether or not they would be accommodating of peers in their class who may have a physical or mental handicap were quite verbal in stating that they would readily accept them. Yet the education system has continued to protect the nonhandicapped children from the handicapped with no ostensible ethical, moral, or educational justification.

One of the major reasons for mainstreaming is founded on financial grounds. It appears that it is economically more feasible to mainstream children and provide support through special education services than it is to initiate new building programs, pay for construction and maintenance, and arrange private transportation systems. Some of the antecedents mentioned as representing the strongest evidence for mainstreaming the EMR have recently been tested. Reports have been published offering objective results of how pilot programs have succeeded. In the states of Washington, Texas, Arizona, Kentucky, and Virginia, successful descriptions of mainstreaming programs have been reported (Birch, 1974). In each of these pilot programs, one of the major organizational patterns aiding mainstreaming was utilizing the support of resource rooms or teachers and whatever additional assistance and personnel were required.

While mainstreaming may positively effect many EMR children, there are those who will derive little benefit from it. While it is evident that there are states that have implemented a successful mainstreaming program, one wonders what the effect of mainstreaming will be upon other populations of retarded children. As an example, the mainstreaming of trainable and subtrainable children might not prove to be advantageous, and, thus, impose a disservice to both the retarded and normal populations. The outcome of a mainstreaming project depends highly upon the attitude of teachers and administrators who are involved in its implementation. One of the key ingredients in the states cited as initiating successful programs was the continual monitoring of the various aspects of the venture. Without constant surveillance, the successes or failures of the program cannot be validated, the changes in behavior or classroom skills are difficult to interpret, and, thus, the effectiveness of the experience is questionable.

SUMMARY

One of the major reasons for educational and behavioral problems in managing a class of retarded children is that their curriculum is not always appropriate. In preparing for a new class the teacher is often faced with files of irrelevant information and obsolete anecdotal records. The teacher, as well as the child, is frustrated when outdated test results are incorporated into plans for teaching. In order to understand what to teach, the educator first needs to know the child. It is, therefore, imperative that some form of assessment be undertaken as soon as possible. This information will directly affect the organization and management of the class and can offer a foundation for reappraisal later in the year.

This chapter has presented an overview of the evaluation, classroom management, and organization necessary in teaching the mentally retarded. Initially, evaluation was discussed as it pertained to the overall schema of classroom management and organization and reasons for its importance were emphasized. The educably mentally retarded, trainably mentally retarded, and severely and profoundly retarded were discussed and synopses of their curricula were outlined. Rates of development and the importance of developmental levels for the mentally retarded were stressed, in addition to recommendations for implementing realistic techniques in the use of educational behavior modification. Suggestions have been offered to the teacher concerning alternatives which exist for persistent classroom problems and how these behaviors may be avoided.

A final area discussed was the mainstreaming of educably mentally retarded children in regular classes, and reasons were advanced for this current trend in special education.

REFERENCES

Alpern, G. D., and C. C. Kimberlin. 1970. Short intelligence test ranging from infancy levels through childhood levels for use with the retarded. Am. J. Ment. Deficiency 75: 65—71.

Ashlock, P., and A. Stephens. 1967. Educational Therapy in the Elementary School. Charles C Thomas, Publisher, Springfield, Ill. 102 p.

Balow, B. 1971. Teachers for the handicapped. Compact. 5:43—46.

Bender, M. 1971. An experiment using a visual method of instruction followed by imitation to teach selected industrial education psychomotor tasks to severely retarded males. (In preparation.)

Birch, J. W. 1974. Mainstreaming: Educably Mentally Retarded Children in Regular Classes. Leadership Training Institute—Special Education. University of Minnesota Press, Minneapolis. 104 p.

Birch, J. W., and G. Stevens. 1955. Teaching exceptional children in every classroom: Reaching the mentally retarded. In J. W. Birch, Mainstreaming: Educably Mentally Retarded Children in Regular Classes, pp. 1—2. University of Minnesota Press, Minneapolis.

Bradtke, L., W. Kirkpatrick, and K. Rosenblatt. 1972. Intensive play: A technique for building affective behaviors in profoundly mentally retarded young children. Educ. Training Ment. Retard. 7:8—13.

Geddes, D. 1974. Physical activity: A necessity for severely and profoundly mentally retarded individuals. In Physical and Recreational Programs for Severely and Profoundly Retarded Individuals. Department of Health, Education, and Welfare, United States Office of Education, Bureau for the Education of the Handicapped, Washington, D. C.

Guskin, S. L., and H. H. Spicker. 1968. Educational research in mental retardation. In N. R. Ellis (ed.), International Review of Research in Mental Retardation. Vol. 3, pp. 217—278. Academic Press, Inc., New York.

Kirk, S. 1972. Educating Exceptional Children. Houghton-Mifflin Company, Boston. 478 p.

Sheppard, D. 1973. Teaching Social Behavior to Young Children. Research Press, Champaign, Ill. 80 p.

Swanson, S., and R. L. Jenkins. 1969. From the other side of the teacher's desk. *In* Discipline in the Classroom, pp. 3–6. National Education Association, Washington, D. C.

Van Til, W. 1956. Better Curriculum—Better Discipline. *In* Discipline in the Classroom, pp. 1–3. National Education Association, Washington, D. C.

Webb, R. C. 1969. Sensory-motor training of the profoundly retarded. Am. J. Ment. Deficiency 74:283–295.

13

Nutritional Deficiency And School Performance

David M. Paige, M.D., M.P.H.

Nutrition is critical to the health, well being, and educational motivation of an individual. The physical, chemical, and physiologic development of the brain and the consequent behavior in all species of higher animals evolves from the continuous interaction of genetic and environmental factors. The role of appropriate nutrition in optimizing this interaction cannot be overemphasized.

Nutrition is operative at many levels. On the most primitive plane, it is essential for survival. Nutrition is directly concerned with the provision of energy and nutrients needed for cellular structures in various metabolic systems. On the most advanced level, it is critical to the realization of the highest form of intellectual performance of which man is capable. Between these two extremes, nutrition is responsible for the pupil's perception of his home and environment, integration with his family, identification with his culture, as well as social and cognitive development.

Aberration from adequate nutrition may be seen in states of hunger, chronic undernutrition, malnutrition, starvation, and death. On the opposite end of the scale, overnutrition may range from slight excesses of acceptable weights to gross obesity, degenerative diseases, metabolic disorders, and death.

To consider the problems of malnutrition in preschool and school age children is, in effect, to summarize the previously poor nutritional experience of these children, for, in reality, the ramifications of malnutrition cannot effectively be conceptualized for any one point in time. To fully comprehend the magnitude of the problem, malnutrition must be considered a continuum; that is to say, an insidious cycle of events, often originating in utero, that continues to take place throughout the individual's life.

Recent preschool and school nutrition surveys suggest that a significant number of students, especially in the lower socioeconomic groupings, have inadequate dietary intake. This less than optimum dietary experience presumably finds its expression in stunted growth, poor weight patterns, possible reduced brain cell size and number, perhaps decreased head circumference, and a variety of other quantifiable biologic and biochemical parameters. This in turn may result in a child who does not effectively relate to his environment. His intellectual performance may be diminished when compared to his appropriately nourished peers. His decreased responsiveness, evidenced by inattention, distraction, tiredness, and evasion, does not permit normal experiences within the classroom, thereby disrupting and reducing the amount of time devoted to learning. Thus, as a consequence of his experiential deprivation, the malnourished child finds his biologic deficits compounded. It is suggested that this group of children who have not had their depressed nutritional status redressed prior to entering school may be amenable to modification by their participation in school food programs.

In order to adequately understand the sequelae of undernutrition and overnutrition, it is imperative to first recognize the significance of growth and development in stimulating, influencing, and moderating the performance of the student.

THE MECHANISMS OF GROWTH

Growth is peculiar to the young of any species. It is characterized by almost infinite detail, great orderliness, and impressive variability. As defined by the National Institute of Child Health and Human Development (Cone, 1968), growth is:

> an increase in size or number . . . growth is a term indicating a multiplication of mass, which may be applied to a proliferation of cells, or to aggregates of cells such as tissues, organs, organisms, etc. It involves intrinsically all reproduction and depends upon a sequence of genetic, constitutional, environmental, nutritional, and endocrine influences.

The National Institute of Child Health and Human Development defines development as the:

> acquisition of an increase in complexity of function whether applied to cell differentiation, morphogenesis of organs, or maturation of an individual organism, and it is molded both by heredity and by experience, i.e., nutritional, biochemical, intellectual, emotional, social, cultural, etc.

In a longitudinal sense, growth may be considered as a form of motion or distance attained over time. It may also be viewed cross-sectionally in increments of growth per unit of time (Cone, 1968). The latter is called the velocity of growth.

It is important to appreciate that growth is not a homogeneous event for all body organs. Rather than a continuously uniform phenomenon, it is distinctly heterogeneous. For example, the head is much larger at birth than other parts of the body but, during the course of growth, it assumes a relatively smaller size proportionate to other body parts such as the chest or abdomen. Despite the differential period of growth for various body organs, overall growth may be viewed as a constant event (Figure 1). Body growth may be conveniently divided into three periods: infancy, early school years, and adolescence.

Cell Growth

As growth has been defined as an increase in the size of an animal or an individual organ, it is important to recognize that organ mass is the result of a continuous accretion of protein and, in some cases, lipids (fatty tissue). Hence, when the rate of net protein synthesis and degradation reach equilibrium, growth ceases.

Winick (1970) points out that since net protein synthesis is linear in all organs during fetal development and for a period of time postnatally, growth would appear to be a homogeneous process. Yet cell number and cell size dictate whether the protein will be found in great numbers of small cells or a fewer number of large cells. Therefore, the quantity of protein would be an imprecise indicator of the nature or characteristics of organ growth.

The initial period of growth is referred to as the stage of *hyperplasia*. The fact that the DNA in the cell nucleus is constant for any diploid cell facilitates the quantitation of cell number. Subsequent to this proliferative period, there is a reduction in cell division as reflected by a decrease in DNA and a corresponding increase in RNA (ribonucleic acid). This intermediate period is termed the stage of *hyperplasia* and *hypertrophy*. Finally, the last period of growth is distinguished by an increase in RNA and cell size, but a constant amount of DNA within the particular organ. This stage of organ development has been called the period of *hypertrophy*. The above three stages constitute organ growth.

Factors Affecting Growth

Among the human host factors commonly associated with nutritional diseases are age and sex, physiologic and pathologic status, habits and customs, genetic background, and psychobiologic characteristics and reactions. Besides the importance of each one of these factors, there are physiologic moments, such as pregnancy, lactation periods, and early childhood, when the human being is particularly vulnerable to nutritional disease. Mothers and children merit separate consideration because they constitute a high risk group. The special risk is connected with the process of growth and development, the distinguishing characteristic of childhood, and, inferentially, the maternity period.

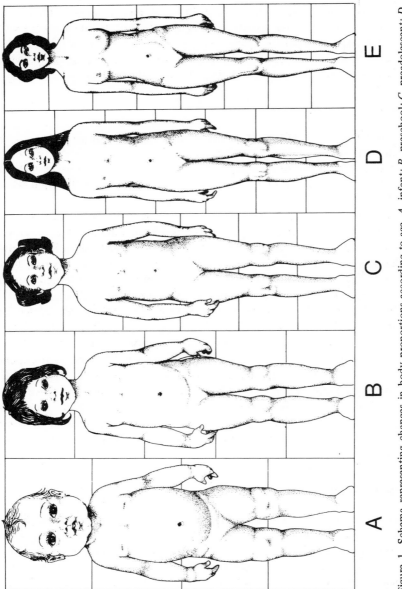

Figure 1. Schema representing changes in body proportions according to age. *A*, infant; *B*, preschool; *C*, preadolescent; *D*, adolescent; *E*, adult. Note in particular the variation in head size.

Since nutritional requirements are directly related to the rate of growth, the younger the child, the greater are the nutritional demands per unit of body weight. Severe malnutrition occurs with particularly high frequency during the early periods of most rapid changes. This is one of the reasons why overt malnutrition develops more rapidly and frequently in young children and is correspondingly rare in adults.

Because nutrition and socioeconomic factors are interrelated, the independent role that nutrition may play in pregnancy outcome has been difficult to evaluate. Nevertheless, a large body of data points to a relationship between the quality of maternal nutrition and the eventual condition of the fetus. Yet it must be remembered that, with severe maternal malnutrition, high rates of spontaneous abortion or infertility frequently result rather than fetal malnutrition per se.

Patterns of Growth

Generic to each organism is its own timetable of growth. While all children travel the same road toward the achievement of maturity, the distance covered and the time taken to reach a given milestone vary from child to child. Therefore, the physical and emotional parameters of any group of children at a given chronologic age will differ widely. The most accurate index of physical growth is represented by plotting height and weight over time to determine whether the child follows his own percentile patterns of growth. The anthropometric determination can be validated when necessary by radiologic examination of the centers of ossification in select bones (see Chapter 5). This technique will provide information regarding the child's bone age which can be compared to his chronologic age to determine what differences, if any, exist.

STUDIES OF ANIMAL GROWTH

An increasingly large number of studies outlining the effect of caloric and protein deprivation in the animal model indicate permanent deficits result from nutrient restriction. Particular attention has been directed to the central nervous system in these investigations.

Winick (1969) has shown that poor nutrition interferes with cell division resulting in permanent defects. He points out that there is a critical period of interference with regard to the effects of poor nutrition on brain growth and development. In the experimental rat model, the most vital period was the first 21 days following delivery. Nutritional insults during this period led to a permanent decrease in brain cell number.

While an organ such as the brain may continue to develop, disturbances of growth by way of nutritional deprivation during the essential period of hyperplasia will lead to a permanent irreversible injury if not remedied during this phase of organ maturation. Nutritional insults which occur during hypertrophy, or the phase of increasing cell size of organ growth, will result in deficits which are reversible through overfeeding.

Martin (1973) noted that caloric deprivation during periods of rapid animal brain growth caused permanent deficits, including diminished brain weight due to a decrease in the number and size of cells in the central nervous system, as well as loss of quantity of DNA and the amount of myelin. Furthermore, Cowley (1968) has reported that, although rats fed low protein diets did not show a loss of ability in learning a maze, the progeny of these study animals, as well as two succeeding generations, evidenced a marked deficiency in learning new tasks. A consistent finding in animal studies indicates that both calorie and/or protein deprivation, coupled with inadequate environmental stimuli, act in a synergistic fashion resulting in a decrease or loss of learning capabilities.

STUDIES OF HUMAN GROWTH

In the human, two-thirds of the brain cells are present at birth and the remaining one-third can be demonstrated to develop from birth to 6–12 months of age (Martin, 1973). Winick and Rosso (1969) suggested the possibility that poor cerebral maturation in infants, as evidenced by decreased DNA content and reflected by a small head circumference, is a function of a compromised postnatal nutritional status. Martin (1973) noted that studies in animals are in agreement that the period of most rapid brain growth is the critical period when poor nutrition may affect the growth and development of the central nervous system. Since the stage of maximum growth of brain size occurs during the first 2 years of life with 80% completion by that time, it is reasonable to assume that the potential exists for a profound effect on further intellectual potential.

Cravioto, DeLicardie, and Birch (1966) have identified several factors which tend to prejudice the growth and development of malnourished children. They suggest that the learning process is hindered due to a decrease in responsiveness of the malnourished child to his environment. In addition, perceptual or cognitive developmental anomalies resulting in long-term disturbances are much more apt to occur during periods of nutritional insult.

Birch and Gussow (1970) have reported that a major consequence of malnutrition is reduced behavioral responsiveness to environmental stimuli. This lowered level of awareness results in less time in which to interact with the environment and, consequently, less time in which to learn. Furthermore, such experiential deprivation can be expected to produce a certain degree of developmental lag. The detrimental influences to the child can be more profound if the so-called critical periods for learning are undermined by nutritional deprivation. Although some of this work can be criticized for not providing an adequate profile of the children prior to their investigation, it certainly points up the potential severity of the problem.

Eichenwald and Fry (1969) conclude that malnutrition in critical periods of early life can affect not only the physical and biochemical profile in children, but also has a profound impact on intellectual potential. The authors point out that poor protein nutrition or synthesis during brain development can result in permanent dysfunction. The neural deficit results in altered mental ability. Inadequate feedings during key periods in utero and infancy may also contribute to inadequate myelination (the lipid sheath covering certain nerve fibers), leading to various neurologic disorders.

It has been theorized that the multifaceted impairment emanating from insufficient nutrition may be responsible for the poor performance of certain societies. Cravioto (1970) has also emphasized the point in his experimental observations that inadequate protein intake during the period of early neurologic development does indeed affect intellectual performance.

Stoch and Smythe (1967), in their study in Cape Town, South Africa, followed a group of undernourished infants for 11 years. They determined that the intellectual performance of these youngsters was exceedingly poor. They proposed that the brains of these children reach maturity at a suboptimal size. The most striking finding was the discovery that 60% of the undernourished children on intelligence testing fell below the level of the lowest child in the control group and only one surpassed the mean. Disparities in backgrounds of the matched groups in regard to family life style, even though they came from similar socioeconomic deciles, tend to bias the study and weaken the conclusions.

Martin (1973), reporting on Mönckeberg's (1968) studies, indicated that 14 marasmic (wasted) infants who had excellent care following hospitalization were found to be below average in height, head circumference, and intelligence at 6 years of age as compared to the normal standards in that country. These suboptimal measurements resulted despite the fact that the mothers of the previously emaciated infants were given nutritional counseling in addition to 20 liters of free milk.

Chase and Martin (1970) studied a group of 19 malnourished children during the first year of life. They were matched as to sociodemographic factors with a group of normal controls. The malnourished experimental children showed significant differences in height, weight, and head circumference when compared to the control children. It appeared that those who were malnourished during the initial 4 months of life or longer experienced the most severe sequelae. In fact, these children showed intelligence and developmental quotients 30 points lower than the control group and 25 points lower than those children who were malnourished for less than the first 4 months of life.

Psychologic testing can be difficult, as well as inaccurate, when infants are to be evaluated. The problems are more acute when examining the malnourished child, who tends to be both nonverbal and reclusive. There remains a crucial need for a psychologic profile for malnourished children and a reliable tool for the assessment of the contribution of an inadequate diet upon intellectual retardation with specific retesting procedures for a sufficient period following the introduction of a wholesome diet.

SCHOOL SURVEYS: PREVALENCE OF POOR NUTRITION

The Ten-State Nutrition Survey (1972) emphasized the prevalence of poor nutrition in many segments of our society. The finding of vitamin A and vitamin C deficiency, rickets (vitamin D deficiency), and iron deficiency anemia high-light some of the results of this survey. The less than adequate nutritional profile is frequently rooted in poverty-stricken or disorganized socioeconomic settings. This fact is observed in multiple preschool and school surveys (Table 1).

Stine, Saratsiotis, and Furno (1967), in review of 842 early admission children to the Baltimore City School system, found that the heights and weights of the students were below those for standard populations of American children and they approximated the measurements of malnourished children from underdeveloped countries. In addition, it was discovered that 25% of the children were below the tenth percentile for head circumference, and that 20% of the black males had suggestive evidence of anemia.

A review of 40 children 3–5 years of age by Crispin et al. (1968) was undertaken to evaluate growth and body composition. There were two groups selected, one of high and the other of low socioeconomic status. The height and weight of the pupils, as well as four other body parameters and three skinfold thicknesses, were measured. The results suggested that growth and nutritional state were superior in the group with the highest socioeconomic background. Kerrey et al. (1968), in a companion study, concluded that the favorable nutritional condition of the higher socioeconomic group is attributed to their nutrient intake.

Christakis et al. (1968) investigated 642 New York City school children between 10 and 13 years of age who lived primarily in tenements. They judged the diets of 73% of the sample to be inadequate. Twice the frequency of excellent dietary histories was reported for children from nonwelfare families. Further-more, children with poor diets were discovered to be anemic. The thiamine, biotin, riboflavin, pantothenic acid, niacin, vitamin B_6, vitamin B_{12}, folic acid, vitamin A, ascorbic acid, and total cholesterol were assayed by Baker et al. (1967) on the same 642 children. It was ascertained that thiamine, biotin, and ascorbic acid were all markedly below the norm for the population when there was inadequate protein intake. In 12% of the subjects, it was considered that the protein intake was inadequate.

Myers (1968), in her study of 322 pupils in the fourth through the sixth grades in a depressed section of Boston, concluded that children living in this area show physical and biochemical abnormalities frequently associated with poor nutrition. Some of the more significant findings included marked dental pathology, gingivitis (inflammation of the gums), and scaling skin. It was

Table 1. Relative Importance of Nutritional Problems[a]

Ethnic Group	Low-Income Ratio States — Iron	Protein	Vitamin A	Vitamin C	Ribo-flavin	Thiamine	Iodine	Growth and Development	Obesity	Age (yr) and Sex (M, F)	High-Income Ratio States — Iron	Protein	Vitamin A	Vitamin C	Ribo-flavin	Thiamine	Iodine	Growth and Development	Obesity
Black	X[b]	O[c]	Y[d]	O	Y	O	O	Y	-[e]	0–5; M,F	Y	O	Z[f]	O	Z	O	O	Y	-
	X	N	Z	O	Y	O	O	Y	-	6–9; M,F	Y	O	N	O	Z	O	O	Y	-
	X	N	N	O	Y	N	O	Z	Z	10–16; F	Y	O	N	O	Z	N	O	Z	Z
	X	O	N	O	Y	N	O	Z	Z	10–16; M	Y	O	N	O	Z	N	O	Z	O
White	Y	O	Z	O	N	O	O	Y	-	0–5; M,F	Z	O	N	O	Z	O	O	Y	-
	Y	O	N	O	N	O	O	Y	-	6–9; M,F	Z	O	N	O	O	O	O	Y	-
	Y	O	N	O	N	N	O	Z	Z	10–16; F	Z	O	N	O	O	O	O	Z	Z
	Y	O	N	O	N	N	O	Z	Y	10–16; M	Z	O	N	O	O	O	O	Z	Z
Spanish-American	Y	O	X	O	Y	O	O	Y	-	0–5; M,F	Y	O	O	O	O	O	O	Y	-
	Y	O	X	O	Y	O	O	Y	-	6–9; M,F	Y	O	O	O	O	O	O	Y	-
	Y	N	X	O	Y	O	O	Z	-	10–16; F	Y	O	O	O	O	O	O	Z	-
	Y	O	X	O	Y	O	O	Z	-	10–16; M	Y	O	O	O	O	O	O	Z	-

[a]Modified from the Ten-State Nutrition Survey, 1968–1970, 1972 United States Department of Health, Education, and Welfare Publication No. (HSM) 72-8132.
[b]X, high.
[c]O, minimal.
[d]Y, medium.
[e]-, not available.
[f]Z, low.

demonstrated that there were marked excesses below the twenty-fifth percentile for height and weight in both blacks and whites within this population of children.

Dibble et al. (1965) reported some preliminary biochemical findings in junior high schools representing three socioeconomic levels. In the first school, the children were mostly black and their fathers were laborers. In the second, the majority of the children were white with most fathers engaged in professional, managerial, and white collar jobs. The third school consisted primarily of white children whose fathers were skilled and unskilled laborers. In the first school, as could be anticipated, the intake of all nutrients was the poorest. Those children were classified as moderately short, and their average weight and hematocrits as a group were the lowest. Furthermore, ascorbic acid (vitamin C) levels in one-third of the children in the predominately black school were below the acceptable range.

Skidmore (1965) studied 75 randomly selected children aged 4–6 years from Head Start Programs, and the following information was revealed: 50% of the children has a source of vitamin C once a week or less, and only 4% had an adequate daily supply; 24% never ate green vegetables; 66% had one glass or less of milk per day; 65% drank a sweetened beverage; and 56% had candy daily. It was concluded that school menus contributed greatly to the daily essential nutrient requirements of these students.

Becker (1959) reported on a population of 1,200 school aged children, predominately white with a small number of blacks and Indians, using 24-hr. recall of diets as the source of nutritional information. Approximately one-third of these children had less than the accepted daily requirement of calories; about 50% were poor in ascorbic acid, 40% in vitamin A, 30% in calcium, and 10% in protein.

It should be pointed out that the values used for interpretation in some of the above cited surveys may vary. Numerous guides are available for evaluating dietary, clinical, and biochemical data. An example is the Manual for Nutrition Surveys (1963) published by the Interdepartmental Committee on Nutrition for National Defense.

EVALUATION OF SCHOOL FEEDING PROGRAMS

The Type "A" School Feeding Program represents a major effort by the United States Department of Agriculture, Child Nutrition Division. The program, as outlined in the Child Nutrition Act of 1966 (P.L. 89-642), is designed to meet the following objectives: to "safeguard the health and well-being of the nation's children and to encourage the domestic consumption of nutritious agricultural commodities and other food;" and to "meet more effectively the nutritional needs of our children."

The inception of the child nutrition programs in the 1930's was an attempt to equitably distribute the farm commodity surplus and to raise or maintain farm prices at reasonable levels. Over the past 40 years the initial thrust of these programs has been significantly modified.

Legislative amendments in 1970 coupled with subsequent revisions served as the needed impetus for free or reduced price meals to needy children. It is estimated, however, that in fiscal year 1975 some 5 million children were not participating in the national school lunch program because they attended schools that did not offer food service. This figure represents approximately 10% of the nation's total school enrollment and accounts for 17% of the nation's schools. However, about one-half of these schools do take part in the special milk program.

The school lunch program which utilizes the type "A" pattern is intended to provide one-third of the recommended daily nutritional requirements for school age children. These nutrients include calories, protein, calcium, iron, vitamin A, vitamin C, riboflavin, thiamine, niacin, and phosphorus. They are generally provided for a 10- to 12-year-old child in the following form: whole milk (1/2 pt.), meat or an alternate (2 oz. of lean meat, fish, or poultry or equivalent quantities of an alternate such as eggs, peanut butter, cheese, cooked dried beans, or peas), vegetables and fruit (3/4 c. of two or more vegetables or fruits or a combination of the two), and bread (1 slice of whole grain or enriched bread or an equivalent quantity of biscuits, rolls, or muffins made of enriched flour), and butter or fortified margarine (1 tsp.).

The school breakfast has three components consisting of milk, fruit or juice, and bread or cereal. It can provide children with approximately one-sixth of the recommended daily dietary allowances for the same reference child at 10–12 years of age (Rosenfield, 1972).

The impact of such a program on the nutritional well being and behavioral activity of the student within the classroom remains uncertain. Additional information is required inasmuch as increasing attention is being directed to the school feeding program as a vehicle by which to rectify the previously poor nutritional status of school children.

Despite the lack of a systematic analysis of school food programs, Mayer (1966) has suggested that the school is the ideal place to upgrade the nutritional profile of malnourished children. In the paper "Focus on Oklahoma Food Habits" (unpublished), the thesis was advanced that those children who regularly consume the type "A" school lunch are better off nutritionally than those who do not. In "A Report of the Dietary Phase of the Chestuee Nutrition Study" by the Tennessee Department of Public Health (1958), it was established that 75% of the 441 rural children surveyed ate a school lunch. This was, in many instances, the most nutritious meal of the day for the child. Other reports tend to lend support to the school food program as an important mechanism for modification of the undernutrition and malnutrition that exists in the preschool and school age population.

Our studies (Paige, 1972) on the impact of school feeding programs showed no significant difference in height, weight, and hematocrits over a 1-year period between participating and nonparticipating students in an organized school feeding program. In fact, over 60% of the pupils in the school feeding program who began the academic year with a low or deficient hematocrit (i.e., evidence of anemia) finished the year with an equally low hematocrit irrespective of whether they were fed in school through the type "A" program or not. These studies also indicated that nutritionally disadvantaged, institutionalized children participating in a school feeding program did no better than those comparably matched school children who were not participating in the school feeding program.

In addition, it was determined that the use of family size and income to determine the student's eligibility for participation in free or reduced price school feeding programs was less than adequate in identifying children who are at nutritional risk. Our study (Paige, 1971) of four schools in a large metropolitan area, in which two of the schools were predominately black and the other two predominately white, indicated that administrative decisions predicated on economic criteria frequently failed to select students evidencing a poor nutritional status judged by biologic indices of anthropometrics and hematocrit. Others (Emmons, Hayes, and Call, 1972) have corroborated the fact that, when one studies elementary school children who qualified for free school lunches on the basis of family size and income, there were nearly three times more ineligible than eligible children who were considered to be nutritionally needy on the grounds of biologic indices. The inability to demonstrate improvement in the nutritional status of the child, however, does not obviate the potential short-term benefits on classroom performance which may result from such programs.

Some European investigators have tangentially addressed themselves to the adequacy of the school feeding program. Both Graefe (1966) in Germany and Miedzybrodska (1968) in Poland advocate improvement in the quality of foods utilized in school feeding programs and report advantageous results to the student when nutritious foods are provided.

It is important when considering school feeding programs that the terms "hunger" and "malnutrition" be defined, inasmuch as frequent confusion exists between the two. Malnutrition may be defined as "the state of impaired functional ability or development caused by an inadequate intake of essential nutrients and calories to provide the long-term needs. Malnutrition results in specific symptoms or conditions such as goiter, anemia, vitamin deficiency, or growth retardation" (Read, 1973). On the other hand, hunger "is a psychologic and physiologic state resulting from insufficient food intake to meet immediate energy needs. It can be easily and immediately relieved with food, whereas malnutrition requires a long rehabilitation period and may have lasting effects. Hunger and malnutrition are not synonymous although they are clearly interrelated" (Read, 1973).

While malnutrition in this nation's school children does not exist to any great degree, hunger may be a much more frequent phenomenon. It should be recognized that while hunger may have psychologic and physiologic components, it does not affect or alter neurologic structure. Hunger may, however, be a factor in modifying or reducing the short-term ability of the student to learn by interfering with his thought processes and activity, resulting in experiential deprivation.

NUTRITION AND CLASSROOM PERFORMANCE

While concern with the interrelationship of hunger and learning is of considerable interest, the few published reports which directly address this issue are equivocal at best and disallow specific inferences to be drawn.

An early summary prepared by Roberts (1927) noted that the "mere provision of the mid-morning snack does not necessarily increase food intake or accelerate gains." She concluded by stating that efforts directed at supplementation should be focused upon the nutritionally needy child.

Other studies (Laird, Levitan, and Wilson, 1931) conducted in grades one, three, or five indicated that nervousness was eliminated in about one-half of the children, with almost 85% showing improvement in excitability, fatigability, perseverance, concentration, and socialization when fed wholesome diets. The control group, which had nothing more than a play period, did not show significant improvement in behavior. On the other hand, well-executed studies have found little difference in IQ or school performance in marginal nutritional problems as seen in populations within the United States.

A carefully organized Canadian study (Tisdall et al., 1951) compared children who lunched at school with others who ate at home. While minimal improvement in growth and other biochemical indices were found in pupils whose noon meals were provided at school, no significant differences in tests of intellectual performance, grades, reading levels, or mathematical skills were found over the 2-year study period. Again, in an Alabama study (Edwards, Lomax, and Grimmett, 1956) conducted over a 6-month period, there were improvements in nutritional parameters, but no effect on intellectual skills could be documented as a result of a special school lunch program.

In Sweden and Norway, where school breakfast programs have been operational for many years, data indicate that more weight was gained by children eating a breakfast rather than a lunch at school. This fact is particularly evident when the breakfast was planned to nutritionally complement the home meals. On the other hand, the children were noted to have a decreased appetite for the evening meal if they had eaten their school lunch (Eeg-Larsen, 1969).

The impact of breakfast programs is currently being examined in the United States. A series of studies conducted at the University of Iowa (Tuttle et al., 1954) were concerned with the effect on school performance efficiency during the late morning if breakfasts were eliminated. Data on 25 boys concluded that the omission of breadfast had no effect in terms of neuromuscular tremor, maximum grip strength, and grip strength endurance. Differences of significance were present, however, with an enhanced maximum work rate and output following a basic breakfast as opposed to a diminished effort during these tasks if the breakfast were withheld. Teacher reports indicated that the students had an improved attitude and school record during the period that breakfast was included. Additional data from these studies imply that there was no difference in late morning efficiency which could be related to variance in the size or content of the breakfast.

These conclusions are further supported by Swedish investigators (Arvedson, Sterky, and Tjernstrom, 1969) looking at students 7–18 years of age who consumed breakfast in school. Work performance, arithmetic test scores, or individual reports of hunger or fatigue were not different for children who were provided breakfasts high in either protein or calories. However, breakfast intakes of less than 400 kcal did produce a negative influence on performance. Thus, the role of school feeding programs on the amelioration of hunger and the altering of certain behavior characteristics obviously requires additional study.

It does appear, however, that there can be little argument with the provision of nutritional support within the school program inasmuch as definitive research results are not required to justify the inclusion of a program which would provide what is considered to be adequate nutrition. The consequences of such programs may or may not result in the desired behavioral or nutritional improvements. Yet this may be a function of the insensitivity of our outcome measures rather than an inability to effect the desired results. In addition, it must be remembered that such programs have an economic impact on the family since they extend the food budget dollar and provide a model for proper eating habits which will become part of the youngster's lifelong pattern of nutrition.

CATCH-UP GROWTH

The ability of children with stunted growth due to poor nutrition to amend their inadequate growth at a later date is still an unsettled issue. It has been suggested that, once specific critical periods of growth have passed, it is difficult, if not impossible, to compensate for undernutrition. Many investigators have hypothesized that nutritional insults which occur during the preschool years are responsible for permanently dwarfed growth. In the animal model, experiments show that nutritional interference imposed shortly after birth and during critical periods of development has permanent and obvious effects on the subsequent growth of the animal. By contrast, malnutrition at a later stage might depress growth only for the duration of the deprivation without altering the ultimate size of the adult animal. However, even in the animal model, the stage of development at which the young animal ceases to be vulnerable to permanent impairment cannot be precisely defined as there tends to be species variability, although the vital period most frequently terminates at the conclusion of the suckling period.

In a growing child, however, evidence is fragmentary and scanty. Most human data on physical growth are handicapped by lack of information on nutrient intake, confounding socioeconomic variables, genetic potential of the subject, scarcity of dietary data, and lack of information concerning health care. The literature for developing, as well as developed, countries appears to suggest that previously malnourished children do not obtain the height, weight, and bone age of children of the same ethnic background but of a higher social class for at least several years.

In studies by Garrow and Pike (1967), malnourished Jamaican children were compared to their immediate relatives. By using a matched pair technique, it was determined that the index malnourished case, examined 2–8 years following discharge from the hospital, was slightly taller and heavier than the nonmalnourished sibling.

Graham and Adrianzen (1972) have systematically addressed the issue of catch-up growth in a population of approximately 200 children and their siblings who were examined longitudinally over many years. This investigation initially called attention to the wide variability in catch-up growth, noting that the children experiencing the most dramatic and impressive recoveries were those who simultaneously encountered dramatic changes in their environmental milieu following rehabilitation from the malnutrition. These workers demonstrated that eight children who experienced distinct improvement in their home environment exhibited marked gains in height beginning as late as the eighty-eighth month of life, and that, at the mean age of 9, they were at the twenty-fifth percentile of the United States Boston-Stuart growth standard.

The results of IQ estimation in this population were varied and no inferences could be drawn nor estimates given as to the intellectual catch-up in this group of children. Graham and Adrianzen (1972) reported, "All we can say is that there has not been an improvement to parallel or match those observed in height and head size. Of the many important factors responsible for measurable intelligence at eight years of age, certainly severe and prolonged deprivation during early life, when at home or in an institution, looms as most impressive."

Graham and Adrianzen (1971) considered the interrelationship of growth inheritance and environment, and concluded that negative environmental factors which result in inadequate nutrition over the critical periods of growth play as significant a role as inheritance in determining the growth and eventual stature of the child. They do note, however, that "Catch-up growth both in height and in head size can go on for many years after a period of severe malnutrition. Head size, and presumably brain mass, may not be selectively affected by severe malnutrition in early life and may remain a function of body mass."

These most important issues must obviously await further definitive research before conclusions can be drawn. It does appear, however, that the potential for rehabilitation and recovery is not as narrow as had previously been considered. This more optimistic suggestion should lend support to the programs aimed at the nutritional enhancement of youngsters within the school situation, particularly in the early grades.

THE INACCURACIES OF PHYSICAL MEASUREMENTS

Widely used tables and graphs for plotting weight, height, and head circumference for the United States population were developed in Boston and Iowa. These standards are based on the measurements of children of Northern European ancestry from about 1930 to 1946 (Cone, 1968). Our data would indicate that the utilization of growth standards generated by a white suburban population generations ago may inadequately express the current growth potential of children. Ignored is the secular trend in physical growth—that is, the long-term tendency toward increases in height, weight, and other body measurements— which have been observed to be occurring in most populations in the United States (Paige, 1975).

To illustrate, the average increase in height for an 8-year-old black male has been 1.49 in. per decade, while weight has increased at an average of about 3.3 lbs. in a similar 10-year period. Parallel increases are observed in females. These secular changes have also led Garn (1962) and Moore (1970) to caution against relying upon obsolete age-size standards for interpreting the adequacy of growth in today's children; the unqualified use of these standards alone may lead to erroneous conclusions.

Our studies indicate that an incomplete picture of the growth of disadvantaged black children considered to be at risk would emerge if school health officials were to continue to simply rely on the percentile growth achieved by these children when indiscriminately compared to nationally used reference standards. At this point in time, the outdated growth standards do not accurately reflect ethnic and cultural differences as well as the secular trends which have taken place over generations.

Despite growth achieved, 22% of the children we studied were diagnosed as having nutritional anemia as evidenced by low or deficient hematocrits. This anemia combines with poor growth and is reflected in higher rates of absenteeism. Such youngsters are clearly at nutritional risk and in need of specific efforts aimed at providing a nutritional headstart (Paige, 1975).

IDENTIFICATION OF CHILDREN AT RISK FOR NUTRITIONAL DISORDERS

The screening procedures which are routinely carried out to identify children who are at risk for nutritional disorders include height, weight, head circumference, triceps skinfold, arm circumference, and certain biochemical indices. In spite of the inconsistent and sometimes obsolete standards of growth for children, careful and repeated measurements of the following parameters remain as the mainstay of the screening process.

Height

Height is a most useful linear measurement and is an important biologic index to the previous nutritional status of the child. Interference during critical periods of growth will manifest itself in stunted height. Abnormal linear growth can be confirmed radiologically by the use of a bone age determination. Length in the case of infants and toddlers and height in older children must be accurately obtained to be of maximum usefulness. The infant or child should be naked or in his undershorts and firmly placed on a measuring board which has a sliding head. Older children should be measured in an erect posture, without shoes, and with heels and feet together against a rigid standard (Figure 2).

Weight

Weight is also an important growth indicator which is more likely to reflect recent changes in nutrient intake. The weight, therefore, may rise and fall on the basis of short-term nutritional practice, habit, or interference, whereas height will reflect more prolonged nutritional disorders (Figure 3).

Weight is the simplest measurement for personnel to obtain as the most reliable overall index of body mass. The concept of weight is also well understood by mothers and represents a practical form of nutrition education. Because of the range of normal variation, isolated readings are of less value than serial determinations. Further, deviations from normal growth can be observed early while visual recordings can be used for health education. It is important to remember from a practical point of view that a standard technique is mandatory when weighing children. The scale should be accurate and weights recorded by trained personnel. The beam and balance must be inspected frequently and the child should be weighed in his underclothes.

Head Circumference

Head circumference has been used in many studies as an approximate indicator of brain size and is most readily utilized in screening procedures carried out in infants and toddlers. It has less reliability and validity in the older toddler and school age youngster (Figure 4).

It must be borne in mind that tall and fat children may have differences in head circumference when compared to short and thin children. Other variables besides skull contents intervene to affect head circumference such as skull thickness and edema or swelling of the scalp and temporal muscles. Thus, prior

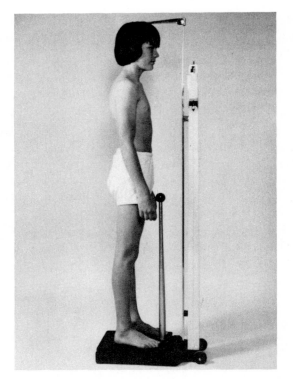

Figure 2. Suggested method of obtaining an accurate height and weight.

to measurement, the examiner must inspect the child's head to ensure a reliable recording. Finally, it must be remembered that the relationship between growth, head size, and intelligence is not always as compact as one might anticipate.

Triceps Skinfold

Triceps skinfold is a measurement of the thickness of the skin in the outer portion of the upper extremity and provides a satisfactory estimate of local fat as well as total body fat. Therefore, it is a reflection of the general health and well being of the youngster. The determination of skinfold thickness is accomplished by special calipers. While it has limited usefulness in some situations, many investigators have urged the inclusion of triceps skinfold measurements in screening for nutritional disorders in children as an indicator to the adequacy of body mass.

Arm Circumference

Arm circumference is primarily a measurement of muscle mass unless the child is obese. In developing countries, there are few overweight children beyond 6 months

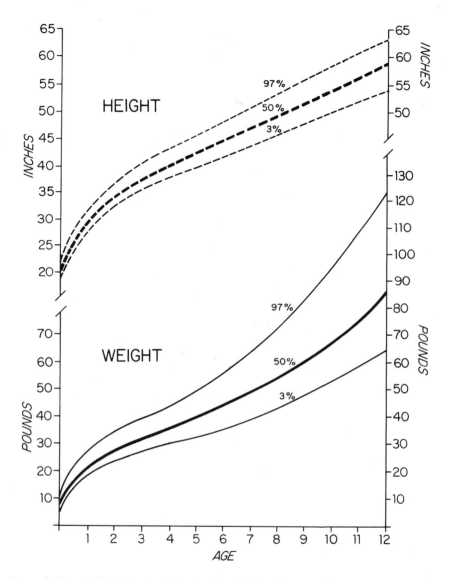

Figure 3. Standard height and weight chart from birth to 12 years of age. In spite of the noted inaccuracies, careful measurements serve as a reliable screening mechanism for children at risk for nutritional disorders.

of age and this makes the measurement an impractical guide. In children, fat contributes only a few millimeters to the total arm circumference. Yet several studies have demonstrated that estimates of wasting correlated well with the measure arm circumference as well as weight deficits in the presence of clinical stigmata of protein calorie malnutrition.

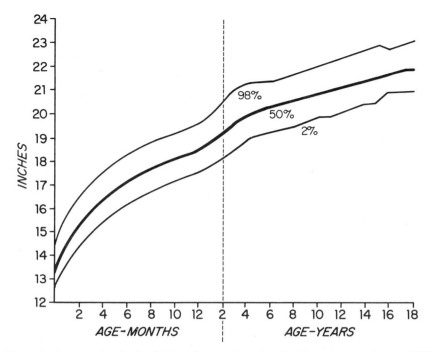

Figure 4. An example of a head circumference chart showing the mean growth curve (50%) as well as the extremes of normal (98 and 2%).

Biochemical Indices

Biochemical indices are frequently used to assess the nutritional status of children. It is appropriate to consider the hypothetical sequence of biochemical events that precedes the appearance of clinical signs of nutrient deficiency.

Initially, as the deficiency evolves, body stores of the nutrients are depleted. This leads to a gradual reduction of the nutrient concentration in the blood and other tissues which ultimately results in a decrease in the urinary excretion of the particular ingredient. The next stage manifests itself as a decrease or modification of nutrients supplied which in turn results in functional impairment. Finally, anatomical lesions characteristic of the clinical disorder appear (e.g., scurvy due to vitamin C lack or rickets secondary to vitamin D deficiency). It is important to note that the entire gamut of these aberrations may arise not only from dietary lack, which is considered a primary deficiency, but from a variety of secondary causes, such as poor gastrointestinal absorption, impaired transport of the substance within the body, or decreased utilization.

Biochemical tests in these instances frequently fall into two categories: measurement of blood or urine levels (e.g., ascorbic acid or vitamin C), with or without the administration of a test or loading dose, and the determination of specific enzyme activity or changes in the levels of certain metabolites. It is important to bear in mind that even though one nutrient is focused upon, one should not infer that simple single deficiencies are present. They are, in fact, relatively uncommon, with multiple states of malnutriture far more frequent. While a detailed review of the biochemical deficiencies which exist in abnormal nutrition is beyond the scope of this chapter, some of the more common deficiencies will be highlighted.

The adequacy of caloric intake at the moment is difficult to assess. Familiar tests such as the basal metabolic rate and the blood sugar level provide some insight into the energy situation, but in reality they do not correlate precisely with the demands or requirements of carbohydrate metabolism. It is fair to conclude, however, that caloric or energy deficiency may exist in children who are fatigued, listless, and unable to concentrate, which may indeed result in poor classroom performance and behavior.

Protein Deficiency

The number of biochemical studies of protein-calorie deficiency is legion and is a discipline unto itself. A foolproof biochemical technique for the detection of marginal states of protein deficiency or for the assessment of dietary protein intake within various school age populations does not yet exist. The measurement of serum protein fractions in the blood such as serum albumin has recently been shown, however, to be an important index of the adequacy of protein nutrition (Baertl, Placko, and Graham, 1974).

Protein deficiency may be responsible for seriously affecting a child's immunity to infectious diseases and, therefore, may be a contributing factor to poor classroom attendance. Antibodies, the mechanism for preventing or combating infections, are protein molecules. If the child is severely protein depleted, the antibody response will be diminished in the face of an acute infection. On a more significant level, protein deficiency can alter cellular growth of certain organs, often resulting in more frequent and acute illnesses.

Iron Deficiency Anemia

Iron deficiency anemia appears to have become more prevalent during the past 20 years. It is difficult to define precisely those factors within society which contribute to the increased incidence of this common type of anemia. At the onset, it should be remembered that iron deficiency anemia is merely a symptom of a more general nutritional and environmental problem. Confusion still exists as to acceptable lower limits of iron nutriture. The Interdepartmental Committee on Nutrition of National Defense (Manual for Nutrition Surveys, 1963) suggests that children 3–12 years of age be evaluated for the degree of anemia, as shown in Table 2 and Figure 5. The World Health Organization (1972) has

Table 2. Interpretation of Hemoglobin and
Hematocrit Levels in Children Aged 3–12 Yrs.

Level	Hemoglobin (g%)	Hematocrit[a] (vol %)
Deficient	10 or below	30 or below
Low	10–10.9	30–33.9
Acceptable	11.0–12.4	34–36.9
High	12.5 or greater	37 or greater

[a]The hematocrit determination is an extremely valuable technique for anemia screening as it requires only a few drops of blood from a fingerstick. The result of the test is immediately available following several minutes of centrifugation.

suggested that a child between the ages of 6 months and 6 years may be identified as anemic if the concentration of hemoglobin is less than 11 g% or the hematocrit less than 33%.

One should, however, avoid the hazard of failing to recognize that those individuals whose hemoglobin and hematocrit levels are above the minimum level may still represent a deficiency state. Diamond (1970) has reported a number of adolescent girls with acceptable hematocrit levels whose lassitude, irritability, and ill-defined symptoms disappeared when iron supplements were added to the diet. A report of the 62nd Ross Conference (Smith, 1970a) on Pediatric Research addressing itself to Iron Nutrition in Infancy has summarized the findings of Diamond as well as the following authors.

Howell (1970a) has studied the interrelationship between iron deficiency anemia and learning disabilities. In 89 iron-deficient children 4–5 years of age, psychometric tests, including the Stanford-Binet, Goodenough Draw-A-Person, and the Gestalt, were within the expected normal range, while tests of attentiveness and ability to focus on, orient to, and sustain interest in a learning task did show marked differences from nonanemic children. When the iron deficiency was corrected, the pattern of attentiveness and learning improved. Sulzer has also recently reported improvement in learning performance and concentration in iron deficient children following specific treatment.

Iron deficiency has been discovered to critically affect all cell systems, as many proteins and enzymes depend upon adequate iron stores for normal function. Iron deficiency also appears to have a promotive role in infection. While previous reports have suggested an adverse relationship, this position has been more recently challenged. Howell's (1970b) study of 761 iron-deficient infants showed no significant difference in the incidence of infection between anemic children and those with normal hemoglobin values. At the present time, the question remains unanswered. Yet it is the consensus of many investigators that problems with increased infection are not a primary concern in iron deficiency anemia (Smith, 1970b).

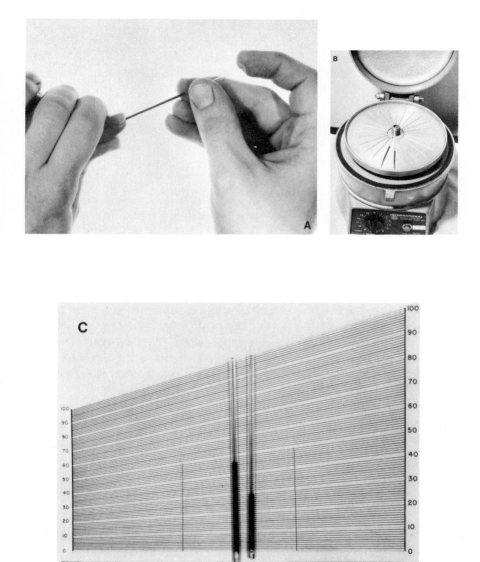

Figure 5. The hematocrit is a precise, rapid method of anemia screening. *A*, the fingertip is pierced with a lancet and the blood collected in a microhematocrit tube. *B*, the tubes are placed in a portable centrifuge and spun for 15 mins., separating the red blood cells from the serum. *C*, the height of the red blood cell layer in the tube is measured on a graph and expressed as the hematocrit. The hematocrit *on the left* (47%) represents a high value and that *on the right* (30%) represents a deficient level or anemia.

Iron deficiency and its effect on growth appears to be another unsettled issue. Previous reports of a strong relationship between iron deficiency and stunted growth have been challenged. Hunter (1970) and Shubert (1970) corroborate each other's findings, showing no difference in weight gain or linear growth in iron deficient and nonanemic groups. It appears that only when iron deficiency becomes so severe as to cause anorexia (loss of appetite) and reduce caloric intake is growth retarded. The growth retardation in this instance must certainly result from the caloric deprivation rather than the anemia per se.

SUMMARY

Early malnutrition has been found to have permanent and profound effects on the eventual intellectual potential and behavior of experimental models. The human implications of poor nutrition are less clear. Yet sufficient data exist to suggest that poor nutrition hinders the growth and development of malnourished children. The effects of early nutritional insults are intensified if they occur during critical periods of growth. Poor nutriture can evidence itself in various degrees. On the most critical level, it can be directly or indirectly responsible for neural impairment. Less dramatically, a reduced nutritional status can result in decreased responsiveness to the environment, thereby interfering with the effectiveness of the school experience, creating learning lags. And at the very least, malnutrition can affect such hard to measure indices as attitude toward school work and performance efficiency. Indirectly, poor nutriture can serve to increase a child's susceptibility to infection.

Catch-up growth, or the remediation of the effects of early malnutrition, has long been held to be only minimally possible. Recent studies, however, have suggested that the ability to compensate at a later date for poor early growth should be given more credence.

Information obtained from the study of nutritional support through school feeding programs affords only basic information. It has been demonstrated that, in many instances, meals provided by such programs may contribute significantly to a child's total food intake. Conclusive evidence, however, does not exist to substantiate the contention that children participating in school feeding programs are necessarily in better health, as could be supported by comparatively better biochemical or anthropometric indices of growth. Neither has there been documented improvement in school performance as measured by contemporary testing instruments. Dietary supplementation does appear, however, to produce a beneficial effect on such behavioral factors as attention span, concentration, and work efficiency.

The identification of the child at risk for nutritional disorders must be included as an important factor in determining the extent and the remediation of malnutrition. Poorly nourished children must be so identified by the careful use of biochemical and anthropometric screening procedures and, subsequently, measured against growth standards which are applicable to the individual child's culture. The use of dated or otherwise inappropriate norms to evaluate a child's nutriture can lead to erroneous conclusions and might exclude many malnourished children from the attention their health status demands.

Finally, it must be remembered that malnutrition all too frequently is only one of a number of contemporaneous factors which may influence the health and subsequent school performance of the child. Often, poor nutriture is the result of a variety of social ills. For a total perspective, malnutrition cannot be viewed apart from the child's entire social and cultural milieu.

REFERENCES

American Academy of Pediatrics Committee Statement. 1973. The ten-state nutrition survey: A pediatric perspective. Pediatrics 51:1095–1099.

Arvedson, I., G. Sterky, and K. Tjernstrom. 1969. Breakfast habits of Swedish school children. J. Am. Dietet. A. 55:257–261.

Baertl, J. M., R. P. Placko, and G. G. Graham. 1974. Serum proteins and plasma free amino acids in severe malnutrition. Am. J. Clin. Nutrition 27:733–742.

Baker, H., O. Frank, S. Feingold, G. Christakis, and H. Ziffer. 1967. Vitamins, total cholesterol and triglycerides in 642 New York City school children. Am. J. Clin. Nutrition 20:850–857.

Becker, B. 1959. Report of a Study of Food Habits in Oklahoma. State Department of Health, Oklahoma City, Okla.

Birch, H. G., and J. D. Gussow. 1970. Illness and medical care of children. In H. G. Birch and J. D. Gussow (eds.), Disadvantaged Children: Health, Nutrition and School Failure, p. 261. Harcourt, Brace and World, Inc., New York.

Chase, H. P., and H. P. Martin. 1970. Undernutrition and child development. New England J. Med. 282:933–939.

Christakis, G., A. Miridjanian, L. Nath, H. S. Khurana, C. Cowell, M. Archer, O. Frank, H. Ziffer, H. Baker, and G. James. 1968. A nutritional epidemiologic investigation of 642 New York City children. Am. J. Clin. Nutrition 21:107–126.

Cone, T. E., Jr. 1968. Physical growth and maturation. In R. E. Cooke and S. Levin (eds.), The Biologic Basis of Pediatric Practice, pp. 1338–1339. McGraw-Hill Book Company, Inc., New York. 1739 p.

Cowley, J. J. 1968. Time, place and nutrition: Some observations from animal studies. In N. S. Scrimshaw and J. E. Gordon (eds.), Malnutrition, Learning and Behavior, p. 218. Massachusetts Institute of Technology Press, Cambridge, Mass.

Cravioto, J. 1970. Complexity of factors involved in protein calorie malnutrition. World Rev. Nutrition Dietet. 14:7–22.

Cravioto, J., E. R. DeLicardie, and H. G. Birch. 1966. Nutrition, growth and neurointegrative development: An experimental and ecologic study. Pediatrics 38:319–372.

Crispin, S., E. Kerrey, H. M. Fox, and C. Kies. 1968. Nutritional status of preschool children. II. Anthropometric measurements and interrelationships. Am. J. Clin. Nutrition 21:1280–1284.

Diamond, L. K. 1970. In N. J. Smith (ed.), Iron Nutrition in Infancy. Report of the 62nd Ross Conference on Pediatric Research, p. 19. Ross Laboratories, Columbus, Ohio.

Dibble, M. V., M. Brin, E. McMullen, A. Peel, and N. Chen. 1965. Some preliminary biochemical findings in junior high school children in Syracuse and Onondaga County, New York. Am. J. Clin. Nutrition 17:218–239.

Edwards, C. H., J. A. Lomax, and G. Grimmett. 1956. Effects of a dietary supplement on height and weight of children. J. Home Econ. 48:363.

Eeg-Larsen, N. 1969. Dietary programmes in school feeding. In G. Blix (ed.), Symposia of the Swedish Nutrition Foundation. VII. Nutrition in Preschool and School Age, pp. 131–136. Almquist & Wiksells, International Booksellers, Uppsala, Sweden.

Eichenwald, H. F., and P. C. Fry. 1969. Nutrition and learning. Science 163: 644–648.

Emmons, L., M. Hayes, and D. L. Call. 1972. A study of school feeding programs. I. Economic eligibility and nutritional need. J. Am. Dietet. A. 61:262–275.

Focus on Oklahoma Food Habits. School Lunch Division, State Department of Education, Vocational Home Economics Department, (Unpublished).

Garn, S. M. 1962. Anthropometry in clinical appraisal of nutritional status. Am. J. Clin. Nutrition 11:418–432.

Garrow, J. S., and M. C. Pike. 1967. The long-term prognosis of severe infantile malnutrition. Lancet 1:1–4.

Graefe, H. K. 1966. Basic problems regarding optimal school lunches. Deutsch. Gesundh. 21:1029–1035.

Graham, G. G., and B. Adrianzen T. 1971. Growth, inheritance and environment. Pediat. Res. 5:691–697.

Graham, G. G., and B. Adrianzen T. 1972. Late "catch-up" growth after severe infantile malnutrition. Johns Hopkins Med. J. 131:204–211.

Howell, D. A. 1970a. In N. J. Smith (ed.), Iron Nutrition in Infancy. Report of the 62nd Ross Conference on Pediatric Research, p. 24. Ross Laboratories, Columbus, Ohio.

Howell, D. A. 1970b. In N. J. Smith (ed.), Iron Nutrition in Infancy. Report of the 62nd Ross Conference on Pediatric Research, p. 30. Ross Laboratories, Columbus, Ohio.

Hunter, R. E. 1970. In N. J. Smith (ed.), Iron Nutrition in Infancy. Report of the 62nd Ross Conference on Pediatric Research, p. 31. Ross Laboratories, Columbus, Ohio.

Kerrey, E., S. Crispin, H. M. Fox, and C. Kies. 1968. Nutritional status of preschool children. I. Dietary and biochemical findings. Am. J. Clin. Nutrition 21:1274–1279.

Laird, D. A., M. Levitan, and V. A. Wilson. 1931. Nervousness in school children as related to hunger and diet. Med. J. Rec. 134:494–499.

Manual for Nutrition Surveys. 1963. 2nd Ed. Interdepartmental Committee on Nutrition for National Defense, National Institutes of Health, United States Government Printing Office, Washington, D. C. 327 p.

Martin, H. P. 1973. Nutrition: Its relationship to children's physical, mental and emotional development. Am. J. Clin. Nutrition 26:766–775.

Mayer, J. 1966. The school lunch program: A factor in children's health. Postgrad. Med. 39:A101–A106.

Miedzybrodska, A. 1968. Trial evaluation of the effect of school meals served according to elaborated standards. Roczn. Panstw. Zukl. Hig. 19:483–490.

Mönckeberg, F. 1968. The effect of early marasmic malnutrition in subsequent physical and psychological development. In N. S. Scrimshaw and J. E. Gordon (eds.), Malnutrition, Learning and Behavior, pp. 269–278. Massachusetts Institute of Technology Press, Cambridge, Mass.

Moore, W. M. 1970. The secular trend in physical growth of urban North American Negro school children. Monogr. Soc. Res. Child. Develop. pp. 62–73.

Myers, M. L. 1968. A nutritional study of school children in a depressed urban district. II. Physical and biochemical findings. J. Am. Dietet. A. 53:234–242.

Paige, D. M. 1971. School feeding program: Who should receive what? J. School Health 41:261–263.

Paige, D. M. 1972. The school feeding program: An underachiever. J. School Health 42:392–395.

Paige, D. M. 1975. Growth in disadvantaged black children. J. School Health 45(3):161–164.

Read, M. S. 1973. Malnutrition, hunger and behavior. II. Hunger, school feeding programs and behavior. J. Am. Dietet. A. 63:386–391.

Report of the Dietary Phase of the Chestuee Nutrition Study. 1953–1958. Nutrition Services, Tennessee Department of Public Health.

Roberts, L. J. 1927. Nutrition Work with Children. University of Chicago Press, Chicago. 639 p.

Rosenfield, D. 1972. Nutrition in U. S. D. A. Child and Family Feeding Programs. Presented at Food Update Eleven, Panel on Nutrition and the Public, April 18, Key Biscayne, Florida. (Unpublished).

Shubert, W. K. 1970. In N. J. Smith (ed.), Iron Nutrition in Infancy. Report of the 62nd Ross Conference on Pediatric Research, p. 31. Ross Laboratories, Columbus, Ohio.

Skidmore, K. 1965. Study of Head Start Preschool Children's Food Habits. Baltimore, Md. (Unpublished).

Smith, N. J. (ed.) 1970a. Iron Nutrition in Infancy. Report of the 62nd Ross Conference on Pediatric Research. Ross Laboratories, Columbus, Ohio. 46 p.

Smith, N. J. (ed.) 1970b. Iron Nutrition in Infancy. Report of the 62nd Ross Conference on Pediatric Research, p. 30. Ross Laboratories, Columbus, Ohio.

Stine, O. C., J. B. Saratsiotis, and O. F. Furno. 1967. Appraising the health of culturally deprived children. Am. J. Clin. Nutrition 20:1084–1095.

Stoch, M. B., and P. M. Smythe. 1967. The effect of undernutrition during infancy on subsequent brain growth and intellectual development. South African Med. J. 41:1027–1030.

Ten-State Nutrition Survey. 1968–1970. 1972. IV. Biochemical. Department of Health, Education, and Welfare Publication No. (HSM) 72-8132. 296 p. (See also American Academy of Pediatrics Committee Statement, 1973.)

Tisdall, F. F., E. G. Robertson, T. G. H. Draka, S. H. Jackson, H. M. Fowler, J. A. Long, L. Brouka, R. G. Ellis, A. J. Phillips, and R. S. Rogers. 1951. The Canadian Red Cross school meal study. Canad. M. A. J. 64:477–489.

Tuttle, W. W., K. Daum, R. Larsen, J. Salzano, and L. Roloff. 1954. Effect on school boys of omitting breakfast: Physiologic responses, attitudes and scholastic attainments. J. Am. Dietet. A. 30:674–677.

Winick, M. 1969. Malnutrition and brain development. J. Pediat. 74:667–679.

Winick, M. 1970. Cellular growth in intrauterine malnutrition. Pediat. Clin. N. Am. 17:69–78.

Winick, M., and P. Rosso. 1969. The effect of severe early malnutrition on cellular growth of human brain. Pediat. Res. 3:181–184.

World Health Organization. 1972. Nutritional Anemias. Technical Report Series, No. 503. World Health Organization, Geneva, Switzerland. 29 p.

14

Minimal Cerebral Dysfunction: Nature and Implications for Therapy

Robert B. Johnston, M.D.

Few handicapping conditions afflicting children require so much interdisciplinary communication but have received so little cooperative professional interaction as the syndrome of minimal cerebral dysfunction (MCD). The physician makes the diagnosis after careful attention to history, physical findings, and ancillary tests and confidently returns the properly labeled package to the educator, whom he assumes will plug the child into the MCD training course. Little does he realize the immensely complicated educational issues that are involved in providing effective remediation programs for these children. On the other hand, equal naïveté is exhibited by the educator who considers soft signs to be the new type of highway billboard that collapses on impact, the electroencephalogram to be the ultimate tool in identifying brain damage, and the MCD child to be an unreachable student who probably is doomed to a life of academic failure and, even worse, drug dependency. These and other misconceptions on both sides of the physician-educator team must be clarified and resolved.

The primary issue as to whether or not there are educational implications for MCD is extremely controversial. Before addressing this complicated issue, it is necessary to define the concept of MCD, the nature and basis of the child's behavior and learning deficits, the methods and pitfalls of the diagnostic process, the therapeutic aspects, and the overall prognosis. In addressing itself to these issues, this chapter will identify and clarify areas of mutual awareness, concern, and interest shared by the physician and educator so that there will be improved communication and cooperation toward the goal of providing better service for the MCD child and his family. An overview approach such as this one cannot

This paper was supported in part through Project 917, Maternal and Child Health Service, United States Department of Health, Education, and Welfare.

detail the many opposing views surrounding the MCD concept. Sufficient references will be cited for further clarification.

INTRODUCTION

For centuries man has been concerned with the nature-nurture controversy concerning the determinants of behavior and learning. Until recently, major emphasis has been placed on nurture, with many environmental influences as primary determinants. Now the pendulum is swinging toward the nature side, with emphasis on the contribution of the brain to behavior and learning disabilities. Since the early work of such investigators as Strauss and Lehtinen (1947), a constellation of specific types of behavior, such as distractability, perseveration, and impulsivity, has been thought to be related to underlying brain dysfunction. Likewise, certain specific types of learning disabilities have been ascribed to brain dysfunction rather than some deficiency in the environment. Thus, these efforts to implicate the brain have resulted in removing the dunce cap of the past and placing the EEG electrode on the head of the deviant student!

Syndrome Identification

A syndrome is defined as a group of symptoms and/or signs that occur together to characterize a given condition. Those individuals falling into a particular syndrome can be homogeneous with little variability from individual to individual, or heterogeneous with many features in common but with some unshared characteristics. If the group is homogeneous, such as persons with Down's syndrome (see Chapter 10), information from previous study and research about the condition—nature, prognosis, and response to therapy—is often applicable to specific individuals within that group. On the other hand, if the group is heterogeneous, it is more difficult to make generalizations about specific members of the group.

The definition of the MCD syndrome indicates a very heterogeneous group of normally intelligent children who have deficiencies in behavioral and/or learning skills thought to be secondary to central nervous system (brain) dysfunction as evidenced by a number of characteristics occurring in isolation or in a variety of combinations (i.e., impaired perception, language development, memory, impulse control and/or motor function) (Clements, 1966).

Identifying Terms

Because this group of children is so heterogeneous and has such a variety of characteristics, it is difficult to find an appropriate title. This obsession with proper labels for these children has been referred to as the "Rumpelstiltskin fixation" (Ross, 1968), referring to the story of the young maiden who could achieve freedom if she could only name her captor. By the same token, there is a misguided impression in certain circles that if these children were only properly labeled their difficulties would be resolved. A short review of some of the proposed labels will outline the problem.

Identification by major trait is ineffective. "Hyperkinetic syndrome" excludes that small percentage who are hypoactive. "Perceptually handicapped" both oversimplifies the condition and eliminates many of those children who are without acknowledged perceptual problems. Eponyms identifying the syndrome by the main or initial investigator (Strauss syndrome) fail to account for the additional characteristics that have been added to this concept since the initial descriptions.

One term that has been popular in the past is minimal brain damage (MBD). The difficulties with this term are many. It conjures up the mental image of a brain that is pocked by scars and holes which, to say the least, is totally inaccurate and unproved. Damage implies a known causative factor, and the idea that the damage cannot be corrected ignores the fact that many of the cases probably represent slow maturation rather than specific brain damage per se. Consequently, in general, the term "brain damage" is quite stigmatizing and implies a negative response to intervention.

Acceptance, although not universal, has been greater for the term minimal cerebral dysfunction. The term "minimal" is relative to the severe forms of brain dysfunction (mental retardation and/or cerebral palsy) and does not refer to the degree of handicap, which is by no means minimal. The term "cerebral" has received some opposition because it refers to cortical areas of the brain and not technically to some of the lower brain centers which have been implicated in certain aspects of this syndrome. The term "dysfunction" allows for a wide range of abnormalities, without limiting the spectrum to anatomic deficits, and permits inclusion of biochemical, physiologic, and maturational factors. One can imagine a massive switchboard with a few lines misconnected without total destruction or disruption of any of its major components.

Because of the lack of actual direct proof of brain damage or dysfunction and because of the stigmatizing effect of these terms, an alternative term which refers to the delayed or irregular maturation (DIM) of the nervous system alone has been suggested. (This is to be differentiated from delayed and underdeveloped maturation giving an eponym of DUM, a label that has been used for centuries.)

The term "psychoneurological learning disability" (Myklebust and Boshes, 1960) has much appeal to the educator since it identifies the learning disability as the common thread among the children in this group. It also emphasizes the educational role in handling the problem, admits to a psychologic and neurologic component, and allows the school system to deal with the disability without the necessity for medical intervention.

The confusion and controversy over the proper designation of this syndrome graphically illustrates the results of multidisciplinary approaches with a failure of interdisciplinary communication. It vividly points out the difficulty, if not impossibility, of allotting one classification to a very heterogeneous group of children. For the purpose of simplification, the designation of minimal cerebral dysfunction will be utilized in this chapter.

DESCRIPTION OF THE ENTITY

Before surveying the many characteristics of this syndrome, the teacher should be forewarned about certain facts. The presence of any one of these character- istics does not necessarily imply MCD for at least two reasons. Many of the findings are developmental in nature, implying normality at a certain age (i.e., short attention span in a 3-year-old, letter reversals in a 6-year-old). Second, the described behavior may well be due primarily to environmental factors (the non-MCD "spoiled child") and not associated with a dysfunctioning nervous system. It is not an uncommon mistake to consider all types of hyperactivity to be the result of MCD. However, diagnosis of MCD is made only after careful observation and analysis of all findings, and should not be based on a few isolated characteristics.

There are many features of this syndrome that may hinder the child's emotional adjustment and academic achievement. An individual child may embody a few or many of these invisible handicaps. Those with many typical characteristics may be responsible for the seasoned educator's request for an early retirement or the student teacher's consideration of an alternate career in fashion design!

For the purpose of chapter organization and not necessarily technical accu- racy, the MCD child may be characterized by looking at deficits in his attention- control functions, as well as in his other nonverbal and verbal learning skills.

Attention-Control Deficits

Attention involves the ability to maintain an orientation to a given subject and requires a number of complex connections within the brain. Control refers to that ability to maintain direction in both physical and mental processes.

Attentional Peculiarities "Johnny is constantly on the go, flipping from one thing to the other, completing none of his assignments and frequently disrupting the class with interruptions. He also has frequent temper outbursts, usually with the slightest provocation." . . . a frustrated teacher.

This child shows many of the difficulties that are symbolic of the group of attention-control deficiencies. His *short attention span* denotes a failure of the physiologic mechanisms to alert and to maintain vigilance on one subject. Casual stimuli such as swinging pigtails or squeaking desks interrupt his attention easily. On the other hand, another child may display *perseveration*—an inability to shift attention from a less important item and a persistence in insignificant motor, verbal, visual, or thought activity, exemplified by repetitive circle drawing, daydreaming, etc. Care must be taken to differentiate plain old boredom with schoolwork from abnormalities in attentional functions by investigating abilities in other settings (i.e., can he attend to Saturday morning cartoons for longer than 15–20 mins.?).

Hyperactivity "My son acts like something inside him will not let him rest. He cannot stand still. He sleeps with one foot next to the floor because as soon as he wakes up he is on the go." ... an exhausted mother.

This characteristic is commonly identified in the MCD child and has several variations. The above "human dynamo" is frequently seen but not caught in the classroom. Mothers of these children often recall excessive movements even while carrying the baby in the womb. Other-types of hyperactive children are the fidgeters, who restlessly shift, tap, rustle, and generally disrupt the structured classroom but are normally active on the playground. Also, there are the stimulus-bound children, whose activity is not excessive but is totally non-directed and inappropriate—the "whirling dervish" whose rushing from one thing to the other virtually destroys the teacher's classroom or the physician's examining room in 2 mins.! This type of driven behavior is thought to be most characteristic of certain types of brain dysfunction. Paradoxically, there is also a small group of children who are less active than normal (*hypoactive*), but who are included in this syndrome because they share many of the other common features of MCD.

Difficulties in control can affect both movement and behavior. The lack of control of impulses (*impulsivity*) leads to many difficulties in lessened frustration tolerance, erratic mood swings, and antisocial behavior. In addition, deficient control and coordination of movements (*incoordination*) leads to clumsy performance, with resultant poor penmanship in the classroom and perennial bench warming on the sports field.

Nonverbal Learning Deficiencies

Many of the deficiencies to be described below share a common basis—the inability to grasp the significant aspects of a situation, whether it be in interpersonal relations, interpretation of drawings, learning a motor skill pattern, or orienting oneself in space. Again, a given child may possess one or a combination of these features (Johnson and Myklebust, 1967).

Social Imperception A child's insensitivity to social pressures may be related to his inability to perceive the situation properly. Some MCD children have difficulty interpreting nonverbal communication—i.e., gesture, scowl, hug, etc.—and, therefore, fail to respond appropriately to these clues. Additionally, antisocial behavior and poor response to discipline may be the result of antihedonism (Wender, 1971). This is defined as a reduced sensitivity to pleasurable or painful social experiences, with the resultant effect that the rewards of a job well done or the criticism for unacceptable behavior do not influence the child's subsequent performance.

Graphic Learning Deficiency   Incompetent learning through pictures may be related to the inability to perceive the "gestalt" or entire picture (i.e., the child may interpret a picture of a square as four unrelated lines, failing to grasp the whole as more than just the sum of its parts). Likewise, the child may focus on one element of the picture and fail to grasp the nature of the entire setting.

Motor Pattern Learning Defect   Although specific aspects of control and coordination may be intact, failure to realize the motor pattern or sequence of movements required to accomplish a motor task is just as debilitating. For instance, a child with this deficit may very well have the ability to hold and loop his shoelace adequately, but cannot orchestrate these movements into a meaningful sequence to ultimately tie a bow. This type of difficulty often generates the impression that "he could do it if he would only try."

Body Image and Spatial Orientation Inadequacy   The development of one's own body image and its orientation in space have been theoretically related to a number of learning problems too complex to detail here. Very simply, a child who is unable to understand the relative position of his body parts—for instance, his fingers—may have extreme difficulty with fine manipulation and writing. If his orientation in space is poor, he could experience difficulty identifying letters whose differences were based primarily on spatial orientation (i.e., b, p, and d).

Verbal Learning Disability

The child's academic career is hampered not only by the above deficits but also by dysfunctions allegedly directly involved in the processes of reading, writing, and arithmetic. These impairments have been generally classified as perceptual handicaps and involve the brain's processing of information received from the senses—vision, hearing, and touch.

Basically, each sensory system must accurately receive and transmit information to the brain, requiring, for instance, a normal visual or hearing apparatus. The brain must then, like a computer, register the information, incorporate it into its fund of past experience, and use it by accurate recording, storage, and recall. Finally, the brain must integrate information from all these sensory modalities through an intersensory network and transmit it to other systems (motor) for proper action or response. For instance, the brain must combine visual information (graphic symbols) with auditory information (phonemic sounds) to identify a word, and then properly coordinate motor activity to vocalize the word (Chalfant and Scheffelin, 1969; and Gofman, 1971).

Obviously, there are many phases of these central processing systems that might be inoperative and produce various types of perceptual handicaps. Commonly noted defects include inability to discern visually significant features from minutiae, letter and word reversals, poor copying skills, inability to remember instructions given verbally, and difficulty in discriminating the differ-

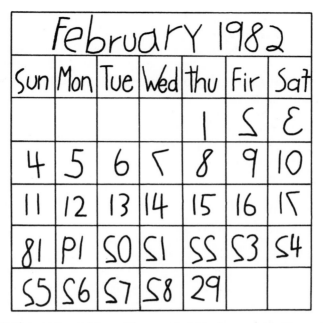

Figure 1. Calendar constructed by a 7½-year-old child of normal intelligence but with a learning disability.

ence between certain closely related sounds. Figure 1 illustrates some of the problems noting the "hopeless entanglement of confusion with visual memory, spatial relations, sequencing, left-right progression, and fine motor skills" (Gofman, 1971).

The concern with perceptual deficiencies as relevant factors in the learning disabled child has reached a high level of popularity but is now being questioned and reexamined by several investigators. On the one hand, Frostig (1972) feels that perceptual problems are basic to learning disabilities and that visual-perceptual exercises enhance overall development. However, there are contradictory findings which would disagree with this viewpoint, since it is not uncommon to find children with visual-perceptual signs who read and learn quite well, and conversely, children with markedly deficient reading skills who have no evidence of perceptual deficits at all (Symmes and Rapoport, 1972). It is essential to be aware of this controversy, but it will not be debated in this short chapter. Reference should be made to other sources (Smith and Marx, 1972).

ETIOLOGY

The physician is vitally interested in determining the causes of MCD in order to establish more meaningful subcategories, improved methods of prevention, and more effective medication strategies.

On the other hand, etiology is not a prime concern to most educators. Yet, despite educator Cohen's cleverly catchy clause, "Etiology be damned," (Cohen, 1973), the educator should have some awareness of the possible causes as part of her understanding of the entity.

Additionally, despite the emphasis on the central nervous system and its role in behavior and learning, it should be recalled that there are yet many other influences that exist, such as innate temperament and psychosocial and psycho-dynamic factors, that play an important function in the evolution of certain behavior and learning disabilities. These, however, will not be detailed in this section.

Insults to the Central Nervous System

The developing and maturing brain is subject to a number of possible insults, especially during certain critical time periods, such as gestation, labor, and delivery. As a result, there is a wide variety of potential impairments that can ensue which are generally termed "the continuum of reproductive casualty" (Knobloch and Pasamanick, 1959). The latter include degrees of brain injury ranging from death through mental retardation and cerebral palsy to MCD (Table 1).

Those insults that primarily interfere with the nutrition and oxygen supply to the brain cells in the fetus may be caused by certain conditions in the mother such as infection, high blood pressure, or bleeding during pregnancy, or by abnormalities limited to the baby, such as prematurity, breathing difficulties, or chemical imbalances. It is most important to realize, however, that not all children who experience such incidents develop evidence of brain dysfunction; nor, on the other hand, do all children with MCD characteristics have a history of such insults.

Table 1. Spectrum of Impairments Noted in Brain Dysfunctions[a]

Function	Degree of Impairment	
	Severe	Minimal
Motor	Cerebral palsy	Cluminess
Sensory	Blindness	Visual imperceptibility
	Deafness	Poor auditory memory
	Loss of sensation	Astereognosis
Intellectual	Mental deficiency	Specific learning disability

[a]Modified after Paine (1962).

It is interesting to note that as a result of recent advances in maternal and newborn care, the severity of the complications associated with birth have lessened; thus, there are fewer casualties at the extreme end of the spectrum (death or profound mental retardation). Yet there does appear to be an increase in those survivors at the opposite pole of the spectrum with characteristic MCD symptoms.

Noninsult Factors

There are several instances where a careful review of the history fails to uncover an incident which may account for the apparent brain dysfunction. Many cases may merely represent the result of a slower rate of central nervous system maturation rather than defective brain development or damage. In certain students, there is a familial or hereditary tendency toward MCD as evidenced by a higher than expected incidence in individual families involving mainly male siblings, parents, and grandparents. It is little consolation for the teacher who has just completed 1 year of frustration with a child with MCD to realize that he has three younger brothers who appear to have similar difficulties coming her way!

Consideration of the fascinating possibility of specific biochemical abnormalities contributing to brain dysfunction will be discussed later in this chapter.

MEDICAL EVALUATION—NEURODEVELOPMENTAL ASSESSMENT

One of the major stumbling blocks to effective communication and cooperation between teachers and physicians is the confusion surrounding the medical assessment of the child with behavior and learning disabilities. The teacher is justifiably perplexed by the contradictory diagnostic impressions given by different physicians. It is not uncommon for an individual child to be evaluated by a number of professionals and to be considered "all boy who will outgrow it," "perfectly normal," "emotionally disturbed," "late bloomer," "perceptually handicapped," "neurotically inhibited," or "brain damaged." These impressions emanate from generally competent physicians who, because of differences in training, interest, and time, view the nature of the problem and the method of assessment in markedly dissimilar ways.

Underlying some of this confusion is a lack of awareness that the assessment of the child with behavior and learning difficulties requires a different, nontraditional approach to testing neurologic function—the neurodevelopmental assessment. Abnormalities noted in this examination are termed "soft signs" and reflect subtle neurologic dysfunction that is inappropriate for the age of the child. Details of these controversial soft signs will be discussed below.

Goals of the Assessment

Figure 2 represents a conceptual model of the relationship between brain function, the clinical neurologic assessment, and behavior and learning dis-

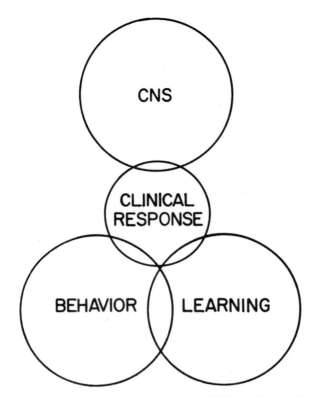

Figure 2. Interrelationships of factors in assessment of MCD. Evidence of faulty clinical responses by the brain may be an associative link to incriminating brain dysfunction in certain behavior and learning disabilities.

abilities. The brain is responsible for mediating behavior and learning. If behavior and learning skills are deficient, it is possible that the underlying cause is a malfunctioning brain. If there were the technical know-how to measure brain function directly—i.e., to determine anatomic, biochemical, or electrical changes involved in the brain's reception and processing of information—it would be unnecessary to examine the child further. For example, if electrical circuits involved in visual reception and processing could be monitored directly, perceptual deficiencies could be elicited and documented without the need for complicated testing. Although preliminary research studies look promising with regard to the auditory and visual evoked potentials (Preston, Guthrie, and Childs, 1974), at the present time there are no direct techniques of measuring brain function. Hence, there is a need for indirect measurements. These indirect measurements involve the brain's competence to perform certain tasks which are classified as clinical responses. Soft signs then represent subtle deficiencies in a number of specific neurologic skills. If the presence of soft signs indicates dysfunction in given areas of the brain, it is theoretically possible that there is an associated dysfunction in anatomically related regions of the central nervous system which ultimately results in behavior and learning disabilities. Therefore, it is through the concept of soft signs that one attempts to find an associative link, rather than a direct link, between brain dysfunction and behavior or learning deficits.

Parameters of Measurement

There is no single test that will indicate overall normal or abnormal brain function. Therefore, assessment of many areas of function is necessary. Unfortunately, there are no reliable neurologic tests to evaluate those areas of the brain that directly mediate behavior or learning. Therefore, the physician is primarily interested in the testable areas of motor, sensory, and laterality skills, while other specialists are more involved in definitive testing of language, perception, and cognition (Gofman, 1971).

With regard to the neurologic assessment, it is important to realize the developmental nature of the skills tested. During the first 14–16 years of life, the brain is constantly undergoing maturation. The dramatic nature of this developmental process is most evident during the initial 5 years of life, as the individual's skills in motor, adaptive, language, and personal social abilities progress at a rapid rate. Less dramatic, but just as important, is the continuation of this maturational phenomenon during the school age years. The child's ability to perform certain motor, sensory, and laterality skills increases as maturation progresses. It is this level of refinement that is assessed in the neurodevelopmental exam. The inadequate performance of a given task is not necessarily abnormal unless it is inappropriate for age. It is not uncommon that certain skills would be normally deficient at one age but undergo improvement due to maturation at a later age. Therefore, it is vital to be aware of what degree of competence is expected for a given task at a given age. In other words, soft signs at any age are not necessarily abnormal. It is this concept that is not well understood and leads to an extreme amount of confusion. The uncertainty concerning the significance of soft signs stems, for the most part, from the lack of appreciation of these developmental considerations.

A brief description of some sample components of the neurodevelopmental exam with examples of soft signs will be discussed below, not with the expectation of making medical diagnosticians out of teachers, but to give some understanding of the complexity of the assessment and to eliminate some of the mystery ascribed to it.

Motor System

Motor skills involve the brain's ability to control body tone and movement. There appears to be a higher incidence of motor problems or clumsiness in children with learning disabilities who have had a history of prior central nervous system insult. Such areas as muscle control, coordination, balance, station, and associated movements are surveyed.

Faulty control and coordination are illustrated by the presence of involuntary twitching movements, unusual posturing when the arms and hands are extended, or abnormal coordination of voluntary rapid finger or arm movements. Most normal 8-year-old children have acquired an adequate degree of proficiency in these spheres.

Balance and station difficulties are characterized by the inability to maintain balance on one foot with the eyes closed, capably walk a straight line heel-to-toe, or preserve the normal swing and posture of the arms during walking or running. Competence in these areas is usually achieved at 7–8 years of age.

Associated movements refer to those involuntary muscle movements that occur at the same time that voluntary movements are taking place in another part of the body. As the brain matures, its ability to progressively inhibit unwanted movements increases. The normal spectrum ranges from an infant who responds to a rattle by total body activity rather than movement of one arm to the adult who is able to focus his response to watch repairing by precise fine finger control without movement of any other part of his body. The presence of associated movements is observed clinically in the resting hand during the time that fine finger movements are occurring in the other hand (sometimes noted during writing assignments) and during rapid alternating movements of the arm. Most children over the age of 9 can inhibit these extraneous movements.

Sensory System

In addition to identifying gross sensations such as heat, pain, or touch, the nervous system, as it matures, begins to integrate sensations in a more complex fashion. These are termed "higher cortical functions" and refer to such skills as simultactgnosia, finger identification, stereognosis, and graphesthesia.

Simultactgnosia is the ability to identify two simultaneously applied touches to different parts of the body (face and hand). Prior to the age of 7, most children will not appreciate the more distal touch (hand). Finger identification concerns both the proper labeling of individual fingers, as well as recognition of their relative position to each other—skills which are usually accomplished by the age of 7–8. Stereognosis refers to the ability to identify an object by feel without seeing it and is tested by utilizing such items as a bottle cap, button, or key. Most children can successfully master this task by 5–6 years. Graphesthesia is another fancy term to indicate the ability to identify symbols such as letters or numbers written by the examiner on the skin (usually on the fingertips), and again is usually perfected by the age of 6.

Laterality Relationships

There are two separate entities within the concept of laterality relationships: lateral dominance (preference) and left-right orientation.

Dominance has received considerable attention in the past. It is thought that as the brain matures it begins to allocate individual functions to specific areas. As a part of its organizational maturation, one side of the brain becomes dominant for language and may be associated with the development of dominance for other skills. The assessment of dominance in hand, eye, and leg preference is readily accomplished. It is usually accepted that a child begins to develop hand preference by 18 months but may be somewhat ambidextrous until the age of 5 years. What is less well accepted, however, is that hand preference, although established, does not stabilize until 9–10 years of age, as pointed out by Belmont and Birch (1965). Thus, during the time from 5 to 9 or 10 years of age, the child may normally vacillate in his hand selection. Eye preference may be established in the eye with the best visual acuity and really has nothing to do with central brain dominance. At any rate, what has been looked for in the past as a sign of normal brain organization is one-sided preference for all lateral functions (i.e., the child prefers to use his right eye, right hand, and right foot for all activities). However, most well-controlled studies fail to show any correlation between the lack of complete dominance and learning disabilities, although this has been a well-accepted legend for years (Stephens, Cunningham, and Stigler, 1967).

Another important aspect of laterality development is that of left-right orientation, referring to the child's ability to identify left and right directions. There is normal sequence of developing these skills, beginning at 6 years and terminating at 10, involving abilities to identify one's own left and right, cross-identify by placing left hand on right ear, for instance, as well as identify left and right on a confronting indivudual. There is some evidence in the literature that this type of difficulty may be associated with reading and writing disabilities because of the basic left-right orientation thought to be necessary for accomplishing these skills (Gofman, 1971).

Ancillary Measurement—The EEG

The role of the EEG in assessing a child with possible MCD needs clarification. To hold that the normal EEG "rules out brain damage" is totally inaccurate and should be abolished from the educator's glossary of terms. To understand the limitations of the EEG, it is necessary to realize that it measures electrical impulses from the outer surface of the brain next to the skull. It has absolutely no ability to identify thinking disorders, perceptual problems, attentional peculiarities, or the wide range of brain processing dysfunctions described above. The EEG may be useful in identifying specific areas of the brain which have abnormal electrical activity related possibly to some underlying damage or malfunction; however, these are not the findings that one usually discerns in the *minimally* involved nervous system.

It is true that certain studies have shown that there is an increased incidence of mildly abnormal EEG's in children diagnosed as MCD compared to apparently normal children. However, the changes are not particularly significant nor are they of diagnostic import. It should be carefully noted that approximately 20% of the normal population has some type of abnormality in their EEG pattern quite similar to those changes observed in some of the MCD children. On the other hand, there are several children with classic MCD symptoms with perfectly normal EEG's. What all this means is that, for an individual case, the EEG is not particularly helpful. If the EEG is normal, brain dysfunction is not ruled out; if it is mildly abnormal, it cannot be differentiated from the identical EEG's that are seen in 20% of the normal population.

Although there are some exciting indications that the use of evoked potentials in EEG research may have relevance in the future to diagnostic and therapeutic endeavors (Preston, Guthrie, and Childs, 1974), it is not widely utilized at this time and should not be confused with the common everyday use of the EEG.

MEDICAL SUPPORT

The physician is not only a diagnostician, case coordinator, and counselor but also a biochemist by virtue of his increasing interest in and use of medication for the amelioration of certain symptoms common to the MCD child. During the past four decades since Bradley's (1937) initial discovery of the quieting effect of Benzedrine on brain-damaged children, this issue has been met with uncertainty by many, enthusiasm by some, and horror by a few. For the educator to cooperate in a medication venture, it is necessary that she understand the underlying rationale, usual treatment regimen, and nature of resistance to this mode of therapy.

Rationale for the Use of Stimulant Drugs

There are several unproved theories (Wender, 1971) as to the manner in which these medications exert their influence. One general hypothesis postulates that there is a deficiency in the brain's ability to inhibit certain activites. For instance, if the brain's filtering mechanism (reticular-activating system), which usually dampens irrelevant incoming stimuli, is defective, attention-control problems described above ensue because of overstimulation. The stimulant drugs then would intensify the filtering mechanism's effectiveness and improve the child's attentional skills by paradoxically reducing the stimuli reaching the brain. A sedative, on the other hand, would decrease the filtering function, resulting in worsening of behavior, a commonly noted clinical experience.

Additionally, there is an area of the brain (limbic system) that may be responsible for setting up the electrical circuits that make one responsive to reinforcement and reward which are basic to learning. Medication that would stimulate this underactive area would allegedly enhance the effect of reward, increasing both social and academic learning.

Basic to all central nervous system functions are the chemical substances (neurotransmitters) that convey messages from one nerve cell to the other. When supposed deficiencies of these chemicals (which currently cannot be measured in the blood) are corrected by medication, there may be an overall increase in the efficiency of certain brain functions. Such medications as Ritalin and Dexedrine are thought to function in this fashion. Megavitamins, on the other hand, do not fall into this category of substances, and their use has not been proved to be effective.

These theories offer certain models from which one can develop treatment strategies with the realization that there has been no substantial proof of one theory or the other at the present time.

Results of Medical Therapy

Interpretation of any study demonstrating the results of medication in MCD must be tempered by at least two important factors. The placebo effect—a positive response to *any* pill—will give falsely positive results if not dealt with by well-structured and long-term studies. Secondly, since there is a variety of conditions concealed under the umbrella of MCD, there are a wide range of responses to the drug, and generalizations concerning its effectiveness for the group as a whole cannot be made.

Results of well-controlled studies of the most commonly used drugs, Dexedrine and Ritalin (Millichap, 1968), indicate that between 60–80% of MCD children have favorable responses, as measured by improvement in hyperactivity, attention span, temperament, or response to discipline. The effect on cognitive skills is more difficult to assess. Conners (1971) suggests that the improvement of controls (better attention) is the essential feature for enhancement of cognition. Others feel that there is a more direct effect with improvements in tests of general intelligence and visual-motor perception (Millichap, 1968).

Since drug effectiveness can be measured by changes in behavior and learning, a number of protocols have been developed to aid the teacher's observations. Davids (1971) identifies areas of hyperactivity, attention span, variability, impulsiveness, irritability-explosiveness, and school work. Conners (1969) categorizes observations into daydreaming-inattention, defiance and aggression, anxiety and fear, hyperactivity, and peer relations.

In conclusion, medication in selected children results in obvious and occasionally "miraculous" improvement in certain of the above-mentioned spheres. Yet there are many apparent failures that act as constant reminders that medication is certainly not the panacea that some would like to believe, and that it must be used in association with other types of supportive counseling and remediation efforts.

Drug Management Regimen

Generally, medication is initiated in small doses, with gradual increases to a maintenance level when maximum benefits are obtained. Since some children respond differently to these medications, it is often necessary to alter the drug type, amount, or timing of dose to determine the appropriate combination.

Additional adjustments may be necessary as time progresses. Although these alterations in the regimen are distressing to the child, parent, teacher, and school nurse, it should be understood that it is not an unusual occurrence and does not necessarily indicate a poor prognosis.

Although there are several medications in use (Wender, 1971), this discussion is limited to Dexedrine and Ritalin. If one of these medications proves to be ineffective, a trial attempt is usually made with the other. In the adult nervous system, both of these drugs result in increased rather than decreased activity. However, in children whose nervous systems have not yet reached maturity, these medications often work paradoxically to diminish the activity level.

Dexedrine is available in a 5-mg tablet which is effective for 3–5 hrs., and a 10-mg spansule with timed release ingredients which usually lasts from 12–18 hrs. Ritalin is made only in tablet form of varying strengths, the most popular of which is the 10-mg tablet which is effective for 3–5 hrs. The long-acting, once-a-day spansule has, unfortunately, not met with outstanding success. Since the tablet form has an effect for approximately 4 hrs., the school's cooperation is necessary for a midday dosage.

The amount of medication required is not proportionate to the degree of dysfunction (i.e., a child on a large amount of medication is not necessarily more neurologically involved than his associate on a much smaller dosage). Unlike drugs such as aspirin which are taken intermittently and on the occasion of a headache or toothache, these medications are prescribed over a long period of time and are not used merely in times of crisis. The stability of the child's response to the medication depends on the gradual cumulative effect of the drug over a period of time, so that "shotgun" therapy at periodic intervals is usually ineffective. These children, like teachers and physicians, are subject to good and bad days. Medication should not be altered each time a disturbance or problem is generated.

Resistance to the Use of Stimulant Drugs

Opposition to medication for MCD children is based on a variety of factors—some rational, others irrational—as discussed below.

Indiscriminate Use All that is hyperactive is not MCD. Medication should be prescribed only after thorough analysis and study of the child. Then follow-up and close supervision in conjunction with a total remediation education program are necessary. Situations where medication is used indiscriminately and independently of other supportive measures are a disservice to the child and his family.

Dependence on Medication Just as in other chronic deficiency conditions, such as diabetes and dwarfism secondary to absent growth hormone that require replacement therapy, there arises a fear that the child will use the medication as a crutch and not develop his own coping abilities in the future. This emotional need of the child should be dealt with, but not at the expense of discontinuing the replacement of his deficiency (insulin, growth hormone, or Ritalin). These medications should not be considered "chemical straitjackets," binding the child to a given chemically induced response. Rather, in many cases, they provide a means by which he can broaden his horizons and choose to respond in a more effective and meaningful way.

Addiction The adult may become dependent or addicted to certain medications associated with the generation of euphoria or "high" feelings. The developing nervous system of children does not respond to the stimulant drugs in that fashion. There has been no evidence of any euphoric effect of these drugs, nor have there been any reported cases of addiction or dependency in the MCD population. Justifiable concerns are raised about older siblings in the household or adolescents in the school who might attempt to confiscate the medication for their personal use.

Side Effects For the most part, the major side effects consist of loss of appetite, sleep disturbances, or indigestion. These are usually evident early in therapy and either diminish or are remediable by altering the dosage. The long-term results of drug therapy are not well identified, as evidenced by several studies presently concerned with the effect on overall height and weight (Safer, Allen, and Barr, 1972). There have been no reported cases of irreversible or severe toxic effects in those children with properly controlled medication regimens.

Misunderstood Goals As mentioned above, often expectations of medication are overinflated in MCD. One should not assume that the child will "fall apart" if he forgot to bring his noontime medication to school, nor should one expect him to be perfectly controlled and unresponsive to family events, school pressures, or the excitement of upcoming holidays while on medication.

EMOTIONAL SUPPORT

Only a brief summary of the many approaches to the psychologic needs of the child with MCD will be considered in this chapter.

Because of his defective attention-control abilities, the child requires a fair degree of imposed, structured environmental controls and limits. An open classroom model, with its wealth of stimulation and lack of structure, is often the undoing of many MCD children.

Secondly, the child needs simple routines with minimal variation. Teachers are encouraged to maintain as much of a routine as possible, and parents are likewise advised to maintain regular patterns of activity each day upon his return from school.

Thirdly, discipline must be firm, consistent, and involve *important* issues. Parental and teacher awareness that some of the offenses are unavoidable and unintentional helps to ease the tension within the home and classroom. The tendency to be constantly "on him" concerning aspects of tidiness, manners, clumsiness, and activity should be tempered with understanding and alleviated by permitting him to isolate himself in his room or gym class and pursue any and all activities that he so desires (i.e., by "getting off his back").

Finally, it is of vital importance that he establish and maintain his self-esteem despite his academic and/or athletic deficiencies. Some outlet and opportunity for success should be used which does not require skills in his deficient areas—scouting, swimming, music, art, stamp, or coin collecting. Both at home and at school attempts should be made to refrain from belittling him or emphasizing his deficiencies to his peers.

EDUCATIONAL SUPPORT

In this section, an overview of the presently utilized treatment models and strategies will be inspected, pointing out the controversial nature and lack of uniform agreement as to the most expeditious method to educationally intervene with the MCD child (for additional information see Chapter 12).

Remediation Models

During the past decade, there have been several classroom models in existence, ranging from complete isolation to total incorporation of the MCD child in the regular classroom.

Self-Contained Classroom   In the self-contained classroom, the child is removed from the regular classroom, given a specially trained teacher and a modified curriculum. In an attempt to decrease interfering stimuli, a specifically designed area utilizing cubicles, carpeting, subdued lighting and colors, as well as non-movable furniture, is arranged for the student.

Disadvantages of this concept arise by virtue of the stigma attached to the isolated child who is different, the subsequent reluctance of the regular classroom teacher to assume teaching responsibility for anyone but normals (role of the special educator), having disabled peers as models of behavior, and, finally, inappropriate mixing of MCD and mentally retarded children.

Resource Rooms   With the utilization of resource rooms, the child remains within his regular classroom and with his normal peers for most of the day. When the class approaches a subject in which the pupil requires individualized attention, he moves to the resource room where specific techniques are utilized to help improve his deficient areas.

Mainstreaming   Under the mainstreaming concept the child remains in the regular classroom. The regular teacher's isolation with these problem children is lessened by the support received from regular visits of a consultant who assists in developing specialized approaches for individual students. In addition to employing specific teaching strategies, adjustments to the child's individual characteristics are implemented. For instance, the child with excess energy may be assigned such tasks as erasing the board, opening the window, or running an errand. The child with poor penmanship may receive oral exams. The child with a short attention span may receive instructions in three 20-min. segments instead of over an uninterrupted hour.

This model, in theory, helps improve the child's worth by lessening the stigma of being different since he is with normal peers and uses them as models of behavior. In practice, however, it sometimes suffers from the variability of teacher ability, lack of classroom control, and inability to satisfy individual needs because of the excessive demands of a large class.

Educational Strategies

Details concerning controversial issues involved in the many approaches to educational remediation should be reviewed in the educational literature since only the basics will be touched upon in this section.

A fundamental approach has been to remediate those deficiencies thought to be underlying the learning disability. For instance, impairments such as the inability to discriminate figure-ground relationships or faulty auditory memory are treated in a particular fashion. Subsequently, many specialized training activities have been devised seeking to rectify those deficits described above, such as visual and auditory imperception, flaws in intersensory integration, and motor incoordination.

Considerable interest and popularity has been associated with perceptual-motor techniques, as evidence by many proponents (Johnson and Myklebust, 1967) as well as opponents (Smith and Marx, 1972; and Symmes and Rapoport, 1972). Additionally, orthoptic measures, which suggest that a given set of eye movement exercises performed regularly by the child will overcome their handicaps, have received poor reviews as to their theoretic soundness or practical effect on perceptual problems (McGrady and McCarthy, 1971) (see Chapter 2). Another approach concerns working with motor and coordination deficits which are associated with learning disabilities. Opponents suggest that the exercise may well improve physical fitness or even motor skills but find little evidence for enhancing learning abilities.

The indirect method of attacking deficient skills thought to be related to learning disabilities is contrasted to the opposite tact which directly approaches the subject that is to be taught. For instance, rather than teaching a child to differentiate a square from a triangle in order to improve his perceptual skills, the direct method would devote time and effort in the use of accepted methods to teach him to read or write, subsequently enhancing his reading and writing skills directly.

The latter approach, being dissatisfied with the conclusion that dyspedagogy is better than no pedagogy at all, berates the teaching profession to engineer more effective technologies in the actual teaching of the three R's. These task-oriented approaches are well outlined by Bateman (1973) and Cohen (1973).

IMPLICATIONS

The MCD child with his admixture of etiologies, maladaptive behaviors, and variable responses to therapy certainly exists. He is very much in our midst. The physician and educator must determine whether all this MCD-related information has any implications to the educator. Does the understanding of this particular entity provide any assistance for the educator in planning effective strategies for remediation, any insight into the child as to his individual needs, or any basis for better communication with the physician, parent, or other members of the therapy team?

. . . For Teaching Strategies

The following are quotations from well-known educators who are active in the field of learning disabilities and indicate the wide diversity of opinion concerning the educational implication of MCD. Johnson and Myklebust (1967) write that: "The findings of the neurologist, electroencephalographer and ophthalmologist are of considerable value to the educator. . . . With assistance of these specialists we have acquired detailed statistical evidence which reveals that classifications on the basis of these findings are directly related to the ways in which the child learns most successfully. Therefore, the educational approach is guided, not alone by behavioral criteria but also by physical findings which disclose the status of the nervous system. Only when both are incorporated can the educational remediation be most beneficial." Cohen (1973) writes that: "Knowledge of etiology is irrelevant to remedial education treatments. Etiology may matter to the M.D. but it is irrelevant to the Ed.D. or Ph.D." Bateman (1973) writes that: "Medical classifications such as MCD are as irrelevant to educational practices as educational classifications are to medical practice."

The issue of efficacy of any therapeutic intervention, be it medical or educational, is clouded by the heterogeneity of the group of children classified as MCD. It is naïve to think that because a child is labeled MCD he will respond in the same manner as any other MCD child. Under this general classification are many varieties of children with various degrees and types of deficiencies who have not at the present time been placed in appropriate subgroups. For instance, diagnostic criteria are not established and maintained from one center to the other. Wender (1971) bases his diagnosis primarily on behavioral aspects and found only one-half of his group of patients to have other evidence of neurologic dysfunction (soft signs).

This classification dilemma, as it relates to treatment, is analogous to the diagnosis and treatment of infectious diseases. All patients with infectious disease demonstrate a number of common symptoms and signs (fever, lethargy, malaise); several, but not all, have cough, sore throat, runny nose, whereas other have vomiting, diarrhea, and abdominal pain. To develop adequate treatment approaches, it is necessary to break down this large heterogeneous group to more homogeneous subgroups that share characteristics such as etiology, symptoms, and response to medication. In this way, precise therapies for specific conditions can be developed (i.e., penicillin for a strep throat but not for a virus-induced diarrhea; dietary restrictions and an antispasmodic for an intestinal irritation but not for a sore throat).

Because the MCD classification does not provide significant subgroup categories, the value of a specific therapy is not being properly evaluated because it is applied to a number of dissimilar conditions. Attempts at classifying trait and/or etiologic subgroups are being made. It is anticipated that, through improved taxonomy, responses to explicit therapeutic approaches such as medication, increased structure, and perceptual training can be more reliably predicted according to the subgroup to which the child belongs. Programs for those who are visually oriented would be divergent from programs for those who are auditorially adjusted. However, in the meantime, there is an urgent need for improvement of our general treatment procedures and symptom alleviation (bed rest, aspirin, and a call in the morning) which are being generated for the entire MCD group by those who are developing improved pedagogic techniques (Bateman, 1973; and Cohen, 1973).

. . . For Understanding the Child

The MCD child is special. He requires understanding and support because of and in spite of his sometimes frustrating antisocial and anger-provoking behavior. Often among his needs is the appropriate use of medication, which should not be regarded as a liability by those who are working with him. Above all, every effort should be made to assist him in developing and maintaining a sustaining self-concept in order to alleviate devastating and persistent emotional problems in the future.

. . . For Professional Communication

The attempt to identify the nature of MCD and to impart the many controversial issues facing the physician and the educator should lead to a greater awareness of each discipline's role and limitations. Rather than the perpetuation of professionals who are "insiders" and "outsiders" (Cohen, 1973), it is time that all groups shed their own perceptual handicaps and nongoal-directed hyperactivity in order to communicate and generate meaningful therapeutic programs for the MCD child.

PROGNOSIS AND CONCLUSION

Very little information is available concerning the ultimate outcome of children with MCD. It is difficult to make predictions for a group of children that is so heterogeneous in composition and handled in such a variety of ways. Some studies are rather pessimistic, whereas others are more encouraging, indicating a good prognosis for obtaining higher education. Of Laufer's (1971) 48 cases, 76% were receiving, or had received, higher education. There was a significant correlation between the length of time on medication and ultimate academic achievement. In general, however, at the present time there is little evidence on which to base a prediction for an individual case. Some children improve, making adequate adjustments; others do not.

Many adults today recall one or two classmates from their grade school years who probably would have been labeled MCD, had the concept been popular then. The challenge that faces the educator and the physician now is the hope that the MCD child of today stands an improved chance of obtaining success as compared to his predecessors.

REFERENCES

Bateman, B. 1973. Educational implications of minimal brain dysfunction. In F. F. de la Cruz, B. H. Fox, and R. H. Roberts (eds.), Minimal Brain Dysfunction, pp. 245–250. New York Academy of Sciences, New York.

Belmont, L., and H. G. Birch. 1965. Lateral dominance, lateral awareness, and reading disability. Child Develop. 36:57–71.

Bradley, C. 1937. The behavior of children receiving Benzedrine. Am. J. Psychiat. 94:577–585.

Chalfant, J. C., and M. A. Scheffelin. 1969. Central Processing Dysfunctions in Children: A Review of Research. NINDS Monogr. No. 9, United States Department of Health, Education, and Welfare, Washington, D. C.

Clements, S. D. 1966. Minimal Brain Dysfunction in Children. NINDS Monogr. No. 4, United States Department of Health, Education, and Welfare, Washington, D. C.

Cohen, S. A. 1973. Minimal brain dysfunction and practical matters such as teaching kids to read. In F. F. de la Cruz, B. H. Fox, and R. H. Roberts (eds.), Minimal Brain Dysfunction, pp. 251–261. New York Academy of Sciences, New York.

Conners, C. K. 1969. A teacher rating scale for use in drug studies with children. Am. J. Psychiat. 126:152–156.

Conners, C. K. 1971. Recent drug studies with hyperkinetic children. J. Learning Dis. 4:478–483.

Davids, A. 1971. Objective instrument for assessing hyperkinesis in children. J. Learning Dis. 4:499–501.

Frostig, M. 1972. Visual perception, integrative functions and academic learning. J. Learning Dis. 5:1–15.

Gofman, H. P. 1971. Learning and language disorders in children. Current Probl. Pediat. 1:3–45 (Part I) (August); 1:3–60 (Part II) (September).

Johnson, D. J., and H. R. Myklebust. 1967. Learning Disabilities. Grune & Stratton, Inc., New York. 336 p.

Knobloch, H., and B. Pasamanick. 1959. Syndrome of minimal cerebral damage in infancy. J. A. M. A. 170:1384–1387.

Laufer, M. W. 1971. Long-term management and some follow-up findings on the use of drugs with minimal cerebral syndromes. J. Learning Dis. 4:518–522.

McGrady, H. J., and J. M. McCarthy. 1971. The eye and learning disabilities. Division for Children with Learning Disabilities Newsletter 2 (1).

Millichap, J. G. 1968. Drugs in the management of hyperkinetic and perceptually handicapped children. J. A. M. A. 206:1527–1530.

Myklebust, H. R., and B. Boshes. 1960. Psychoneurological learning disorders in children. Arch. Pediat. 77:247–256.

Paine, R. S. 1962. Minimal chronic brain syndromes in children. Develop. Med. Child Neurol. 4:21–27.

Preston, M. S., J. T. Guthrie, and B. Childs. 1974. Visual evoked responses in normal and disabled readers. Psychophysiology 11:452–457.

Ross, A. O. 1968. Conceptual issues in the evaluation of brain damage. *In* J. K. Khanna (ed.), Brain Damage and Mental Retardation, pp. 20–43. Charles C Thomas, Publisher, Springfield, Ill.

Safer, D., R. Allen, and E. Barr. 1972. Depression of growth in hyperactive children on stimulant drugs. New England J. Med. 287:217–220.

Smith, P. A., and M. A. Marx. 1972. Some cautions on the use of the Frostig test: A factor analytic study. J. Learning Dis. 5:357–362.

Stephens, W. E., E. S. Cunningham, and B. J. Stigler. 1967. Reading readiness and eye hand preference patterns in first grade children. Exceptional Child. 33:481–488.

Strauss, A. and L. Lehtinen. 1947. Psychopathology and Education of the Brain Injured Child. Grune & Stratton, Inc., New York. 206 p.

Symmes, J. S., and J. L. Rapoport. 1972. Unexpected reading failure. Am. J. Orthopsychiat. 42:82–91.

Wender, P. H. 1971. Minimal Brain Dysfunction in Children. Wiley-Interscience, New York. 242 p.

15

Teacher Awareness Of Common Psychiatric Disorders In Children

Alejandro Rodriguez, M.D., and Gregory C. Fernandopulle, M.D.

It is a matter of common experience that, in spite of how objective and mature people attempt to be, initial meetings often form a lasting impact on those who encounter one another. This may further lead, at times, to erroneous impressions and the formation of certain judgments which could, in various ways, alter future relationships.

Several factors, such as physical features, style of clothing, hygienic appearance, manner of greeting including the handshake, general behavior, and ethnic or religious background contribute on occasion to influence first impressions. At times this impression may be communicated to the other individual nonverbally. This subconscious rejection could possibly trigger a similar reaction from the second individual, thus tainting and even obstructing all or at least a portion of future communication between these two individuals.

This chapter opens with a precautionary note because, if there is an awareness of these pitfalls, it is relatively simple to be more objective in formulating precise judgments. This chapter will deal with some common emotional problems of children of varying ages, with suggestions as to what behaviors warrant immediate attention. In spite of the hazards described earlier, the teacher is certainly in an excellent situation to notice latent behavioral deviations in children, and it is with this goal in mind that an attempt will be made to describe some common areas of difficulty in school age children.

THE INTERVIEWING PROCESS

The Initial Interview with the Child

The first meeting between the teacher and the child may or may not occur in the classroom. Since the initial interview usually inaugurates a prolonged dialogue and relationship between teacher and child, it may be useful to review segments of it at this time. A very important aspect of the interview is the recognition and establishment of individuality. To this end, the proper cognizance of the child's name takes precedence. "What would you like us to call you?" is one way in which the child may express his desires and often avoids undesirable nicknames which are usually emotionally charged and frequently oriented toward infantilization or embarrassment of the student.

A brief period spent separately with each child at the beginning of the school year usually provides the foundation for a meaningful, continuing relationship. A few more inquiries concerning where he lives, how and with whom (especially to younger children) he comes to school, and a benign nonthreatening check on his knowledge of the days of the week, date, concept of time and people at home, are very useful baselines to acquire.

In short, the teacher is performing a brief mental status examination regarding some of the pupil's concepts, orientation to person, place, and time, as well as some aspects of reality testing. By this simple exercise, good rapport is readily established. The child also gains the notion that the adult is in charge (which relieves him of considerable anxiety and, thereby, provides more freedom with which to work), while also determining very clearly the boundaries between teacher and child. The factors stated above are very instrumental in demonstrating confidence between the teacher and the student, and are necessary ingredients for a good learning environment in a given educational system. Once this foundation is substantiated, it is infinitely easier for the teacher to be more sensitive to the presence or emergence of emotional pathology.

Interview with the Parents

The parents may on occasion request an interview with the teacher. This could be due to several reasons, some of which include failing grades, complaints by the child to the parents concerning uncomfortable situations with peers or teachers, recurrent suspensions, apparent lack of or excessive homework, and too many extracurricular activities. Should this be the case, it is prudent to allow the parents to initiate the conversation.

If, on the other hand, the teacher arranges for the interview, it is usually good judgment to present the problem gradually and discretely, allowing the parents adequate time to assimilate it. Often parents, as well as educators, use denial, intellectualization, and projection when confronted with anxiety-provoking circumstances, genuinely unaware they are doing so. Knowledge of these simple practices of human behavior are very useful in understanding and communicating, especially in times of a crisis.

It is desirable for both parents to be present at all meetings with the school staff, and it is most beneficial if such a request is made very clearly. This should be true even if the parents are separated, divorced, or remarried, since a child generally functions best if both parents are equally responsible, responsive, and concerned. Often this message is not communicated succinctly, especially to the father who is generally willing to come to a school meeting concerning his child, if adequate time is given to make necessary arrangements. One out of three fathers at our child psychiatry clinic respond during work hours if appropriately contacted (e.g., by a letter or telephone call).

The ability to communicate with both parents jointly also affords the teacher an opportunity to note which of the parents is more talkative, observant, and objective, perhaps providing clues as to the possible source of a child's behavior. On occasion, when parents are given the opportunity to mutually discuss their child with a teacher, common inconsistencies on their part are realized which may be contributing to the deviant behavior of the child.

As in any interview, it is useful to determine and reinforce the positive aspects of the parents' behavior to bolster their own self-esteem. It is desirable, as far as possible, to avoid discussing the destructive aspects of the child's problem as "being beyond repair at this stage." At times, parents appear to be unaware of the particular behavior described. This could be due in part to the normal protective reaction of the parents toward their child, aside from the infrequent case of detachment and lack of interest. This necessary and useful protective behavior is often lacking with foster parents and, on occasion, they must be taught to regard this as a normal parental attitude. A useful way to conclude the interview is to reinforce the positive features of the child's behavior, as well as those of the parents.

Hopefully, Parent–Teacher Association (PTA) meetings can be utilized constructively as a platform for more communication with parents. Parents can then establish social rules for their children in a given neighborhood (e.g., curfew hours, age for smoking, and social functions), rather than permitting children to set regulations they are often not competent to make. In essence, the ideal PTA may act as a forum for all parents to have a more enriching experience, exchange of ideas, and the establishment of standards which make parenthood, growing up, and teaching much more exciting and rewarding endeavors.

SYMPTOMS OF EMOTIONAL DISORDERS AT VARIOUS DEVELOPMENTAL STAGES

Some of the problems or symptoms suggestive of an underlying emotional disturbance according to age groups will be enumerated so that the teacher can assist in the detection and prevention of certain psychiatric disorders. Many of these symptoms overlap, however, and are not limited to the age specified.

Preschool and Kindergarten

Mild Many children entering a nursery school or kindergarten class for the first time will display certain behaviors which are usually transient and of little consequence. The educator should be aware of the broad range of motor and speech development and emotional behavior which normal children of this age group can show. The deviations from the norm discussed below are considered of minor significance, particularly if they subside as the child matures.

Poor motor coordination as manifested by clumsiness in holding, carrying, or throwing objects, constant dropping of articles, walking as if the child had "two left feet," and general awkwardness in movement are all extremely common symptoms, and usually abate within a few years.

Persistent speech problems, particularly stammering, especially when excited, angry, or under any other stress; constant loss of certain words while speaking; and repetition of adjectives, verbs, nouns, and pronouns may occur at times when the child is under duress, or even spontaneously.

Excessive timidity may be within normal limits for children at this stage. Girls may be especially timorous, more so if they are from certain types of homes where being adventurous is equated with exposing oneself to danger. If a child appears to be progressively restricted, passive, and almost cowardly, referral to a physician for a thorough evaluation is warranted. Specific fears, such as terror of monsters, fire engines, and "spookies," are normal as children generally grow out of these fears. If, however, these trepidations persist and restrict a child, a significant underlying emotional disorder may be their cause.

Perpetual problems with food idiosyncrasies, such as excessive eating, attempts at starvation, constant vomiting, eating nonedible material (e.g., crayons, paper, plaster from the wall, play dough, or chalk), or an aberration of bowel or bladder function, such as constant wetting, diarrhea, or constipation, soiling or leaking feces (encopresis), are all entities that necessitate early investigation if persistent and progressive.

Constant temper tantrums and infantile crying are very common phenomena in preschool children. Up to a certain point, such behavior may be passed off as normal, especially if there are signs of improvement following a few weeks of consistent handling (e.g., child left alone or a privilege is withheld or withdrawn). If, however, these temper outbursts are also associated with a reduced attention span, a changing personality, easy distractibility, and poor class performance, a more intensive investigation is required.

Many children indulge in such exercises as thumb sucking or rocking when anxious, but, as they mature, these behaviors diminish. If a child tends to regress to these infantile mannerisms often at very mild provocation, closer observation will prove useful.

Total lack of interest in other children may range from complete isolation to taking a controlling position where the child will communicate only if others acquiesce to his wishes. This is common with children who have no siblings, or where a young child lives with many adults. Should this symptom persist for months, a referral is almost imperative.

Severe Severe emotional disorders rarely evolve spontaneously in the preschool child. More commonly, there is a preceding history of minor psychologic disturbances which may have been ignored. The following discussion of severe symptoms can certainly represent specific psychiatric conditions, but may also suggest the presence of a medical or neurologic illness. Thus, careful evaluation by a physician is obligatory.

Excessive lethargy or hyperactivity are two extremes of behavior which should be considered as pathologic unless proved otherwise. Lethargic pupils may especially tend to escape notice, particularly if they are reasonably intelligent, since they cause very little trouble in class. Some of these children benefit from medication, while others could be incubating a more serious condition requiring sophisticated investigation and management.

If a child in nursery school or kindergarten is noncommunicative or demonstrates little or no speech, a severe emotional problem, neurologic disorder, or physical illness is usually present.

The need to use the toilet constantly for evacuation of the bowels, once an infectious process has been ruled out, is serious enough for immediate referral.

A tic is a repetitive, often purposeless movement, usually involving a small group of muscles (e.g., shrugging one's shoulders, blinking, or facial grimaces). These are best evaluated by the physician during the early stages if they tend to persist. Ritualisms are repetitive acts which vary from those displayed by a child in a given sequence (e.g., sit down, walk on the right side of the desk, clean the chair, look about, sit down again), to a long list of rituals involving most or all one's actions. If observed over a prolonged period, these are best investigated by a child psychiatrist.

Most teachers are familiar with impulsive, destructive behavior which is oftentimes uncontrolled and explosive and which can lead to significant injury. This may be the presenting symptom of a more serious illness.

Elementary School

Mild Anxiety and oversensitivity to new experiences, such as school, separation, rejection, changing relationships, and group pressure, are, to a certain degree, within normal limits for this age group. Many of the conditions which follow can be observed from time to time in the normal pupil, especially when confronted by a novel experience or a taxing responsibility. Occasionally, these minimal deviations in behavior are the forerunner of a significant learning disability or, in some cases, mental retardation.

Lack of attentiveness and apparent disinterest in learning are common presenting features of increased anxiety, depressive reactions, or minimal brain dysfunction, all of which require treatment. Loss of appetite or weight, excessive eating, aches and pains, digestive problems, and other somatic complaints—if persistent, and especially if seen to exacerbate under duress—are symptoms implying possible psychiatric or medical problems.

Acting out, lying, stealing, temper outbursts, and inappropriate social behavior may inhibit the normal learning process. If these behaviors persist, an attempt at correction should be made. Destructive tendencies, such as the tearing of books and breaking pencils or classroom furniture, usually signify underlying emotional pathology.

Inability or unwillingness to do things for oneself is at times the result of being "babied" excessively. Occasionally, this behavior satisfies the need to control the environment, which could be detrimental to a child's work in class. Difficulties and rivalry with peers, siblings, and adults with constant fighting may be a sign of constant frustration at home as well as at school. On the other hand, moodiness, withdrawal, few friends, and other forms of isolation, if long-lived, also require careful investigation. At times, modification of the environment may prove useful (e.g., one-to-one games, small groups, as well as less aggressive activities).

Severe The emergence of severe emotional behavioral disturbances in the elementary student necessitates immediate investigation and appropriate management. Early intervention is the key to therapy. Most psychiatric symptoms can mimic a serious organic disease (e.g., destructive behavior and headaches may result from a brain tumor rather than a personality disorder). A careful physical examination must, therefore, precede the initiation of psychiatric therapy.

Extreme withdrawal, apathy, depression, grief, and self-destructive tendencies are symptoms of a depressive reaction, which is certainly serious in nature and warrants professional attention. Excessive and uncontrollable antisocial behavior, such as aggression, destruction, chronic lying, stealing, and intentional cruelty to animals, suggests a serious character disorder.

Complete failure to learn, speech difficulties, and stuttering become more serious in the elementary age group and require immediate investigation. Severe ritualisms, including detailed movements and repetition of certain words, hand movements, and touching several objects in order, intimates mental retardation or psychotic behavior.

Sexual exhibitionism, sexual assaults on others, removal of clothes and undergarments in public, and attempts at any type of sexual advance could be due to several causes, including exposure to pornography or witnessing overt sexual behavior by others.

Extreme somatic complaints such as a poor appetite, loss of weight, sudden excessive gain in weight, constant menstrual cramps, headaches, and abdominal pain may be the precursor of a significant psychiatric disturbance. Of course, an organic cause should be considered as well.

Junior High and High School

Mild Emotional problems are inordinately common in the teen-aged student. Fortunately, most of the upsets are rather minor and short-lived. During this stage of life, a myriad of physiologic, environmental, and emotional adjustments occur. It is little wonder that this age group is so vulnerable to the stresses of maturation.

Apprehension, fears, and guilt may be related to such areas as sex education (e.g., menstruation and sexual development of breasts and axillary and pubic hair). Constant preoccupation with sex may be manifested by daydreaming, diminishing grades, or occasional sexual acting out. Inability to substitute or postpone satisfaction is a worrisome sign. These individuals constantly seek immediate pleasure-producing experiences, usually completely ignoring the rights of others. Their reality testing often is poor and they live in a dreamworld of their own.

Defiant, negative, impulsive, or withdrawn behavior indicates pathology, if persistent for several weeks. Frequent somatic complaints, as described earlier, or denial of an existing illness (e.g., playing football immediately after a serious injury) suggests a certain degree of anxiety or immature reasoning. Difficulties in learning at this age are often due to an inability to adjust to increased anxiety.

Severe Complete withdrawal is an extremely serious symptom characterized by isolation and the refusal to communicate except with selected individuals. School performance is obviously retarded. Acts of delinquency, asceticism, ritualism, or overconformity usually result in poor grades, suspension, and isolation. Presistent anxiety resulting in phobias and inhibitions is detrimental to the pupil and must be managed by a psychiatrist.

Recurrent hypochondriasis, including headache, abdominal pain, and backache, is often associated with stressful situations such as exams, debates, and other forms of competition.

Sexual aberrations, including open masturbation and the tendency to wear clothes usually worn by the opposite sex, signify a serious underlying emotional disorder, and referral for a psychiatric investigation is suggested.

The behavior described in the above section of this chapter should, of course, be taken in the proper context; the lies of a 4-year-old child could be benign fantasies, but the lies of a 14-year-old may be dishonesty or may even suggest delusional thought processes.

COMMON MAJOR PSYCHIATRIC DISTURBANCES

Hyperactivity

Hyperactivity is often part of a more complex syndrome known as minimal cerebral dysfunction. Impulsivity, temper tantrums, inability to be content with circumstances that please others, low frustration tolerance, and short attention span frequently associated with a learning disorder are some of the primary symptoms of this condition (see Chapter 14).

If hyperactivity is identified at the nursery school level, prior to the accumulation of secondary behavior problems caused by repeated negative experiences, a relatively short treatment plan will probably suffice. These children often benefit very promptly from one of the central nervous system stimulant medications. This form of therapy also serves to differentiate the hyperactive pupil from the emotionally depressed student whose hyperactivity is initiated at a later age and who is not responsive to this form of medical therapy.

The hyperactive child identified in the first or second grade has usually already suffered the consequences of a poor attention span, resulting in retarded reading, comprehension, or arithmetic skills. These children require coordinated treatment very often in the form of medication, special assistance in school, and a more organized life style at home.

The hyperactive third or fourth grader commonly has more deep-seated difficulties, including aggression, anger, and guilt. He also is usually involved in stealing, lying, and acts of cruelty. Medication at this stage ameliorates some of the motor symptoms, but, in addition, the child is in need of extensive emotional support to cope with the associated problems. Some children with all of these characteristics, including a poor academic record, appear prominently in adolescent clinics or as delinquents in the juvenile courts. As a consequence, these patients are often labeled "borderline personalities" and may at times require prolonged inpatient hospital management.

Stealing

The importance of stealing is difficult to evaluate when it occurs at an early age, especially in children from a low socioeconomic group, where a sense of ownership is not clearly defined for several practical reasons. Clothes, toys, books, and other items all become common property; hence, the concept of "I own this," as defined by a more affluent child, does not exist in lower socioeconomic groups.

At the nursery school level, the teacher should be sensitive to and recognize stealing; it is a common phenomenon, but usually of only short duration. In the first and second grades, thieving assumes more importance as it is often associated with other behavior problems. Later on, at the third, fourth, and fifth grade levels, stealing is very rarely an isolated symptom. At this stage, abstract thinking is usually well established and character traits firmly formulated; hence, stealing becomes a more pronounced and significant symptom. By adolescence, stealing definitely becomes a fixed behavioral pattern, and a problem of dire consequence for the person concerned, as well as for society.

Lying

For the child in nursery school or kindergarten, lying can rarely be differentiated from fantasy which is a normal behavior for children of this age. In the first and second grade, the superego or conscience becomes more clearly established so that beyond the age of 9 or 10, repetitive, dishonest, or deceitful behavior portends a significant character disorder. Because lying is associated with other difficulties as the child grows older (as in stealing), a thorough evaluation, followed by a treatment program, is essential in order to deal with the innumerable conflicts which may be troubling the child.

Cruelty

Cruelty is a premeditated action in order to obtain pleasure through hurting or damaging other people or animals. This act must be distinguished from impulsive behavior, such as when a child spontaneously engages in an activity which may injure a pet or friend. Cruelty may be reinforced by parents, especially fathers, who deplore "sissy" traits surfacing in their son's behavior. At times parents encourage cruelty by ignoring it, thus strengthening this abnormal behavior. Identification at kindergarten and elementary school levels is most important to prevent these children from becoming involved in more destructive activities which may, at times, result in harm to peers and infringement of the law.

Firesetting

Firesetting may potentially result in great hazards to the child, to the family, as well as to the neighborhood. The fascination for fire among children is a universal phenomenon. A major accomplishment for many children is the mastery of producing a flame by striking a match. This feat occurs when imitation skills can be combined with the acquisition of fine coordinated motor development. When a youngster learns that this newfound skill annoys the parent, he may on occasion contest them with his "weapon," particularly when things "do not go his way." In this situation, it is recommended that matches be removed from the home, and, if necessary, the parents may equip themselves with lighters. In certain households, it may be necessary to remove knobs from the stove or resort to other similar measures until the attraction for fire diminishes.

Sometimes, in an older child, preoccupation with fire is a good diagnostic clue to mental retardation (e.g., an 8-year-old boy functioning consistently in most areas at a 3- or 4-year level), especially if the child is from a family with an abundance of fire hazards within the home.

Intensive institutional treatment is necessary for some cases. Unfortunately, as demonstrated by many investigators, prolonged inpatient therapy may not avert persistent acts of arson.

Speech Problems

Delay in the onset of language is not rare, even in intelligent children. An overprotected, overindulged child may lag behind in speech as in most other aspects of development. Interaction with the child by the teacher during nursery school or kindergarten may point out the immaturity of a particular pupil. Specific steps initiated at this time to correct the abnormal parent-child relationship (on occasion encompassing the psychiatrist as well as educator) are usually extremely beneficial.

Other common causes of delayed speech are as follows: elective mutism, deafness, aphasia, mental retardation, and autism. An elective mute is readily identified. These children generally do not communicate with or talk to adults, but do so with parents, siblings, and often with classmates, once friendship has been established. These children are very difficult to treat, and, thus, require considerable understanding and patience, especially from the school. Excellent communication between the teacher, parents, and physician or therapist is a prerequisite for successful management.

The deaf mute child emerges when deafness occurs as the result of infection, trauma, or some other injurious mechanism after speech was well established. The lack of response to sound provides suspicion for further investigation and a thorough audiometric examination is needed (see Chapter 3).

A mentally retarded child commonly presents to the professional with a lag in speech development, but the total absence of language at the termination of the kindergarten year is very rare, if retardation is the only cause. In the severely retarded child, associated delay in related gross and fine motor, as well as cognitive developmental milestones, assist in confirming the diagnosis.

The autistic child, as Kanner (1972) points out, ignores parents, children, and all human contact; i.e., he disregards social customs or obligations and responds only to those experiences which stimulate him at a given time. This, in short, is similar to a path of least resistance. The autistic child tends to follow this pattern, even after segments of speech have developed (see Chapter 11).

On occasion, children with severe language aberrations are initially difficult to characterize on account of similar underlying behavioral traits, particularly their destructive play and unruly attitude. The latter is particularly evident in differentiating the aphasic child and the autistic patient. Therefore, close observation in a specialized setting may be required prior to establishing a definitive diagnosis. This sequence of events is of paramount importance as therapy is unique for each specific speech problem.

School Phobia

School phobia has been defined as a reluctance to attend school. This is usually due to separation anxiety of pathologic proportions involving parents (usually the mother) and the child. Both parent and child attempt to satisfy their unresolved needs by remaining in close proximity to each other.

Several symptoms have been observed to accompany school phobia. Nausea, vomiting, loss of appetite, abdominal pain, headache, paleness, and bronchial asthma are most common. These complaints are not present on weekends and holidays, and miraculously disappear if the child is allowed to remain at home. At times these students also have specific fears which include teachers, bullies, strangers, bus rides, and kidnappers. They are sensitive, clinging, and dependent pupils who display considerable difficulty in parental separation, especially from the mother. Once these children are in school, most of the symptoms disappear.

The above definition, which suggests the pathogenesis of school phobia to be the result of separation difficulties, is more applicable for the kindergarten or early elementary school child. Their mothers are unusually overprotective and so demanding that they impress one as using the child to satisfy their own unfulfilled emotional needs. Quite often, their mothers were school phobics and dropouts with separation difficulties from a young age.

The fathers are often incapable of supporting the mother's anxiety when the children show these behaviors. They are generally passive, isolated, distant individuals who require assistance in the understanding of the cause of their youngster's symptomatology and gentle guidance in the redevelopment of an intelligent and compassionate relationship with their child.

Mothers may utilize several excuses or mechanisms (poor weather, the child's symptoms of nausea or abdominal discomfort) to reinforce the school phobia. At times, the parent may displace her anxiety on a teacher or another student, shifting the blame on them for her child's behavior.

Treatment for the younger child consists basically of reducing the parental anxiety, obtaining school cooperation, and consistently demanding that the child return to school. Even in extreme cases, results from this approach have been very satisfactory.

In the older child or young adolescent, school phobia assumes more serious proportions. Very often, the fears cover up greater psychopathology, such as personality disturbances or neurotic and psychotic disorders; hence, these children require a more sophisticated evaluation. The prognosis worsens as the child gets older. It is not uncommon for this child to be hospitalized in order to initially work out some aspects of the separation. He may restart the schooling process while still in the hospital, and, upon discharge, school classes are reintroduced in cooperation with the teacher, physician, and the student.

Truancy

The school phobic must be clearly differentiated from the malingerer, and the child who is a truant. The truant student prefers to roam the streets rather than attend classes or remain at home. He shows little or no anxiety when he is found to be absent from school.

Management of these pupils involves a thorough evaluation of the child and the family situation, including investigation of the methods of supervision of the child in general. Improper school placement, general indifference or total neglect by parents, and very inconsistent expectations are common contributory causes.

TREATMENT MODALITIES

Emotional turmoil and disturbances of behavior have always been a feature of the human species. Listening and appropriate counseling have been the mainstay of therapy throughout the ages. Empathy, understanding, and the facilitation of communication persist as the major therapeutic tools to this day. In years past, the clergy or senior members of the community provided the framework for a treatment program in a home setting where the role of the parent was clearly established.

With time, the interpretation and significance of various behavioral patterns have undergone remarkable change. Some of Freud's concepts have had their impact on the educational system as well as the family unit. Adler, a disciple of Freud's, has particularly elaborated upon the inferiority complex. These impressions of man's psychologic composition, coupled with many social changes, have contributed significantly to produce a relatively new type of parent, depicted most concisely as *the confused parent*. A hallmark of these adults, during encounters with their offspring, is that saying "No" will literally damage the child. They confuse understanding with acceptance, limit setting with rejection, and love with always saying "Yes." Some parents also find it most difficult to accept the idea that toleration of frustration is a major milestone of maturation and formation of one's personality. If all impulses are immediately fulfilled, as most people would like, the process of growing up is markedly hampered.

The treatment plan depends upon many factors, including the age of the student, family dynamics, severity and duration of the disorder, and the availability of skilled professionals to provide long-term care. Common modalities utilized for therapeutic purposes include psychotherapy, behavior modification, and the use of specific drugs.

Psychotherapy

During the last several decades, many new methodologies of treatment for the emotionally ill have been developed. Some of these are discussed briefly.

Individual psychotherapy consists of patient treatment sessions at least once a week lasting approximately 1 hr. for a period of time. The emphasis is directed toward an improved conceptualization of one's own feelings and thought processes. Significant change cannot occur until the patient has developed a comprehensive framework in the understanding of his personal and emotional responses over a significant portion of his life.

Group therapy stresses the interpersonal process. Many problems common to children can be solved, or at least improved to a considerable degree, by the simple technique of common discussion and mutual trust. The ultimate success of this method depends upon the complexity of the problem, the type of group, and the skill and approach of the therapist.

Family therapy focuses chiefly on family interaction with a view to changing the pathologic patterns by the direct participation of the entire family with the therapist, usually over an extended period of time.

Behavior Modification

This treatment method deals specifically with the manipulation or change of observable behavior of an individual. Therefore, this treatment regimen differs significantly from psychoanalysis or psychoanalytically oriented management, which tends to focus on feelings and thoughts.

The basis of behavior modification is learning theory. The schools of Pavlov and Watson utilize conditioning, on the grounds that interrelationships between circumstances and responses develop as a function of the manner in which the situational stimuli are presented. Many psychologists and psychiatrists are proponents of reinforcement theory, where positive and negative reinforcements are used in an attempt to modify behavior.

These principles are taught in several schools throughout the country, whereby reward and/or prearranged punishment are used to advantage in a well-organized setting. It has been possible to integrate practical and workable schedules which can readily be employed by most teachers. In essence, behavior modification produces an opportunity within the classroom for the student to win tokens for, perhaps, paying attention in class, improving scholastic achievement, and interacting usefully with peers and teachers. These tokens can later be exchanged for candy, recreational activities, games, or whatever the child wishes within the bounds of the system. This type of positive reinforcement is much more widely used than negative reinforcement. An example of the latter consists of mild electroshocks to reduce or abolish potentially harmful headbanging (using a special skull cap) in emotionally disturbed children or the utilization of a specialized alarm system at night to help bedwetters.

This mode of therapy is certainly proving useful in given situations. However, whether it should be employed exclusively or in association with other treatment techniques has not been adequately evaluated. In addition, although the short-term results of behavior modification are often impressive, long-range benefits suggest that reappraisal of this treatment regimen is in order.

Medication

The child psychiatrist may utilize drug therapy for the management of a specific disorder, sometimes in combination with the treatment programs outlined above. All pupils who are on a pharmacologic agent require careful and frequent reassessment. There are three basic families of drugs which are commonly employed: stimulants, tranquilizers, and antidepressants.

Stimulants may produce dramatic improvement in the child with hyperactivity and a short attention span, common symptoms of the minimal cerebral dysfunction syndrome (see Chapter 14). Many educators and parents have been properly concerned about possible addiction or other undesirable effects of these drugs. Fortunately, to date, addiction has not occurred in spite of the fact that many children have been treated with central nervous system stimulants for prolonged periods.

The major tranquilizers (e.g., Thorazine) are highly effective in the management of severely disturbed children and adolescents, especially for the treatment of schizophrenia and organic brain disorders. Minor tranquilizers (Equanil, Miltown, Valium, and Librium) may be utilized for the amelioration of certain types of anxiety.

Antidepressants (e.g., Tofrānil and Elavil) may be prescribed by the physician for the management of depression. Occasionally, this group of drugs is valuable in the treatment of extreme hyperactivity unresponsive to stimulants.

CONCLUSION

The participation of the educator in the delivery of mental health services to the community is extensive, as well as important. The school provides for a child—as work and occupation do for an adult—a situation whereby certain needs are met and maximal learning occurs, if conditions are appropriate.

Until a few years ago, the identification of the student with the teacher began in grade one at 6 or 7 years of age. With the advent of nursery and kindergarten education, and, more recently, of day care centers, this process starts at an even younger age. Thus, the teacher's role in developing a child's personality assumes even greater proportions.

Educators are no longer confined to the traditional classroom. They are becoming important members of the team in pediatric hospitals, providing an education for the patients, as well as assisting in diagnosis and treatment. In outpatient clinics, the school counselor provides assistance, not only in diagnosing the scholastic problem, but also in helping with appropriate placement if necessary, as well as giving adequate feedback to the therapist.

Two other areas where teachers provide excellent services are in sheltered homes for certain children and in special education programs. In sheltered homes where children are excluded from the public schools, the educator can play a major role in being sensitive to these particular students and in providing the necessary structure for them to learn with a minimum of anxiety. The role of the teacher as a special educator has been dealt with elsewhere in this text (see Chapter 1).

All of the roles which have been attributed to the educator, as a sensitive observer, provider of an organized structure, limit setter, helper in diagnosis and in treatment, place the teacher in a unique and exciting position in that she, more than any other professional (and, in some cases, parents), is responsible for molding the life of her pupils.

SUGGESTED READING

Bakwin, H., and R. M. Bakwin. 1972. Behavior Disorders in Children. 4th Ed. W. B. Saunders Company, Philadelphia. 714 p.

Fraiberg, S. H. 1959. The Magic Years: Understanding and Handling the Problems of Early Childhood. Charles Scribner's Sons, New York. 305 p.

Freedman, A. M., and H. I. Kaplan. 1967. Comprehensive Textbook of Psychiatry. The Williams & Wilkins Company, Baltimore. 1,666 p.

Kanner, L. 1972. Child Psychiatry. 4th Ed. Charles C Thomas, Publisher, Springfield, Ill. 735 p.

Rodriguez, A., M. Rodriguez, and L. Eisenberg. 1959. The outcome of school phobias. Am. J. Psychia. 116:540–544.

Senn, M. J. E., and A. J. Solnit. 1968. Problems in Child Behavior and Development. Lea & Febiger, Philadelphia. 268 p.

Wender, P. H. 1971. Minimal Brain Dysfunction in Children. Wiley-Interscience, New York. 242 p.

Glossary

Abscess—a cavity filled with pus

Acquired—nongenetic, produced by external forces or influences

Acuity—keenness of vision or hearing

Adipose—of or relating to fat

Air studies—the introduction of air into the cerebrospinal fluid spaces for evaluation of brain anatomy

Amblyopia—decreased vision without apparent change in the eye structures

Ambulation—the act of walking or moving about

Amnesia—loss of memory

Amphetamine—a drug which acts as a central nervous system stimulant

Analgesic—a class of drugs used for the relief of pain

Ancillary—supplementary, additional

Anemia—a condition in which blood is deficient in the quantity of hemoglobin or the number of red blood cells or both

Anomaly—a variance from the normal

Anoxia—a severe reduction in the normal concentration of oxygen within the body

Antacid—a drug that counteracts or relieves gastric (stomach) acidity

Anterior—situated before or toward the front

Anthropometric—relating to the study of human body measurements, especially on a comparative basis

Anticonvulsant—a drug utilized to treat and prevent convulsions

Antidepressant—a drug used to elevate the mood of a depressed individual

Arthritis—inflammation of the joints due to infectious, metabolic, or constitutional causes

Assay—a biologic analysis to measure the quantity or purity of a substance

Asymptomatic—presenting no subjective evidence of disease

Barbiturate—a drug that depresses central nervous system function; a useful anticonvulsant

Benign—nonmalignant, nonrecurrent

Bilateral—affecting both sides

Bilirubin—bile pigment formed by the disintegration of red blood cells

Binocular—relating to the use of both eyes

Brain stem—that section of the brain which includes the vital centers for heart and respiratory rate as well as the control of consciousness

Carbohydrate—sugar, starch, or cellulose

Cataract—an opacity or density of the eye lens

Cerebrospinal fluid (CSF)—the fluid which surrounds and bathes the brain and spinal cord

Chemotherapy—the treatment of a disease by chemicals or drugs

Chorionic gonadotrophin—a substance formed in the placenta which stimulates the gonads

Chromosome—a rod-shaped body within the cell nucleus which contains the germ plasm that transmits hereditary characteristics

Chronic—marked by long duration or frequent recurrence

Chronologic age—the actual age of the individual

Circumscribed—restricted to a limited space

Comatose—a state of unconsciousness

Compliance—the act or process of following a drug treatment or weight reduction program

Conception—the act of becoming pregnant; the state of being conceived

Congenital—existing at or dating from birth

Constitutional—relating to the entire body rather than a particular organ

Cortex—the outer or external layer of the brain; gray matter

Cyanosis—a bluish discoloration of the skin resulting from poor oxygenation

Cycloplegia—the loss of the eye's ability to constrict the pupil

Decibel—a unit of hearing; one decibel is the least intensity of sound at which any given note can be heard

Degradation—the act of reducing a chemical or compound to smaller units

Delirium tremens—alcoholic withdrawal characterized by anxiety, trembling, hallucinations, and excessive agitation

Diploid—double in appearance or arrangement, especially of the basic chromosome number

Diplopia—double vision due to weakness or paralysis of the eye muscles

Distal—at the end of an extremity or organ

Dura—thick, membranous protective covering of the brain

Dwarfism—a condition characterized by short stature, less than average height

Dysplastic—referring to abnormal development or growth

Echolalia—the repetition of words or sentences by an individual, often without understanding

Ectopic—out of place or position

Edema—swelling, collection of abnormally excessive amounts of fluid

Electroencephalogram (EEG)—the recording of electrical currents originating in the brain by means of electrodes placed on the scalp

Emaciation—a wasted or malnourished state

Embryogenesis—the development of a new organism by means of sexual reproduction

Encephalopathy—a process which damages or interferes with brain function
End organ—the organ responsible for a particular function
Enzyme—a substance which accelerates or catalyzes specific chemical reactions within the organism
Epicanthus—a vertical fold of skin on either side of the nose which covers the innermost portion of the eye
Epidemiologic—pertaining to the incidence, distribution, and control of disease
Epiphysis—the end of a bone where the majority of growth takes place
Ergot—a drug used for the treatment of migraine headaches
Esotropia—deviation of the eye toward the nose
Etiology—the cause of a disorder or condition
Exchange system—a diabetic diet which allows the trading of one item of food for another (e.g., a slice of bread for a serving of potatoes)
Exogenous—outside the body or organ
Exophoria—outward deviation of the eye

Fetus—a developing organism; in the human, the period after the third month of intrauterine development
Flaccid—weak, soft, or loose
Focal neurologic signs—neurologic abnormalities restricted to one portion of the body
Footcandle—the amount of illumination produced by a standard candle at a distance of 1 ft
Fovea (of the retina)—a small pit in the retina which provides the clearest vision because of the concentration of a group of nerve cells called cones
Fricatives—the sounds produced by a voiceless breath escaping through the larynx or vocal tract

Generic—characteristic of an entire group or class
Germ cell—the cell of origin which develops into the primitive embryo
Gestation—the period of pregnancy
Global—universal, comprehensive
Glucose—a sugar
Goiter—a visibly enlarged thyroid gland
Gonadal dysgenesis—defective development of the testes or ovary
Gustatory—pertaining to the sense of taste

Habilitation—the process of enhancing an individual's capabilities to the greatest potential
Hallucination—a sense perception not founded upon objective reality
Hallucinogen—a drug or chemical which produces hallucinations
Heart murmur—a sound produced due to the abnormal flow of blood, usually the result of a heart defect
Hematocrit—a measure of red blood cell volume
Hemoglobin—the oxygen-carrying component in the red blood cells
Hepatitis—inflammation of the liver
Hereditary—genetically transmitted from parent to offspring
Hormone—a chemical substance formed in one part of the body which has a specific action on an organ located in another site
Hydrocephalus—an enlargement of the head due to an abnormal collection of cerebrospinal fluid
Hyperventilation—deep breathing
Hypochondriasis—overconcern about one's health

Hypogonadal—pertaining to the decreased function of the sex glands
Hyposensitization—the process of decreasing sensitivity, usually by providing the patient with gradually increasing quantities of the offending substance
Hysterectomy—surgical removal of the uterus (womb)

Iatrogenic—induced by the physician
Immunity—the ability to resist a certain disease or infection
Intracranial—situated within the skull
Intramuscular—within the substance of a muscle
In utero—within the uterus

Karyotype—the chromosome number and composition
Keratoconus—a conical protrusion of the cornea
Kernicterus—excessive serum levels of bilirubin resulting in brain damage

Lactation—the secretion of milk
Lesion—a pathologic disruption of tissue or a loss of a part
Limbic system—a highly complex, phylogenetically old portion of the brain which is thought to be involved with emotion control

Macula—the anatomic area of the retina which provides the clearest vision
Malady—an illness, usually of a chronic type
Malaise—a vague sensation of discomfort
Malignancy—cancer, a tumor with invasive properties
Malingerer—one who feigns an illness
Malocclusion—improper closure of the teeth
Mastoid—the bony prominence located behind each ear
Maturation—the process of becoming fully developed
Medial—toward the middle
Menarche—the onset of menstruation
Meningitis—infection of the brain and its covering membranes
Menses—the monthly flow of blood from the female genital tract
Metabolism—the sum of chemical and physical activity which creates and destroys cells
Milestone—a significant point or event in development
Monoarticular—limited to one joint
Morphogenesis—the development and establishment of form
Mortality—the ratio of deaths to a total population in a given time or place
Multidisciplinary—pertaining to the cooperative participation by several professional groups
Musculoskeletal—referring to muscles and the bony skeleton
Myelin—a fatlike substance which envelops certain nerve fibers or tracts
Myopia—near-sightedness

Neonatal—pertaining to the initial month of life
Nephrosis—a kidney disease which is characterized by fluid retention
Neuromuscular—pertaining to the peripheral nerves and muscles
Neurotic—pertaining to a functional nervous disorder without demonstrable physical lesion; or an emotionally unstable individual
Nystagmus—abnormal jerky eye movements

Occipital—pertaining to the back or posterior part of the head
Ocular—pertaining to the eye
Olfactory—pertaining to the sense of smell
Organ—a part of the body with specialized function (e.g., digestion, respiration)

Organic—originating within the body and affecting the function of the individual
Orthodontics—the dental specialty which is concerned with malocclusion of the teeth
Orthoptics—the prescription of eye movement exercises for the treatment of various visual defects including muscular imbalance
Ossification—the formation of bone
Osteotomy—the cutting of a bone by a surgeon
Ototoxic—a drug which damages the hearing mechanism, resulting in deafness
Ovum—the female reproductive cell, the egg

Pallor—paleness
Pancreas—a gland which lies behind the stomach; it produces digestive enzymes and insulin
Pathogenesis—the sequence of events leading to the development of a disease
Pathology—the study of structural changes within the body caused by disease
Phobia—excessive fear
Phoneme—a member of the set of the smallest units of speech that serve to distinguish one utterance from another
Photophobia—abnormal intolerance of light
Physiology—the study of body and organ function
Placenta—the organ that unites the fetus to the uterus for the provision of various nutrients
Poliomyelitis—a viral disease which causes inflammation and destruction to areas within the spinal cord which innervate muscles
Posterior—situated in back of or behind
Postnatal—pertaining to the time following birth
Postural drainage—the process by which the patient is assisted in clearing sputum and secretions from the lungs by positioning on first one side and then the other
Premorbid—the state or appearance prior to the onset of disease
Prenatal—pertaining to the period existing before birth
Prepubertal—preceding puberty
Presbyopia—far-sightedness
Progeny—offspring, children
Prognosis—a forecast as to the eventual outcome of a disease
Prophylatic—pertaining to the prevention of or the warding off of a disorder
Prosthesis—an artificial device to replace an absent portion of the body
Proximal—nearest to the center
Psychoactive—a central nervous system stimulant
Psychosis—mental illness
Pyogenic—the production of pus

Quadriceps—the groups of muscles on the upper or anterior surface of the thigh

Radiologic—relating to the use of x-rays for diagnosis or use of radiation in treatment
Refractive errors—the imperfect deviation of light by the eye so that the image is distorted by the time it reaches the retina
Regional enteritis—a localized area of inflammation within the small intestine
Regression—progressive decline or loss of skills
Reticular activating system—the portion of the brain which is concerned with the level of consciousness
Retina—the innermost membrane of the eye; it is the perceptive structure of the eye and is connected to the brain by the optic nerve

Rhinitis (allergic)—inflammation of the nose caused by an allergy
Rickets—a bone-deforming disease of children caused by a deficiency of vitamin D
Rooting reflex—the infant's primitive instinct to seek a nipple or food source
Rote—memorization with little comprehension
Rubella—German measles

Salivation—excessive flow or production of saliva
Schizophrenia—a psychotic disorder characterized by flights of ideas, disordered thought processes, and a loss of reality reasoning
Scurvy—vitamin C deficiency resulting in weakness, anemia, bleeding tendency, and spongy gums
Secondary sexual characteristics—sexual features unrelated to the genitalia, such as the beard in a male
Sensorium—the level or state of alertness or consciousness
Sequelae—the permanent consequences of an injury or disease
Shunt—the bypassing of an obstruction within the brain by redirecting the cerebrospinal fluid into the heart or peritoneal cavity through a plastic tube
Sibilants—the "s," "z," "ch," "zh," or "j" sounds
Sign—objective evidence of a disease
Sinusitis—a sinus infection, the air cavities within the cranial bones
Somatic—relating to the body
Spasticity—increased tone and stiffness of the muscles
Sphincter—a ring of muscle which serves to open and close an orifice
Squint—crossing of the eyes
Station—the position assumed while standing
Stereopsis—the perception of objects in relief and not as all in one plane
Strabismus—imbalance of the muscles of the eyeball, resulting in a squint
Stupor—partial loss of consciousness, near coma
Subclinical—pertaining to a condition which is inapparent by the usual tests
Symptom—the patient's perception of a change from normal which may indicate the presence of disease
Synovitis—inflammation of the synovial membrane, the lining of the joint cavities
Synthesis—the production of a substance
Systemic—affecting the entire body

Taxonomy—classification
Tay-Sachs disease—a lethal degenerative disease of the central nervous system, particulary among Ashkenazic Jewish children
Tetanus—an acute disease which causes severe spasms and rigidity in certain muscles (lockjaw)
Topical—pertaining to a drug or substance which is applied to the skin
Transplantation—the transfer of an organ or tissue from one person (or place within the body) to another
Tremor—shaking, shivering, or trembling
Triceps—the muscle along the back of the upper arm
Trimester—a period of 3 months

Umbilical—relating to the navel
Unilateral—one-sided

Vasectomy—sterilization in the male by surgical excision of the vas deferens (the tube connecting the testis and ejaculatory duct)
Virus—an infective agent responsible for a great number of diseases including the common cold. The virus is smaller than most bacteria and is capable of multiplication only within a living cell
Void—to urinate or empty the bladder

Index